Analysis of Complex Arrhythmias—A Case Based Approach

Editors

MELVIN M. SCHEINMAN
FRED MORADY

CARDIAC ELECTROPHYSIOLOGY CLINICS

www.cardiacEP.theclinics.com

Consulting Editors

RANJAN K. THAKUR
ANDREA NATALE

December 2012 • Volume 4 • Number 4

ELSEVIER

1600 John F. Kennedy Boulevard • Suite 1800 • Philadelphia, Pennsylvania 19103-2899

http://www.theclinics.com

CARDIAC ELECTROPHYSIOLOGY CLINICS Volume 4, Number 4
December 2012 ISSN 1877-9182, ISBN-13: 978-1-4557-4889-1

Editor: Barbara Cohen-Kligerman
Developmental Editor: Teia Stone

Cardiac Electrophysiology Clinics (ISSN 1877-9182) is published quarterly by Elsevier Inc., 360 Park Avenue South, New York, NY 10010-1710. Months of issue are March, June, September, and December. Subscription prices are $191.00 per year for US individuals, $277.00 per year for US institutions, $100.00 per year for US students and residents, $214.00 per year for Canadian individuals, $309.00 per year for Canadian institutions, $273.00 per year for international individuals, $331.00 per year for international institutions and $143.00 per year for Canadian and foreign students/residents. To receive student/resident rate, orders must be accompanied by name of affilliated institution, date of term, and the signature of program/residency coordinator on institution letterhead. Orders will be billed at individual rate until proof of status is received. Foreign air speed delivery is included in all Clinics subscription prices. All prices are subject to change without notice. **POSTMASTER:** Send address changes to Cardiac Electrophysiology Clinics, Elsevier Health Sciences Division, Subscription Customer Service, 3251 Riverport Lane, Maryland Heights, MO 63043. **Customer Service: 1-800-654-2452 (US and Canada). From outside of the US and Canada, call 314-477-8871. Fax: 314-447-8029. E-mail: JournalsCustomerService-usa@elsevier.com (for print support); JournalsOnlineSupport-usa@elsevier.com (for online support).**

Reprints. For copies of 100 or more of articles in this publication, please contact the Commercial Reprints Department, Elsevier Inc., 360 Park Avenue South, New York, NY 10010-1710. Tel.: 212-633-3812; Fax: 212-462-1935; E-mail: reprints@elsevier.com.

Printed and bound by CPI Group (UK) Ltd, Croydon, CR0 4YY

Transferred to digital print 2012

Contributors

CONSULTING EDITORS

RANJAN K. THAKUR, MD, MPH, MBA, FHRS
Professor of Medicine, Director, Arrhythmia Service, Thoracic and Cardiovascular Institute, Sparrow Health System, Michigan State University, Lansing, Michigan

ANDREA NATALE, MD, FACC, FHRS
Executive Medical Director, Texas Cardiac Arrhythmia Institute, St David's Medical Center, Austin, Texas; Consulting Professor, Division of Cardiology, Stanford University, Palo Alto, California; Adjunct Professor of Medicine, Heart and Vascular Center, Case Western Reserve University, Cleveland, Ohio; Director, Interventional Electrophysiology, Scripps Clinic, San Diego, California; Senior Clinical Director, EP Services, California Pacific Medical Center, San Francisco, California

GUEST EDITORS

MELVIN M. SCHEINMAN, MD
Professor of Medicine, Section of Electrophysiology, Division of Cardiology; Shorestein Chair in Cardiology, University of California San Francisco Medical Center, San Francisco, California

FRED MORADY, MD
McKay Professor of Cardiovascular Disease, Professor of Medicine, University of Michigan Health System, Ann Arbor, Michigan

SECTION EDITORS

NITISH BADHWAR, MBBS, FACC, FHRS
Director, Cardiac Electrophysiology Training Program, Associate Professor of Medicine, Associate Chief, Cardiac Electrophysiology Section, Cardiology Division, Department of Medicine, University of California, San Francisco, San Francisco, California

RAIMUNDO BARBOSA, MD
Chief, Coronary Center, Hospital de Messejana Dr. Carlos Alberto Studart Gomes, Fortaleza, Ceará, Brazil

EDWARD P. GERSTENFELD, MD
Chief, Cardiac Electrophysiology, Associate Professor of Medicine, Melvin M. Scheinman Endowed Chair in Cardiology, Cardiology Division, Department of Medicine, University of California San Francisco Medical Center, San Francisco, California

BYRON K. LEE, MD, MAS
Associate Professor of Medicine, Director of the UCSF Cardiac Electrophysiology Laboratories and Clinics, Division of Cardiology, Department of Medicine, Cardiac Electrophysiology and Arrhythmia Service, UCSF Medical Center, University of California, San Francisco, San Francisco, California

GREGORY M. MARCUS, MD, MAS
Associate Professor of Medicine, Electrophysiology Section, Division of Cardiology, University of California, San Francisco, San Francisco, California

FRED MORADY, MD
McKay Professor of Cardiovascular Disease, Professor of Medicine, University of Michigan Health System, Ann Arbor, Michigan

WILLIAM NELSON, MD
Director of Cardiology, St. Joseph Hospital, Denver, Colorado

ANDRÉS RICARDO PÉREZ-RIERA, MD, PhD
Chief of Electrovetorcardiography, Disciplina de Cardiologia, Faculdade de Medicina do ABC, Santo André, São Paulo, Brazil

RONN E. TANEL, MD
Associate Professor of Clinical Pediatrics, Section of Electrophysiology, Division of Pediatric Cardiology, Department of Pediatrics, UCSF School of Medicine, UCSF Medical Center; Director, Pediatric Arrhythmia Center, UCSF Benioff Children's Hospital, San Francisco, California

ZIAN H. TSENG, MD, MAS
Associate Professor of Medicine in Residence, Cardiac Electrophysiology Section, Cardiology Division, University of California, San Francisco

AUTHORS

RYAN G. ALEONG, MD
Cardiac Electrophysiology, University of Colorado Anschutz Medical Campus, Aurora, Colorado

NITISH BADHWAR, MBBS, FACC, FHRS
Director, Cardiac Electrophysiology Training Program, Associate Professor of Medicine, Associate Chief, Cardiac Electrophysiology Section, Cardiology Division, Department of Medicine, University of California, San Francisco, San Francisco, California

RUPA BALA, MD
Assistant Professor of Medicine, Hospital of the University of Pennsylvania, Philadelphia, Pennsylvania

RAIMUNDO BARBOSA, MD
Chief, Coronary Center, Hospital de Messejana Dr. Carlos Alberto Studart Gomes, Fortaleza, Ceará, Brazil

ROYCE L. BARGAS, DO
Section of Cardiac Electrophysiology, Division of Cardiology, University of Colorado School of Medicine, Aurora, Colorado

SETH R. BENDER, MD
Fellow in Clinical Cardiac Electrophysiology, Division of Cardiology, Department of Medicine, Cornell University Medical Center, New York, New York

JIM W. CHEUNG, MD, FACC, FHRS
Assistant Professor of Medicine, Division of Cardiology, Department of Medicine, Weill Cornell Medical College, New York, New York

AMAN CHUGH, MD
Associate Professor, Department of Internal Medicine, Cardiovascular Center, University of Michigan Health System, Ann Arbor, Michigan

MARC W. DEYELL, MD, MSC
Electrophysiology Section, Hospital of the University of Pennsylvania, Philadelphia, Pennsylvania

RYAN FOLEY, MD
Resident, Internal Medicine, University of Colorado Anschutz Medical Campus, Aurora, Colorado

FERMIN C. GARCIA, MD
Electrophysiology Section, Hospital of the University of Pennsylvania, Philadelphia, Pennsylvania

EDWARD P. GERSTENFELD, MD
Chief, Cardiac Electrophysiology, Associate Professor of Medicine, Melvin M. Scheinman Endowed Chair in Cardiology, Cardiology Division, Department of Medicine, University of California San Francisco Medical Center, San Francisco, California

LEA EL HAGE, MD
Section of Electrophysiology, Division of Cardiology, University of California San Francisco, San Francisco, California

FREDERICK T. HAN, MD
Assistant Professor, Internal Medicine, Clinical Cardiac Electrophysiology Fellow, Section of Electrophysiology, University of Utah Health Sciences Center, Salt Lake City, Utah; Division of Cardiology, University of California San Francisco Medical Center, San Francisco, California

RUSSELL R. HEATH, MD
Electrophysiology Fellow, Section of Cardiac Electrophysiology, Division of Cardiology, University of Colorado School of Medicine, Denver, Anschutz Medical Campus, Aurora, Colorado

KURT S. HOFFMAYER, PharmD, MD
Section of Electrophysiology, Division of Cardiology, University of California San Francisco, San Francisco, California

BHARAT K. KANTHARIA, MD, FRCP, FAHA, FACC, FESC
Division of Clinical Cardiac Electrophysiology, The University of Texas Health Science Center at Houston, Houston, Texas

DAVID F. KATZ, MD
Electrophysiology Fellow, Cardiac Electrophysiology, Cardiology Division, University of Colorado Denver, Anschutz Medical Campus, Aurora, Colorado

RAKESH LATCHAMSETTY, MD
Clinical Lecturer, Department of Internal Medicine, Brighton Health Center, Brighton, Michigan

BYRON K. LEE, MD, MAS
Associate Professor of Medicine, Director of the UCSF Cardiac Electrophysiology Laboratories and Clinics, Division of Cardiology, Department of Medicine, Cardiac Electrophysiology and Arrhythmia Service, UCSF Medical Center, University of California, San Francisco, San Francisco, California

WALTER LI, MD
Clinical Cardiac Electrophysiology Fellow, Section of Electrophysiology, Division of Pediatric Cardiology, Department of Pediatrics, UCSF School of Medicine, UCSF Benioff Children's Hospital, University of California San Francisco Medical Center, San Francisco, California

GREGORY M. MARCUS, MD, MAS
Associate Professor of Medicine, Electrophysiology Section, Division of Cardiology, University of California, San Francisco, San Francisco, California

FRED MORADY, MD
McKay Professor of Cardiovascular Disease, Professor of Medicine, University of Michigan Health System, Ann Arbor, Michigan

WILLIAM NELSON, MD
Director of Cardiology, St. Joseph Hospital, Denver, Colorado

DUY THAI NGUYEN, MD, FHRS, FACC
Assistant Professor of Medicine, Section of Cardiac Electrophysiology, Division of Cardiology, University of Colorado, Denver, Anschutz Medical Campus, Aurora, Colorado

ANDRÉS RICARDO PÉREZ-RIERA, MD, PhD
Chief of Electrovetorcardiography, Disciplina de Cardiologia, Faculdade de Medicina do ABC, Santo André, São Paulo, Brazil

MARWAN M. REFAAT, MD
Electrophysiology Fellow, Cardiac Electrophysiology Section, Division of Cardiology, Department of Medicine, University of California San Francisco Medical Center, San Francisco, California

ROBERT W. RHO, MD, FHRS, FACC
Sutter Pacific Medical Foundation, Atrial Fibrillation and Complex Arrhythmia Center, San Francisco, California

EMILY RUCKDESCHEL, MD
Adult and Pediatric Cardiology Fellow, University of Colorado, Denver, Anschutz Medical Campus, Aurora, Colorado

WILLIAM H. SAUER, MD
Associate Professor of Medicine, Section of Cardiac Electrophysiology, Cardiology Division, University of Colorado School of Medicine, Denver, Anschutz Medical Campus, Aurora, Colorado

MELVIN M. SCHEINMAN, MD
Professor of Medicine, Section of Electrophysiology, Division of Cardiology, Shorestein Chair in Cardiology, University of California San Francisco Medical Center, San Francisco, California

RAPHAEL K. SUNG, MD
Section of Electrophysiology, Division of Cardiology, University of California San Francisco, San Francisco, California

RONN E. TANEL, MD
Associate Professor of Clinical Pediatrics, Section of Electrophysiology, Division of Pediatric Cardiology, Department of Pediatrics, UCSF School of Medicine, UCSF Medical Center; Director, Pediatric Arrhythmia Center, UCSF Benioff Children's Hospital, San Francisco, California

WENDY S. TZOU, MD, FHRS
Assistant Professor of Medicine, University of Colorado, Denver, Colorado; Section of Cardiac Electrophysiology, Division of Cardiology, University of Colorado School of Medicine, Aurora, Colorado

VASANTH VEDANTHAM, MD, PhD
Assistant Professor of Medicine, Cardiac Electrophysiology Section, Cardiology Division, University of California San Francisco, San Francisco, California

Contents

Foreword: Learning from Others **xvii**

Ranjan K. Thakur and Andrea Natale

Preface: Complex Arrhythmia Cases **xix**

Melvin M. Scheinman and Fred Morady

Disorders of Impulse Formation and Conduction

William Nelson, Section Editor

Abnormalities of Impulse Formation and Conduction **469**

William Nelson

Pitfalls in the interpretation of an electrocardiograph (EKG) include overinterpretation, computer error, and technician error. It is essential that previous tracings be included in the interpretation of the current EKG. Patients should be instructed not to move during EKG recording. The clinician should insist on 12-lead tracings, with 3 rhythm strips at the bottom; single leads are often misleading. Complex arrhythmias require a logical stepwise approach, which can be provided by using a ladder diagram.

Acute Myocardial Infarction

Andrés Ricardo Pérez-Riera and Raimundo Barbosa, Section Editors

Acute Myocardial Infarction Case Histories **479**

Andrés Ricardo Pérez-Riera and Raimundo Barbosa

Through a series of 9 case examples, the reader is asked to diagnose abnormalities in ECG tracings and correlate them with symptoms. Abnormalities include location of Q waves and ST elevation vectors.

Supraventricular Tachycardia

Nitish Badhwar, Section Editor

Supraventricular Tachycardia **493**

Nitish Badhwar

The section in this issue on supraventricular tachycardia (SVT) focuses on difficult cases of atrioventricular nodal reentrant tachycardia, Wolff-Parkinson-White syndrome with recurrent atrioventricular reentrant tachycardia despite multiple ablations, nodofascicular SVT and tachycardia-induced cardiomyopathy associated with double fire, permanent reciprocating junctional tachycardia, and atrial tachycardia. Emphasis is placed on the use of diagnostic maneuvers to make the appropriate diagnosis and on appropriate ablation strategy in patients with recurrent SVT.

signals, and pacing maneuvers. This section is devoted to case reports that demonstrate how these tools can be used to successfully ablate several different complex flutters.

A 70-year-old man presented with repeat atrial flutter 2 years after apparently successful cavotricuspid isthmus (CTI) ablation for typical atrial flutter. An electrophysiology study was then performed, and CARTO electroanatomic 3-dimensional mapping of the tachycardia was consistent with typical flutter. However, entrainment mapping from the lateral and mid CTI revealed postpacing intervals greater than 30 milliseconds more than the tachycardia cycle length. Entrainment mapping from the septal CTI and coronary sinus ostium was in the circuit. A diagnosis of intraisthmus reentry was made and successful ablation was achieved with termination, with radiofrequency ablation directly outside the coronary sinus ostium.

Partial anomalous pulmonary venous return is a relatively uncommon congenital heart disease that may require surgical correction. Atrial arrhythmias are common after surgical correction of congenital heart disease. This article reports a case of intra-atrial reentrant tachycardia following surgical repair of partial anomalous pulmonary venous return and successful catheter ablation. Knowledge of the patient's congenital anatomy and surgical correction, as well as a combination of entrainment and electroanatomic mapping, helped to efficiently define the tachycardia mechanism and to identify the culprit area sustaining the tachycardia.

A 40-year-old man with a history of tetralogy of Fallot and multiple cardiac surgeries presented for mapping and ablation of an incessant atrial tachyarrhythmia. Activation and entrainment mapping in conjunction with an electroanatomic mapping system defined the mechanism of the tachycardia as a dual-loop incisional reentry atrial flutter around previous atriotomy scars in the lateral right atrium. A line of ablation lesions transecting the critical isthmus of both loops of the dual-loop circuit successfully terminated the atrial flutter.

A 67-year-old man without prior heart disease presented with atrial flutter, with a 12-lead electrocardiogram (ECG) suggestive of typical atrial flutter. The patient underwent electrophysiology study and was found to have atypical atrial flutter, with entrainment mapping indicating likely left-sided flutter. Transseptal puncture was performed, and entrainment mapping within the left atrium suggested a circuit close

to the right common pulmonary vein. This case highlights several key findings, including left-sided flutter mimicking typical flutter on 12-lead ECG and the need for careful, high-density mapping in the region of interest to avoid missing a critical area of reentrant arrhythmia.

A 55-year-old man was referred for ablation of symptomatic typical counterclockwise atrial flutter. Concealed entrainment from the cavotricuspid isthmus (CTI) and electroanatomic CARTO activation mapping confirmed the arrhythmia to be typical CTI-dependent atrial flutter. During radiofrequency ablation, a regular irregularity in the tachycardia cycle length (ie, cycle length alternans [250 and 210 milliseconds]), but with the same activation sequence in the right atrium, and fixed cycle length at 250 milliseconds in the left atrium were subsequently noted. This report addresses potential mechanisms and explanations for the cycle length alternans that may be observed during ablation of cavotricuspid isthmus–dependent atrial flutter.

depolarization occurred when the ring catheter was positioned in the left inferior pulmonary vein and a decapolar catheter was in the coronary sinus. Caution should be used with further ablation.

Is This a Good Target Site for Ablation of an Atrial Tachycardia? **575**

Aman Chugh and Fred Morady

This article describes the case of a 68-year-old woman who was referred for atrial tachycardia following a catheter ablation procedure. The tachycardia terminated despite the fact that the pacing stimulus did not result in atrial capture. This finding is very specific for identifying a critical site in a reentry circuit.

Pulmonary Vein Isolation in a 63-year-old Man with Paroxysmal Atrial Fibrillation **577**

Rakesh Latchamsetty and Fred Morady

Pulmonary vein isolation was performed in a 63-year-old man with paroxysmal atrial fibrillation. Electrograms were recorded during antral ablation around the right superior pulmonary vein. It is important to recognize that sometimes with pacing enough decremental conduction occurs into the pulmonary vein to cause conduction block.

Arrhythmias in Repaired Congential Heart Disease

Ronn E. Tanel and Zian H. Tseng, Section Editors

Introduction to Pediatric Arrhythmias **579**

Ronn E. Tanel

This article introduces the section devoted to pediatric arrhythmias. Because intra-atrial reentrant tachycardia is especially common in patients who have had a Fontan operation for single-ventricle physiology or a Mustard or Senning operation for transposition of the great arteries, anatomic considerations and surgical techniques are particularly important to understand when planning an invasive electrophysiology procedure in such a patient.

Intra-Atrial Reentrant Tachycardia in an Adult with Ebstein Anomaly **581**

Walter Li and Ronn E. Tanel

A 42-year-old woman with Ebstein anomaly of the tricuspid valve and multiple prior cardiac surgical interventions presented for electrophysiologic study and catheter ablation of chronic atrial arrhythmias. Electroanatomic mapping and entrainment pacing demonstrated a reentrant mechanism with a site critical to the maintenance of the tachycardia at the septal cavotricuspid isthmus (CTI). Radiofrequency ablation at that site resulted in a change in the activation pattern to that of typical CTI-dependent atrial flutter. The patient was treated with a linear set of ablation lesions in the usual location between the inferior vena cava and the tricuspid valve annulus.

Atrial Flutter 23 Years After Classic Fontan **587**

Kurt S. Hoffmayer and Nitish Badhwar

A 25-year-old man with tricuspsid atresia treated with Blalock-Taussig shunt at 6 months then subsequent Fontan at 2 years presented with atrial flutter. An electrophysiology study was performed, and an electroanatomic map was created that was consistent with a macro-reentrant atrial flutter, with an early-meets-late configuration. Long fractionated potentials were seen in the mid superior right atrium, and

ventricular tachycardia in the setting of atrial fibrillation. Dual tachycardias in patients with implantable cardioverter-defibrillators (ICDs) are common, and studies have reported that up to 10% of ventricular tachyarrhythmias detected by ICDs are preceded by supraventricular tachycardia. It is imperative to distinguish ventricular from supraventricular tachyarrhythmias seen in stored ICD electrograms, as it has significant implications for appropriate ICD programming and use of medical and catheter ablation therapy.

Difficulties in Implantable Cardioverter-Defibrillator Programming **641**

Walter Li and Ronn E. Tanel

This article presents a case of supraventricular tachycardia in a patient with an implantable cardioverter-defibrillator (ICD). Interrogation of an ICD following a device discharge should begin with an evaluation of the current programming, because inappropriate device programming is a common cause of inappropriate shocks. One common pitfall is programming the ventricular fibrillation or ventricular tachycardia detection criteria within the physiologic range of heart rate, particularly in younger patients.

Infra-Hisian Atrioventricular Block **645**

Wendy S. Tzou, Ryan Foley, Duy Thai Nguyen, and Ryan G. Aleong

This article reports the case of a 72-year-old woman with a history of hypertension and hyperlipidemia who presented with episodes of presyncope and 2:1 atrioventricular (AV) block, with alternating left and right bundle branch block. The patient underwent dual-chamber pacemaker implantation. Mechanisms for AV block are discussed.

Inappropriate Discharges After Implantable Cardioverter-Defibrillator Placement **651**

Walter Li and Ronn E. Tanel

This article presents the case of a 16-year-old male with an implantable cardioverter-defibrillator who sustained shocks. He was diagnosed with lead dislodgment likely attributable to twiddler syndrome. The patient's device was revised and the lead replaced, and he made a complete recovery.

New Irregular Rhythm in a Patient with Baseline Left Bundle Branch Block **655**

Marwan M. Refaat and Byron K. Lee

This article reports the case of a 63-year-old man with nonischemic idiopathic cardiomyopathy and baseline left bundle branch block (LBBB) who was fitted with an implantable cardioverter-defibrillator (ICD). The patient was managed for fatigue and episodes of palpitations 4 months after placement of the ICD. This case illustrates the physiology described previously in a patient with an LBBB who is detected to have a near normal QRS complex rhythm.

Index **659**

CARDIAC ELECTROPHYSIOLOGY CLINICS

FORTHCOMING ISSUES

March 2013
Arrhythmias in Athletes
Domenico Corrado, MD, PhD,
Cristina Basso, MD, PhD, and
Gaetano Thiene, MD, *Guest Editors*

June 2013
Mapping of Atrial Tachycardias Post-Atrial Fibrillation Ablation
Ashok J. Shah, MD, Michel Haissaguerre, MD,
and Shinsuke Miyazaki, MD, PhD, *Guest Editors*

September 2013
Remote Monitoring and Physiologic Sensing Technologies and Applications
Samuel Asirvatham, MD,
K. L. Venkatachalam, MD, and Suraj Kapa, MD,
Guest Editors

RECENT ISSUES

September 2012
Contemporary Debates and Controversies in Cardiac Electrophysiology, Part II
Ranjan K. Thakur, MD, MPH, and
Andrea Natale, MD, *Guest Editors*

June 2012
Difficult Decisions in Clinical Electrophysiology—A Case Based Approach
Mark C. Haigney, MD, and
Adam Strickberger, MD, *Guest Editors*

March 2012
Long QT Syndrome
Silvia G. Priori, MD, PhD, *Guest Editor*

ISSUES OF RELATED INTEREST

Cardiology Clinics August 2012 (Vol. 30, No. 3)
Cardiovascular Disease in Pregnancy
Gagan Sahni, MD, and Uri Elkayam, MD, *Guest Editors*
Available at: http://www.cardiology.theclinics.com/

Interventional Cardiology Clinics October 2012 (Vol. 1, No. 4)
STEMI interventions
Sameer Mehta, MD, *Guest Editor*
Available at: http://www.interventional.theclinics.com/

Foreword
Learning from Others

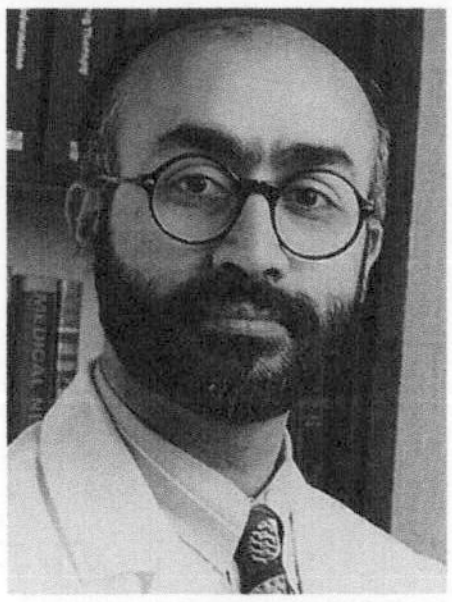

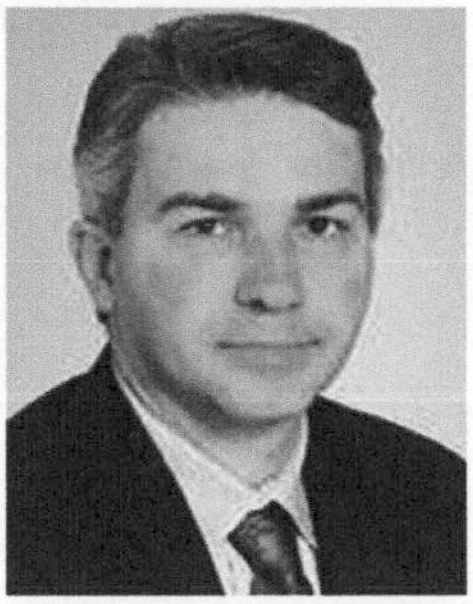

Ranjan Thakur, MD, MPH, MBA, FHRS   Andrea Natale, MD, FACC, FHRS
Consulting Editors

While a fool does not learn from his experience, an intelligent man does;
But, a wise man learns from the experience of others.

—From Sanskrit Proverb

The practice of cardiac electrophysiology requires not only a thorough understanding of established knowledge and new research findings but also a deliberate application of the known principles to solve difficult electrophysiologic puzzles in the laboratory, making clinical decisions under uncertainty and continuously learning from experience.

Although the principles can be absorbed by reading, learning when, how, and which principles are most appropriate for solving a particular problem comes only through deliberate practice, which involves getting it wrong sometimes, learning from that experience, and learning from others as well. Fellowship training under the watchful eyes of good teachers helps establish the core knowledge, but the learning process must continue lifelong. Case studies, the analysis of difficult ECGs and electrograms, while anecdotal or empirical, allow us the opportunity to learn from the experience of others.

We are delighted that Dr Melvin Scheinman and Dr Fred Morady accepted our invitation to edit this issue of the *Cardiac Electrophysiology Clinics*. Both are well-known researchers and teachers. Dr Morady was once Dr Scheinman's fellow at the University of California San Francisco. It is pleasing to see that the "teacher" and the "taught" have come together to share their wisdom. They have assembled a group of colleagues who are similarly experienced clinicians and good teachers to present interesting cases with a message so that all of us can learn from their experience.

Electrophysiologists with varied levels of experience, from fellows to seasoned clinicians, will find this issue useful for learning, reviewing, and teaching others.

Ranjan Thakur, MD, MPH, MBA, FHRS
Sparrow Thoracic and Cardiovascular Institute
Michigan State University
1200 East Michigan Avenue, Suite 580
Lansing, MI 48912, USA

Andrea Natale, MD, FACC, FHRS
Texas Cardiac Arrhythmia Institute
Center for Atrial Fibrillation at
St. David's Medical Center
1015 East 32nd Street, Suite 516
Austin, TX 78705, USA

E-mail addresses:
thakur@msu.edu (R. Thakur)
andrea.natale@stdavids.com (A. Natale)

Card Electrophysiol Clin 4 (2012) xvii
http://dx.doi.org/10.1016/j.ccep.2012.10.001

Preface
Complex Arrhythmia Cases

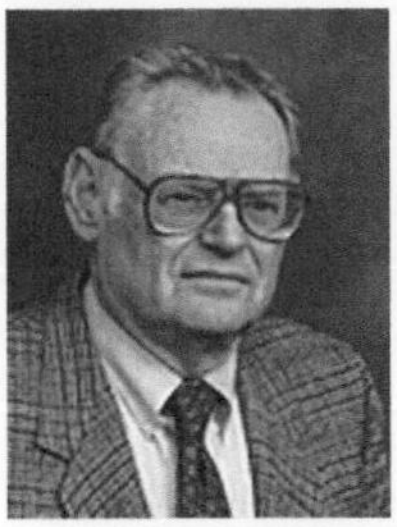
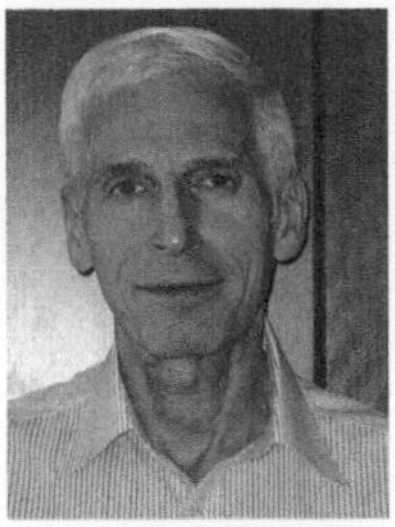

Melvin M. Scheinman, MD   Fred Morady, MD
Guest Editors

We have decided to embark on the second monograph consisting of case studies in electrophysiology and clinical electrophysiology. This was done because of the unexpected and heartening response to the first monograph. The initial effort 3 years ago grew out of a conviction that cardiac rhythm specialists enjoy the challenge of evaluating tracings and matching wits with the authors. This need was felt to be especially important as more and more cardiac journals have chosen to either omit or strictly limit acceptance of case reports.

This issue contains entirely fresh cases gleaned from colleagues from all over the country, and we are grateful for the effort and time expended to provide these case gems. In addition, we have changed the format in that we added an article related to the diagnoses and localization of acute myocardial infarction using a vectorial approach.

We are indebted to our master teacher, Dr Riera, for providing both the excellent case material and the conceptual framework for using this exciting approach to diagnoses of myocardial infarction. Similarly, we thank Dr Nelson for his erudite and clear-cut elaboration on the problem of electrical impulse formation and conduction disturbances.

The issue would not have been possible without the diligent and careful editing by the section editors who spent many hours selecting and clarifying case content. Finally, our sincere thanks are extended to Barbara Cohen-Kligerman of Elsevier for her encouragement and diligence in keeping this project on schedule.

Melvin M. Scheinman, MD
Electrophysiology Service
500 Parnassus Avenue, Suite 433
San Francisco, CA 94143-1354, USA

Fred Morady, MD
University of Michigan Health System
1500 East Medical Center Drive
Ann Arbor, MI 48109, USA

E-mail addresses:
scheinman@medicine.ucsf.edu (M.M. Scheinman)
fmorady@med.umich.edu (F. Morady)

Card Electrophysiol Clin 4 (2012) xix
http://dx.doi.org/10.1016/j.ccep.2012.10.002
1877-9182/12/$ – see front matter

Abnormalities of Impulse Formation and Conduction

William Nelson, MD

KEYWORDS

• Conduction • Electrocardiograph • Arrhythmia • Impulse formation

KEY POINTS

- Pitfalls in the interpretation of an electrocardiograph (EKG) include overinterpretation, computer error, and technician error.
- It is essential that previous tracings be included in the interpretation of the current EKG.
- Patients should be instructed not to move during EKG recording.
- The clinician should insist on 12-lead tracings with 3 rhythm strips at the bottom; single leads are often misleading.
- Complex arrhythmias require a logical stepwise approach, which can be provided by using a ladder diagram.

The electrocardiograph (EKG) remains an important and informative component of cardiac evaluation. Some abnormalities can be determined only by EKG (eg, arrhythmias); some can be diagnosed (eg, myocardial infarction); and others can be suggested when a specific pattern is seen (eg, pericarditis).

A first approach to EKG interpretation can be provided by observations that are available at a glance:

- Are there regular R-R cycles?
- Are P waves present with normal PR intervals?
- Is the frontal plane axis normal?
- Are significant Q waves absent?
- Is there appropriate precordial R wave development and QRS transition?

If all of the observations are present, then the tracing is normal, a conclusion that requires only a few seconds.

In an approach to EKG interpretation, there are several "Commandments," which should be emphasized.

COMMANDMENT 1: THOU SHALT NOT OVERINTERPRET THE EKG

The range of normal is broad and clinical circumstance must dictate the importance of a particular EKG observation. The late Dr H.J.L. Marriott phrased it nicely: "Many an unfortunate individual is limping his apprehensive way through life maimed by the unkind cut of EKG misinterpretation."

COMMANDMENT 2: BEWARE THE MISCHIEVOUS MACHINE

The current 3-channel EKG is an excellent device and most of the problems of yesteryear have been removed. The modern mischief is the EKG analysis provided by the computer. Computer errors are frequent and can be disastrous to both patient and doctor (**Fig. 1**).

COMMANDMENT 3: BEWARE OF TECHNICIAN ERRORS

Even the most conscientious and dedicated technician can record tracings with misplaced electrodes (**Fig. 2**).

St. Joseph Hospital, 1835 Franklin Street, Denver, CO 80218, USA
E-mail address: subscriptions@nelsonsekgsite.com

Card Electrophysiol Clin 4 (2012) 469–478
http://dx.doi.org/10.1016/j.ccep.2012.08.035

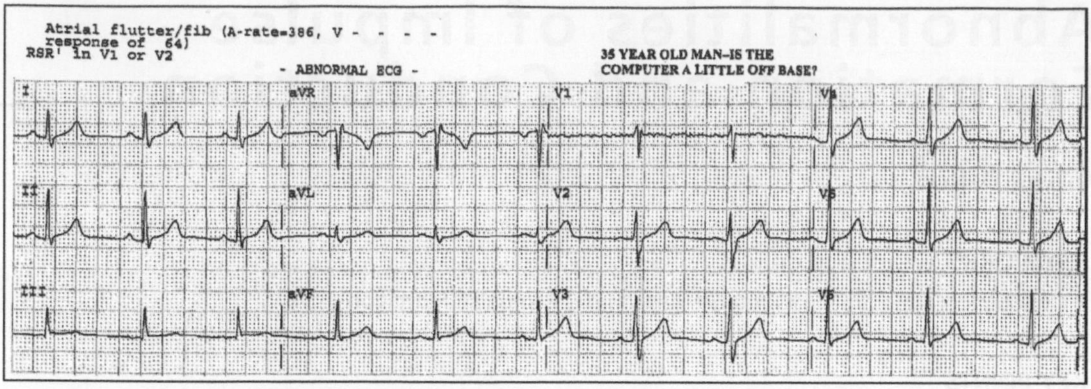

Fig. 1. This young man was referred because of the computer interpretation of his EKG. A glance indicates that the tracing is normal. Clearly, the computer is seriously in error.

COMMANDMENT 4: THOU SHALT NOT INTERPRET THE EKG WITHOUT REFERENCE TO PREVIOUS TRACINGS

It is essential that previous tracings be included in the interpretation of the current EKG. Seeming minor differences in 2 tracings may indicate a significant new abnormality.

COMMANDMENT 5: BE CAUTIOUS OF THE CAPRICIOUS PATIENT

It is prudent to instruct the patient about the fifth EKG commandment, which specifies that moving, wiggling, coughing, or hiccupping during EKG recording is *verboten* (**Fig. 3**)!

COMMANDMENT 6: ASSIDUOUSLY AVOID RHYTHM STRIPS

Insist on 12-lead tracings, with 3 rhythm strips at the bottom. Single leads are often misleading , as is apparent in the strips in **Figs. 4** and **5**.

The sinus node is provided at birth and many keep it as the dominant pacemaker for a lifetime. Other pacing sites are available in the atrium and atrioventricular (AV) junction. They may appear as a normal event if the sinus node defaults or may be a result of abnormal function of the ectopic site. The most common arrhythmias encountered are provided in **Box 1**.

COMMANDMENT 7: LEARN TO USE LADDER DIAGRAMS

Simple arrhythmias are easily analyzed and are obvious at a glance (eg, atrial or ventricular premature beats). Complex arrhythmias require a logical stepwise approach, which can be provided by using a ladder diagram. With practice, one becomes more confident and more frequently correct in a quick analysis in an acute situation. Many ladder diagram analyses are included in the remainder of this article. To save space, most

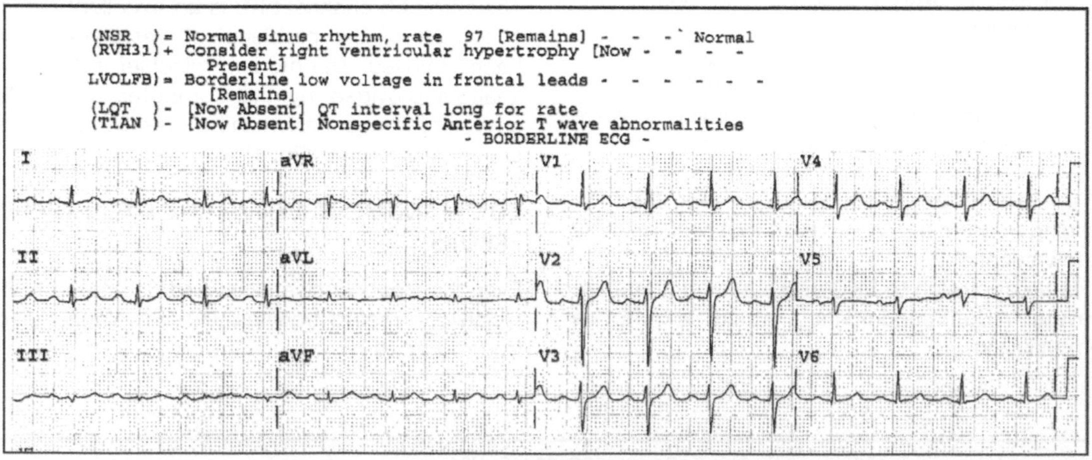

Fig. 2. The computer has not recognized the precordial lead error of the "treacherous technician." Looking carefully: lead V5 is really V1; V3 is V2; V2 is V3; V4 is correct; V1 is V5; V6 is correct. With this rearrangement, the precordial leads are normal and there is no evidence of right ventricular hypertrophy.

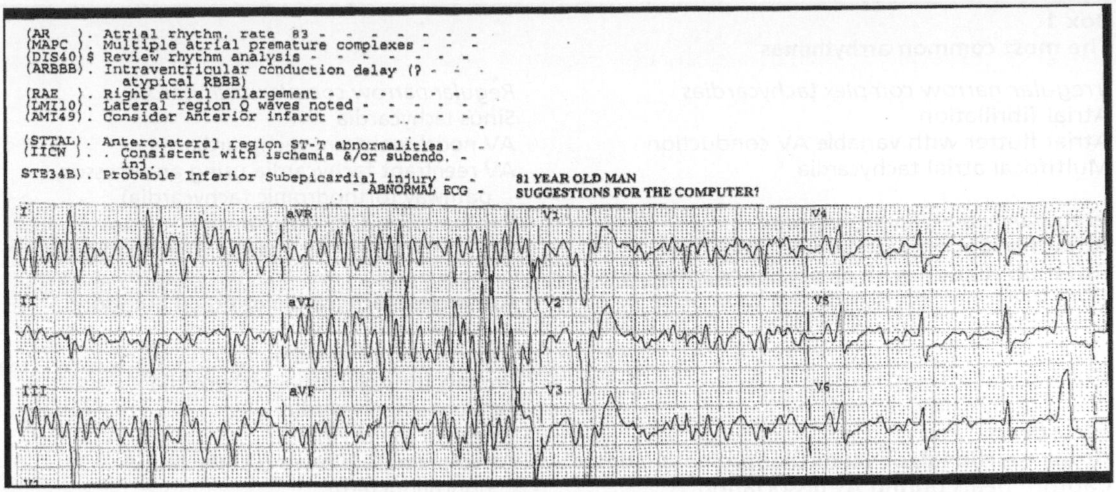

Fig. 3. None of the computer diagnoses is correct. The patient's movements have created sufficient artifact so that the tracing cannot be interpreted.

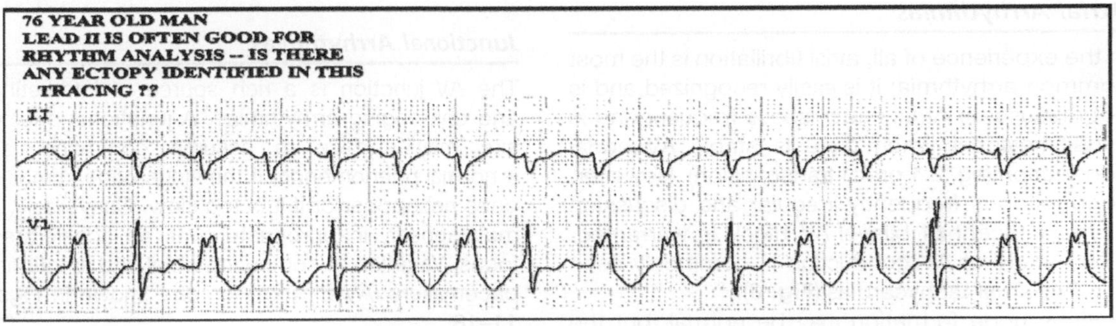

Fig. 4. The morphology of the QRS complexes is the same in lead II, but in lead V1, the pairs of ventricular premature contractions are obvious.

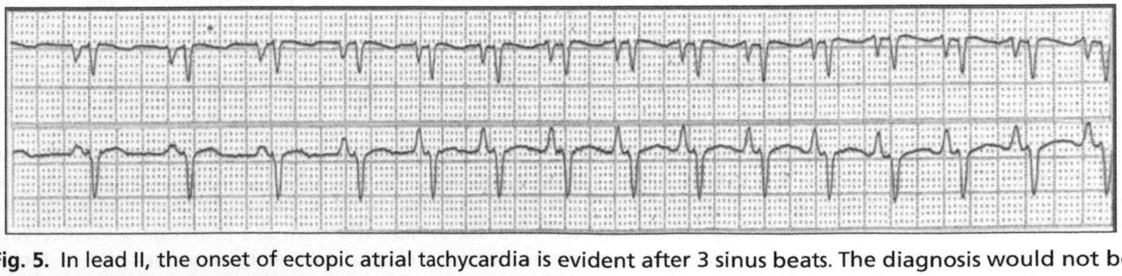

Fig. 5. In lead II, the onset of ectopic atrial tachycardia is evident after 3 sinus beats. The diagnosis would not be possible in the simultaneous V1 strip.

Box 1
The most common arrhythmias

Irregular narrow complex tachycardias	*Regular narrow complex tachycardia*
Atrial fibrillation	Sinus tachycardia
Atrial flutter with variable AV conduction	AV nodal reentrant tachycardia
Multifocal atrial tachycardia	AV reentrant tachycardia using an accessory pathway (orthodromic tachycardia)
Irregular wide-QRS tachycardias	*Regular wide-QRS tachycardias*
Atrial fibrillation with bundle branch block	Supraventricular tachycardia with bundle branch block
Atrial fibrillation with an accessory pathway	Antidromic tachycardia using an accessory pathway
	Ventricular tachycardia
	Primary (ectopic) atrial tachycardia
	Junctional tachycardia
Early beats	*Pauses in the rhythm*
Atrial, junctional, or ventricular premature beats	Atrial premature beats (conducted or nonconducted)
Capture beats during AV dissociation	Ventricular premature beats (with or without retrograde conduction)
Reciprocal beats	Type 1 or 2 AV block
	Sinoatrial exit block
	Concealed junctional extrasystoles

are presented with single rhythm strips, which were obtained from 12-lead tracings.

Atrial Arrhythmias

In the experience of all, atrial fibrillation is the most common arrhythmia; it is easily recognized and is not discussed. Atrial flutter is less frequent and is usually evident when there is stable AV nodal conduction (eg, 2:1 or 4:1 transmission). However, conduction is frequently irregular and discussion of the concept of bilevel AV block is warranted. This variety of AV conduction is commonly seen in other atrial tachycardias (**Fig. 6**).

Sinus node formation may be normal, but the stimulus may not conduct to the right atrium (an abnormality termed sinoatrial exit block) (**Figs. 7–10**).

Junctional Arrhythmias

The AV junction is a rich source of interesting and challenging arrhythmias. A junctional pacing site may surface to assume command, as a normal phenomenon, if the sinus node stimulus does not appear or if it is too slow. Conversely, it may appear, inappropriately, as an accelerated focus. Varieties of competing atrial and junctional pacemakers (AV dissociation) are shown in **Figs. 11–18**.

Fig. 19 is an example of "Up the down stairs."

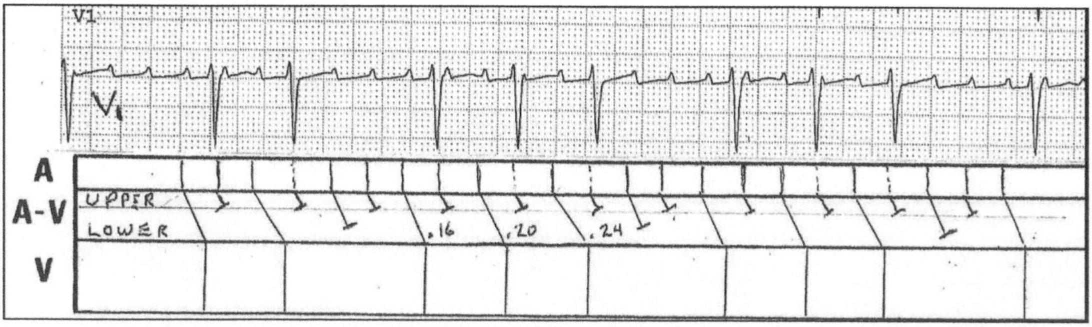

Fig. 6. Concept: alternating impulses do not transmit beyond the upper level. Those capable of transmission into the lower level may conduct on a 1:1 basis (which would be an effective ratio of 2:1 conduction of all potential stimuli). As depicted in the diagram, half of the stimuli of atrial flutter block in the upper level; the remainder may all be conducted, or, as seen, may be transmitted in a 3:2 or 4:3 ratio with the prolonging PR intervals, ending in a blocked impulse (typical Wenckebach phenomenon). Perpendicular lines represent site of block. The numbers are recorded in hundredths of a second (ie, .16 = 160 ms).

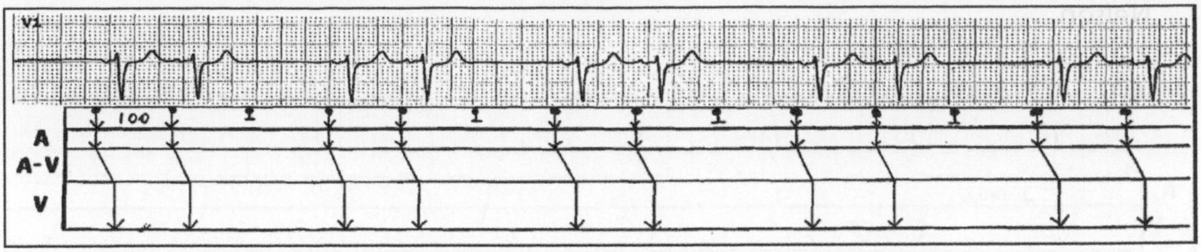

Fig. 7. In the example in this figure, the evident group beating could be atrial bigeminy with a lengthy postextrasystolic pause. However, the P wave morphology is constant. The manifest P-P cycle recurs, with a missing P wave every third beat. This is an example of type 2 sinoatrial exit block.

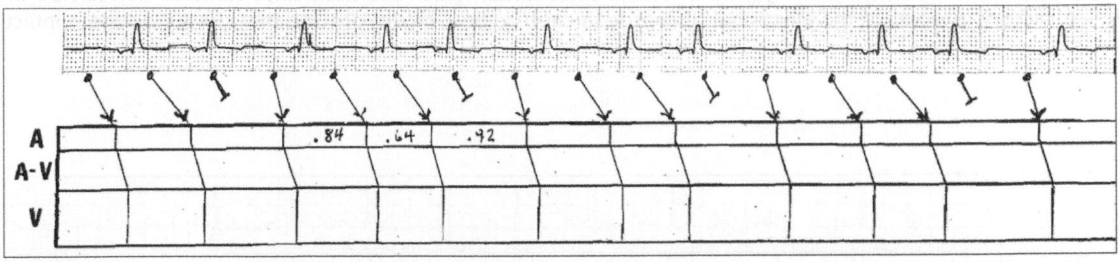

Fig. 8. The repetitive QRS pattern and the missing P waves serve as an alert to sinoatrial exit block. To determine the true sinus rate, the evident R-R cycles are measured. The sum, including the dropped beat, is 2.40 seconds (.84 + .64 + .92 = 2.40). Because this figure represents 4 sinus node discharges, the true sinus interval = .60 seconds–rate = 100/min. The ladder diagram depicts the gradual prolongation of the impulses exiting the sinus node. This is an example of type 1 exit block.

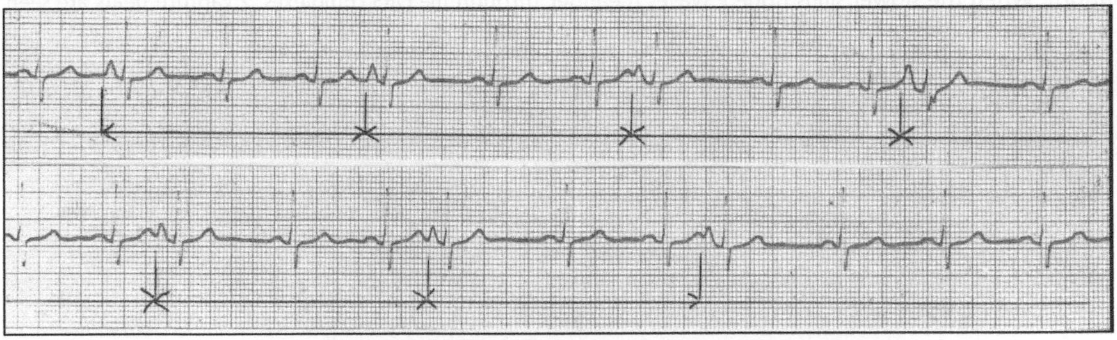

Fig. 9. The numerous atrial premature contractions are evident. A glance suggests that they recur at regular intervals, and such is the case. The measurements provided are from a millimeter ruler and identify the rhythmical discharge of an atrial parasystolic focus, existing independently and in competition with the sinus node activity. The parasystolic site is not altered by sinus discharge, termed entrance block, but if its timing placed it in the refractory period of a sinus node discharge, it would not appear, which is termed exit block. This rhythm was consistent during 5 years of observation. X represent APCs.

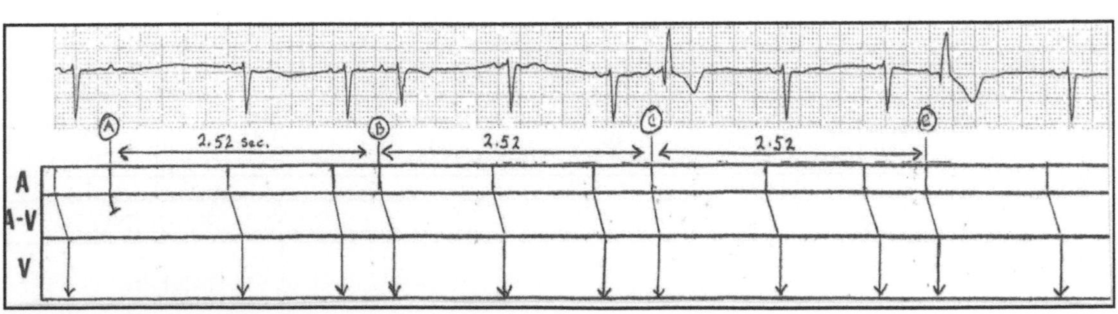

Fig. 10. The timing of the recurrent APCs is constant, with an interectopic interval of 2.5 seconds. This finding identifies an independent atrial parasystolic focus. The result of its discharge is interesting. Stimulus A is so early that the conducting system is refractory and it is not conducted. Stimulus B is normally conducted. Stimuli C find the right bundle refractory and are aberrantly conducted with right bundle branch block.

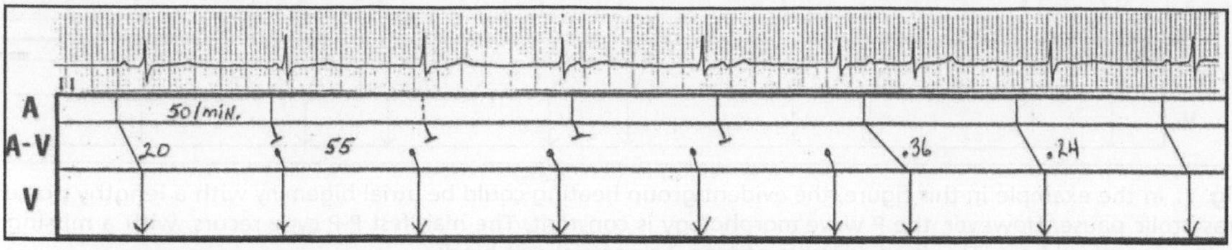

Fig. 11. The problem is sinus bradycardia, which permits a slightly faster junctional focus to assume command (an example of AV dissociation by default of the sinus node). When the tardy sinus stimulus wanders beyond the refractory interval of the junctional discharge, a capture beat occurs, proving that the AV bridge is intact.

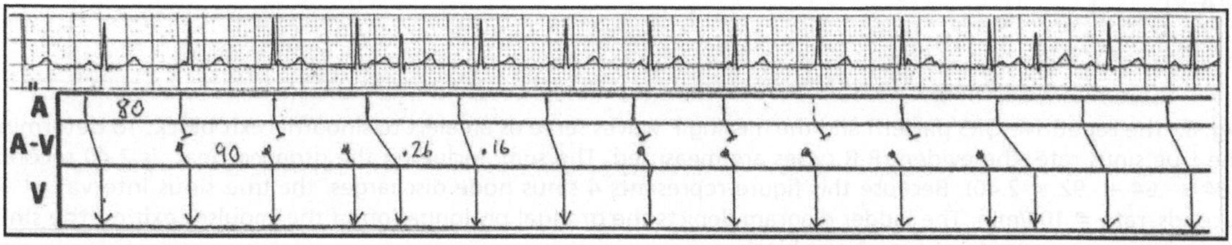

Fig. 12. An accelerated junctional focus at 90/min is in command (an example of AV dissociation caused by usurpation). When the slower sinus node P waves meander through the QRS complexes, 2 capture beats are seen.

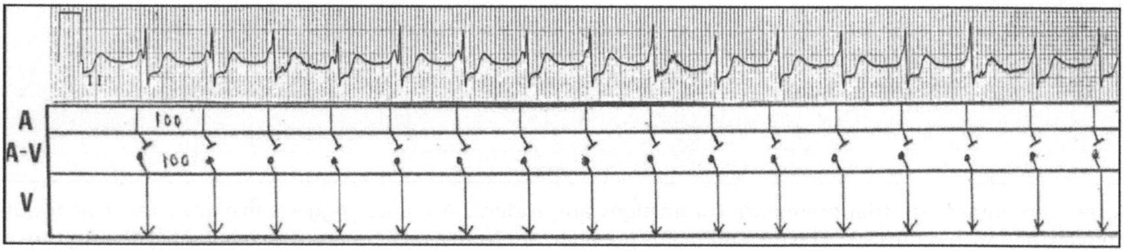

Fig. 13. An accelerated junctional focus at 100/min is competing with the sinus node at the same rate (an example of isochronic AV dissociation caused by an accelerated junctional focus).

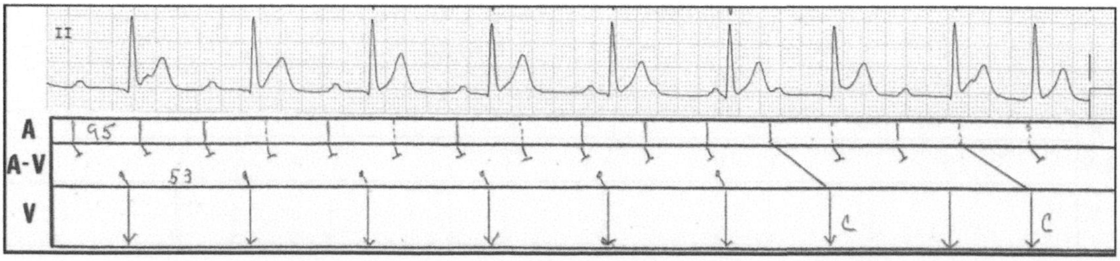

Fig. 14. The sinus rate of 95/min should keep it the dominant pacemaker. However, some degree of AV block prevents transmission and a junctional focus at 53/min appears. This finding represents AV dissociation caused by AV block. That the AV bridge is intact, but depressed, is shown by the 2 capture beats. This arrhythmia is common with drugs that decrease AV nodal conduction. C, capture beats.

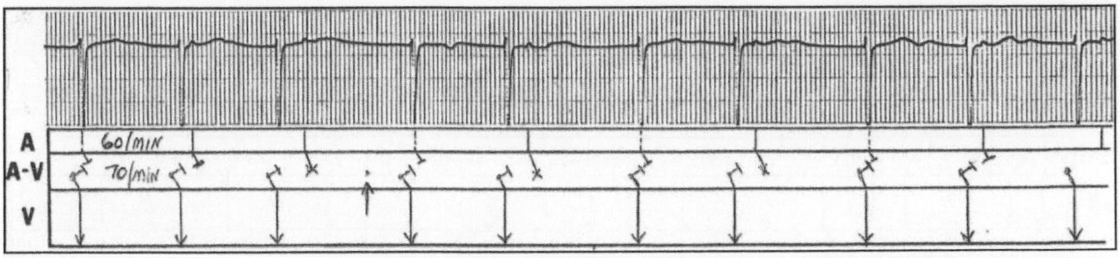

Fig. 15. Sinus P waves are evident at 60/min, but a competing junctional pacemaker at 70/min is in command. The competition of the 2 sites leads to AV dissociation caused by usurpation by the junctional focus. Sinus P waves never succeed in conduction but show the phenomenon of concealed anterograde conduction. When the P wave reaches just the right point in the refractory period established by the junctional discharge, it is able to penetrate to reach the home of the ectopic junctional focus and dislocate its timing. The expected appearance of the junctional discharge is shown at the arrow, but it has been reset and occurs later.

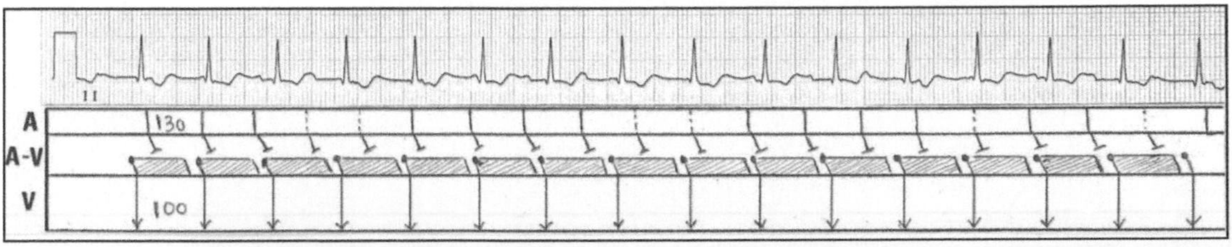

Fig. 16. There is a regular sinus tachycardia at 130/min, which is in competition with an accelerated junctional focus at 100/min, resulting in AV dissociation. Some degree of AV block must be present, or the faster sinus node would be in command of ventricular activation. However, although none of the atrial impulses conduct to the ventricle, there is probably little AV block. The major problem in AV transmission is likely caused by the refractory wake that is repetitively established by the discharge of the junctional focus. The resulting window of opportunity for conduction is small, and functionally nonexistent. Dr Marriott provided a descriptive term for this arrhythmia: block-acceleration dissociation.

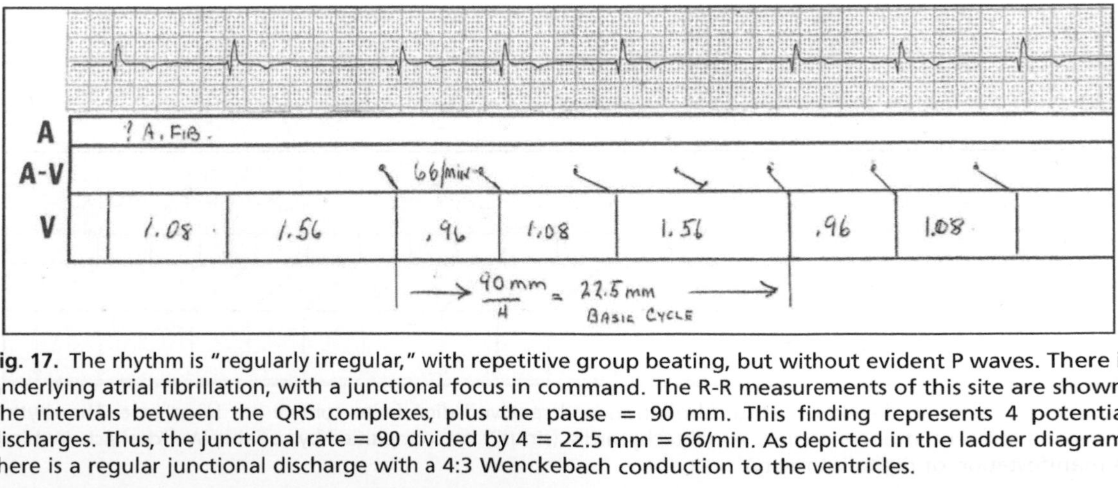

Fig. 17. The rhythm is "regularly irregular," with repetitive group beating, but without evident P waves. There is underlying atrial fibrillation, with a junctional focus in command. The R-R measurements of this site are shown. The intervals between the QRS complexes, plus the pause = 90 mm. This finding represents 4 potential discharges. Thus, the junctional rate = 90 divided by 4 = 22.5 mm = 66/min. As depicted in the ladder diagram, there is a regular junctional discharge with a 4:3 Wenckebach conduction to the ventricles.

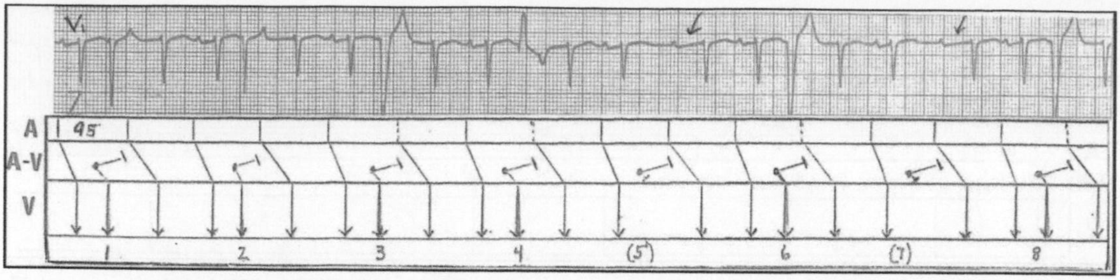

Fig. 18. At first glance, this seems to be simply sinus rhythm at 95/min with multiple, multiform, single VPCs; however, it is an example of concealed events. The alert that something strange is happening is provided by the sudden prolongation of the PR interval for 2 atrial stimuli (*arrows*). The solution is provided in the ladder diagram. An independent ectopic focus is hiding in the AV junction. Its rate is 48/min and it competes with the atrial impulses. Depending on the timing of these junctional stimuli in the refractory period of the preceding depolarization, the junctional stimuli may be conducted:

1. Almost normally (1 and 2)
2. With left bundle branch block aberration (3, 6, and 8)
3. With right bundle branch block aberration (4)
4. May not be conducted but reveal themselves only by causing prolongation of the conducted atrial impulses (5 and 7) This phenomenon has been termed concealed junctional extrasystoles. A difficult arrhythmia!

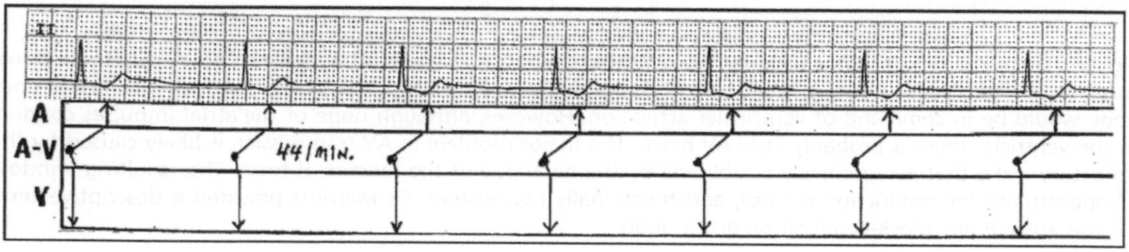

Fig. 19. The junctional stimulus may not only conduct anterograde to the ventricle, it may transmit the impulse retrograde to the atrium. This process resets the sinus node, slowing its discharge and allowing the junction to continue to escape and remain in command.

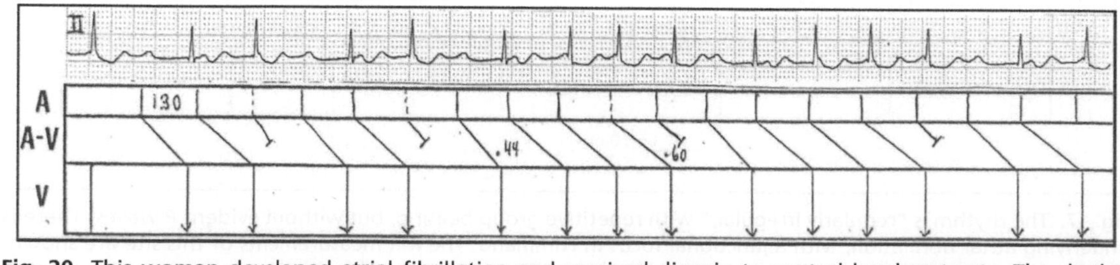

Fig. 20. This woman developed atrial fibrillation and received digoxin to control her heart rate. The rhythm above was present after conversion. Atrial tachycardia (sinus?) is accompanied by variable Wenckebach AV block (a manifestation of digitalis toxicity).

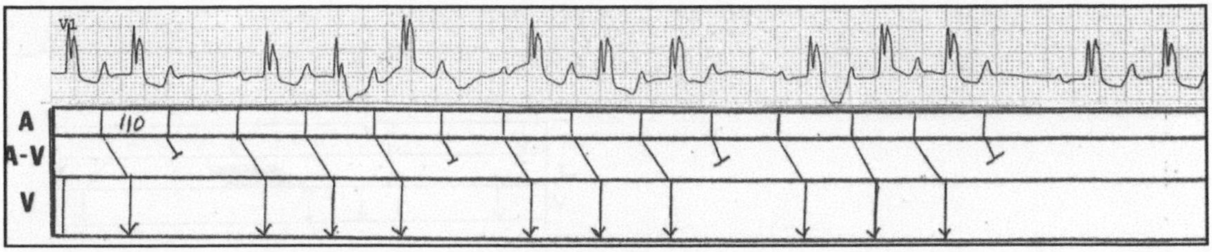

Fig. 21. This man has sustained inferior, posterior, and lateral wall infarctions. His V1 lead shows his conduction abnormality of right bundle branch block. Sinus impulses at 130/min are conducted with a constant PR interval with ratio of 4:3 transmission. An example of type 2 infranodal block.

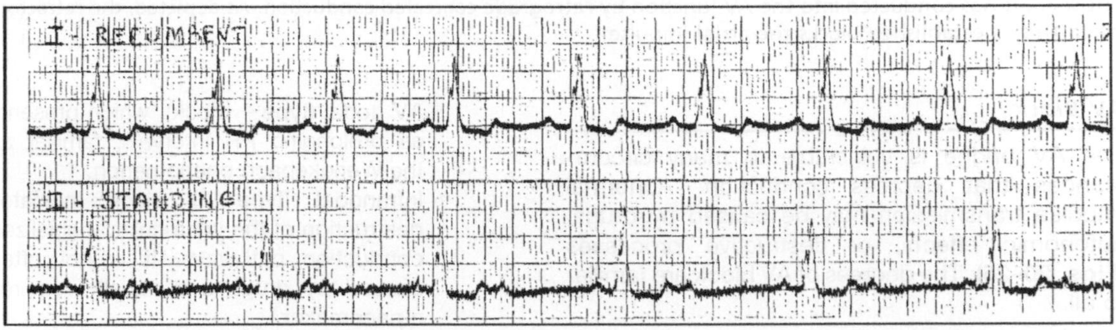

Fig. 22. When there is 2:1 conduction of an atrial stimulus, the problem may be nodal or infranodal. This symptomatic man has an abnormally prolonged recovery after impulse conduction. At a sinus rate of 70/min, he conducts 1:1. When he stands, his heart rate increases to 90/min, 2:1 block begins, and his effective rate falls to 45/min: a reason for his symptoms.

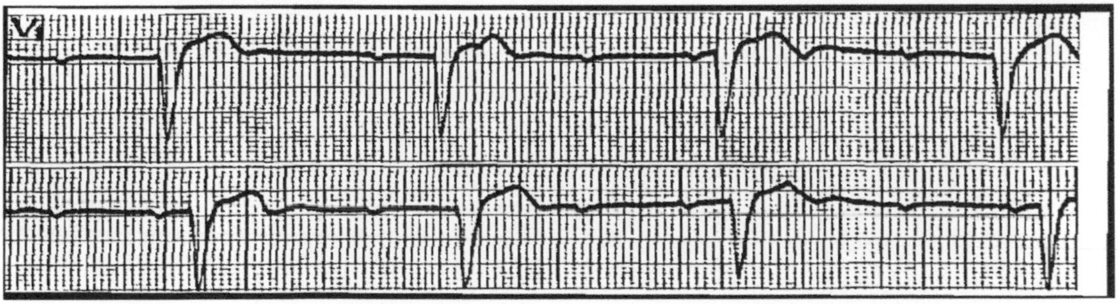

Fig. 23. Third-degree AV block is manifested by complete dissociation of atrial and ventricular events, but the escape pacemaker should be slow (less than 45/min) and usually a wide QRS complex indicates its ventricular origin. There should be no AV conduction, with P waves having ample opportunity for conduction (ie, not an isochronic relationship of P and QRS) (see **Fig. 13**).

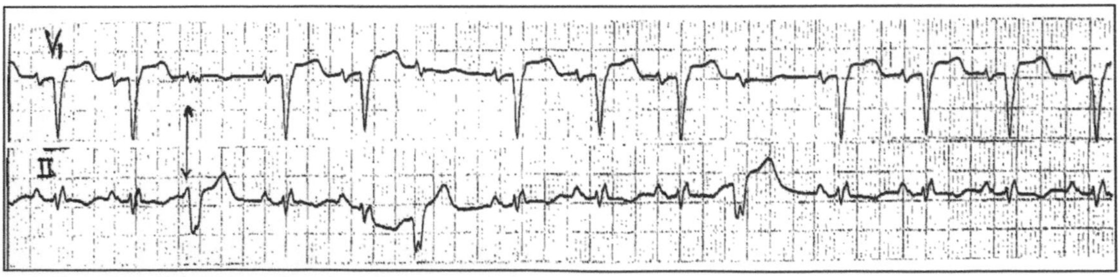

Fig. 24. A potential fooler regarding apparent AV block. Given only the V1 lead, the recurring blocked P waves would be concerning. The simultaneous lead II reveals that the apparent P waves are really VPCs, which are isoelectric in the top lead. Reminder: beware of single rhythm strips! Arrow reflects simultaneous recordings in the 2 leads.

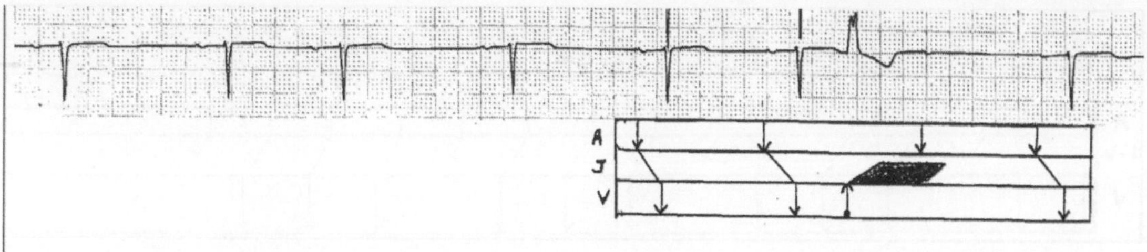

Fig. 25. There is variability of a slow sinus discharge with a prolonged PR interval. A single P wave is not conducted. Did first-degree suddenly proceed to second-degree AV block? The problem is caused by the VPC. Although not seen, it has conducted into the AV junction by retrograde concealed conduction. As depicted, the refractory wake that is established blocks the atrial impulse.

AV Block

The AV bridge is vulnerable to many circumstances that depress conduction. Abnormal impulse transmission may be caused by drugs, autonomic effects, or destructive processes (**Figs. 20–25**). The degrees of AV block are familiar to all.

- First-degree is not a block but a delay, because all atrial stimuli are conducted, albeit with a prolonged PR interval.
- Second-degree may be
  - AV nodal (type 1 block), which presents as prolonging PR intervals, familiar as the Wenckebach phenomenon.
  - Infranodal (type 2) block indicates destruction of the ventricular specialized conduction pathways. It is not often caused by drugs and usually requires a pacemaker.
- Third-degree indicates complete failure of conduction caused by AV block. Block-acceleration dissociation may prevent conduction of all atria impulses (see **Fig. 15**).

Acute Myocardial Infarction Case Histories

Andrés Ricardo Pérez-Riera, MD, PhD[a,*],
Raimundo Barbosa, MD[b]

KEYWORDS

• Myocardial infarction • ST elevation • Diagnosis • Treatment

KEY POINTS

- A pattern of inferior myocardial infarction with ST elevation in lead II greater than lead III suggests occlusion of the left circumflex coronary artery.
- Distal left anterior descending coronary artery occlusions may result in an injury vector directed inferiorly (ST elevation in the inferior leads) and anteriorly.

CASE 1

A 70-year-old black man was admitted with typical clinical picture of an acute coronary syndrome (ACS). He died after 4 hours with pulseless electrical activity. What is the ECG diagnosis (**Fig. 1**)?

ECG Diagnosis

1. Atrial fibrillation.
2. ST segment elevation in aVR, and V1.
3. ST segment elevation in aVR > V1 (Because ST segment deviation vector is directed to upward and rightward, toward aVR lead).
4. Ischemic evidence in posterobasal region: depression of the ST segment in inferior leads and from V4 to V5.
5. Depression of ST segment in V6 > ST segment elevation in V1.

Frontal plane injury vector points toward aVr (**Fig. 2**). Horizontal plane injury vector directed to right and posterior (**Fig. 3**).

Final Diagnosis

The final diagnosis is left main coronary artery occlusion.

CASE 2

A 78-year-old white woman was admitted to the emergency room with clinical picture of acute coronary syndrome.

She underwent primary angioplasty with stent placement in the culprit right coronary artery. Additionally, the angiogram showed a significant proximal obstruction in the left anterior descending coronary artery (LAD). The strategy was then to carry through an elective angioplasty at a later time. After 3 weeks, she returned with several episodes of angina and acute pulmonary edema. After stabilization of the clinical picture the patient underwent successful angioplasty of the LAD.

Fig. 4 shows the ECG 1 at admission <12 hours after pain onset.

WHAT IS YOUR DIAGNOSIS?

ECG Diagnosis

1. Sinus tachycardia, QRS axis −30°.
2. Leads III and aVF show ST segment elevation (subepicardial injury current), mirror image of V1 to V4 (ST depression conspicuous in V2).

Summary

Acute inferior posterior myocardial infarction.

[a] Disciplina de Cardiologia, Faculdade de Medicina do ABC, Santo André, São Paulo, Brazil; [b] Coronary center, Hospital de Messejana Dr. Carlos Alberto Studart Gomes, Fortaleza, Ceará, Brazil
* Corresponding author.
E-mail address: riera@uol.com.br

Card Electrophysiol Clin 4 (2012) 479–491
http://dx.doi.org/10.1016/j.ccep.2012.08.009

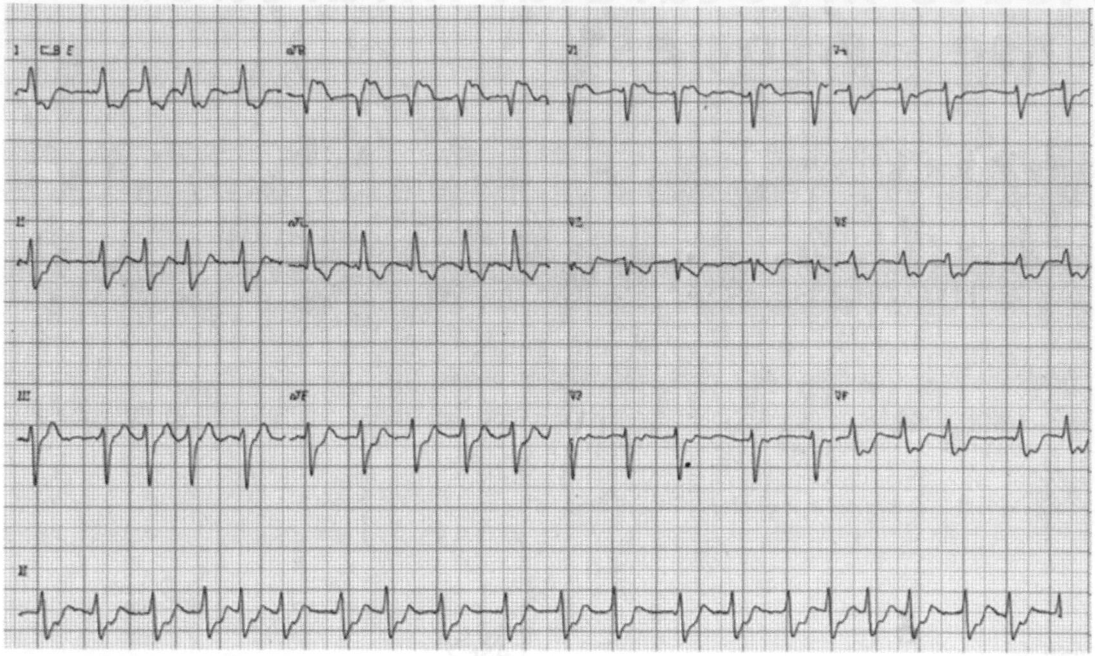

Fig. 1. ECG of patient in case 1.

Fig. 5 is an ECG performed during her second anginal episode.

ECG Diagnosis

1. Sinus tachycardia, extreme left axis deviation (QRS axis –70°).
2. QRS duration 115 ms, qR pattern in I and aVL, rS pattern in II, III, and aVF.
3. SIII > SII followed by minimal ST segment elevation upward convex (subepicardial injury current is present as well as left anterior fascicular block (LAFB).

Prominent anterior forces: qR pattern in V2 with (R wave = 25 mm) followed by rS pattern from V3 to V6 is compatible with left septal fascicular block (LSFB). LSFB is recognized by initial small q waves in anterior precordial leads followed by large terminal forces in the same leads.

Summary

Left bifascicular block: LAFB + LSFB Injury current in inferior leads, initial r wave in all inferior leads.

LAFB may mimic LVH, because SIII >15 mm with inverted T wave in ≥1 of the left sided leads I, aVL, V5, and V6.

Fig. 6 is an ECG recorded on the third day after successful stenting of the LADe.

ECG Diagnosis

Prominent anterior forces (LSFB) has disappeared.

CASE 3

A 46-year-old man presented with a history of 12 hours of anterior precordial chest pain (**Fig. 7**). The next day, the patient returned with precordial pain associated with hemodynamic instability (**Fig. 8**).

ECG Diagnosis

1. Anterior myocardial infarction in acute phase: ST segment elevation from V1–V3 (injury) followed by negative symmetric T wave (subepicardial ischemia).
2. Left posterior fascicular block (LPFB) right inferior axis noted.
3. Complete right bundle branch block (CRBBB).
4. Bifascicular block (LPFB + CRBBB).

Second ECG on the Following Day

1. LAFB.
2. CRBBB.
3. Bifascicular block (LAFB + CRBBB).
4. Anterior myocardial infarction in acute phase: ST segment elevation from V1 to V3 (injury) followed by negative symmetric T wave (subepicardial ischemia).

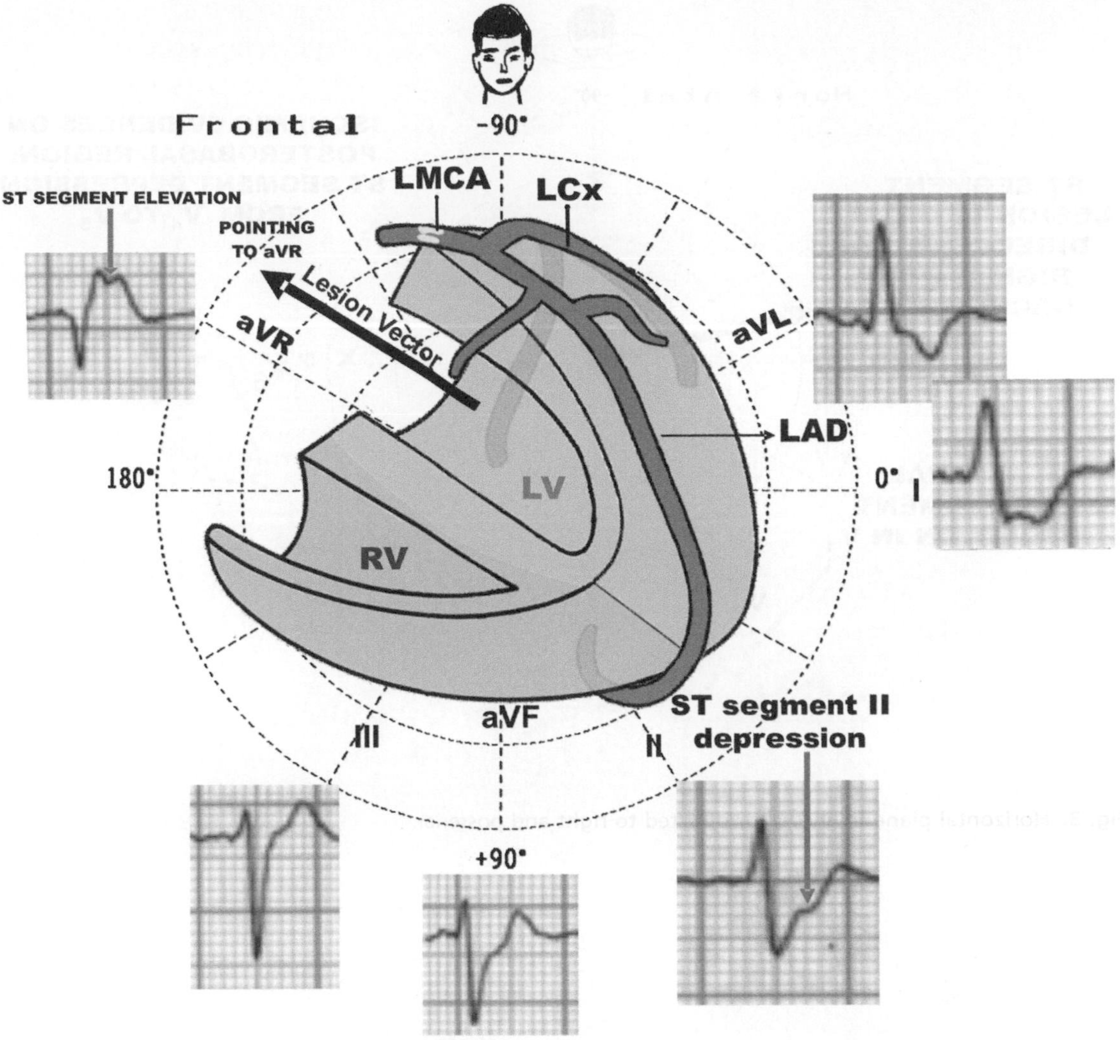

Fig. 2. Frontal plane injury vector points toward aVr.

Third ECG: The Same Night

1. Third-degree atrioventricular block (**Fig. 9**)
2. Extensive anterior myocardial infarction.

Summary

Alternating left fascicular block (LPFB and LAFB) and RBBB = trifascicular block, which evolved into complete atrioventricular block. This case illustrates severe intraventricular conduction disorder after acute anterior myocardial infarction.

CASE 4

A 49-year-old man was admitted to the emergency room with pain with and hypotension (**Figs. 10** and **11**).

ECG Diagnosis

1. ST-segment elevation in inferior leads. III > II suggests a right coronary occlusion.
2. ST-segment elevation in V_4R followed by positive T wave is indicative of right ventricle involvement.

CASE 5

Tracings were recorded in the emergency room during chest pain in a 67-year-old woman (**Fig. 12**).

ECG Diagnosis

ST elevation in the inferior leads with reciprocal changes in the precordial leads, ST segment elevation is now present in the anterolateral leads.

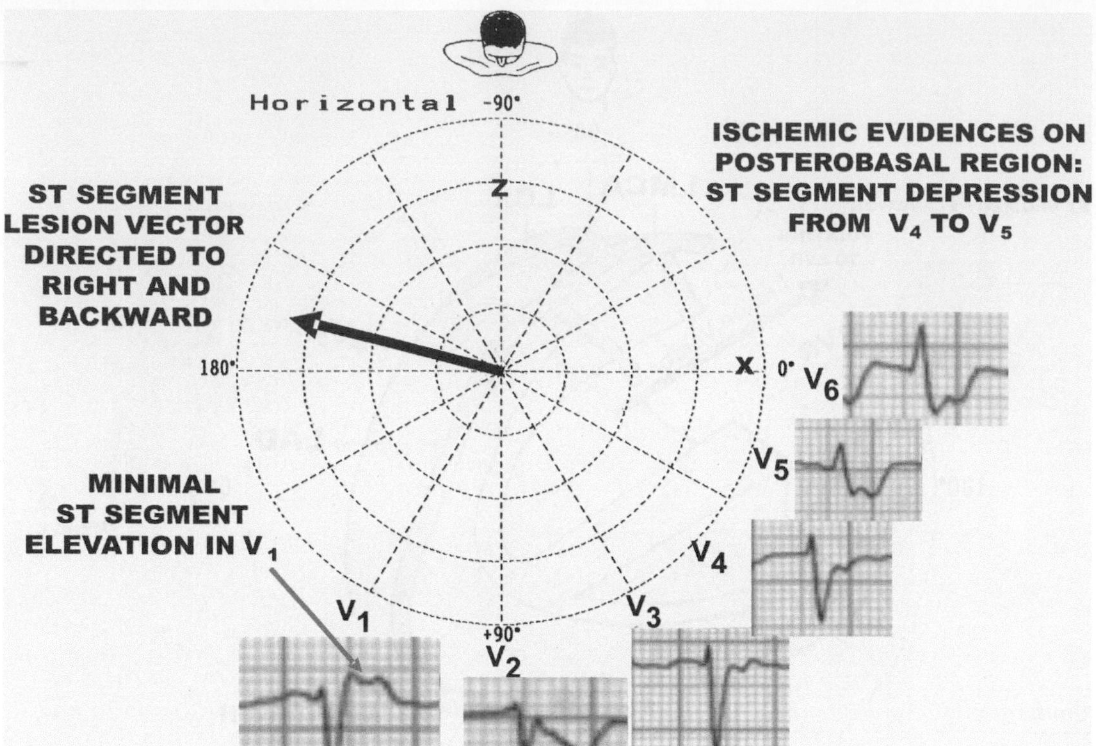

Fig. 3. Horizontal plane injury vector directed to right and posterior.

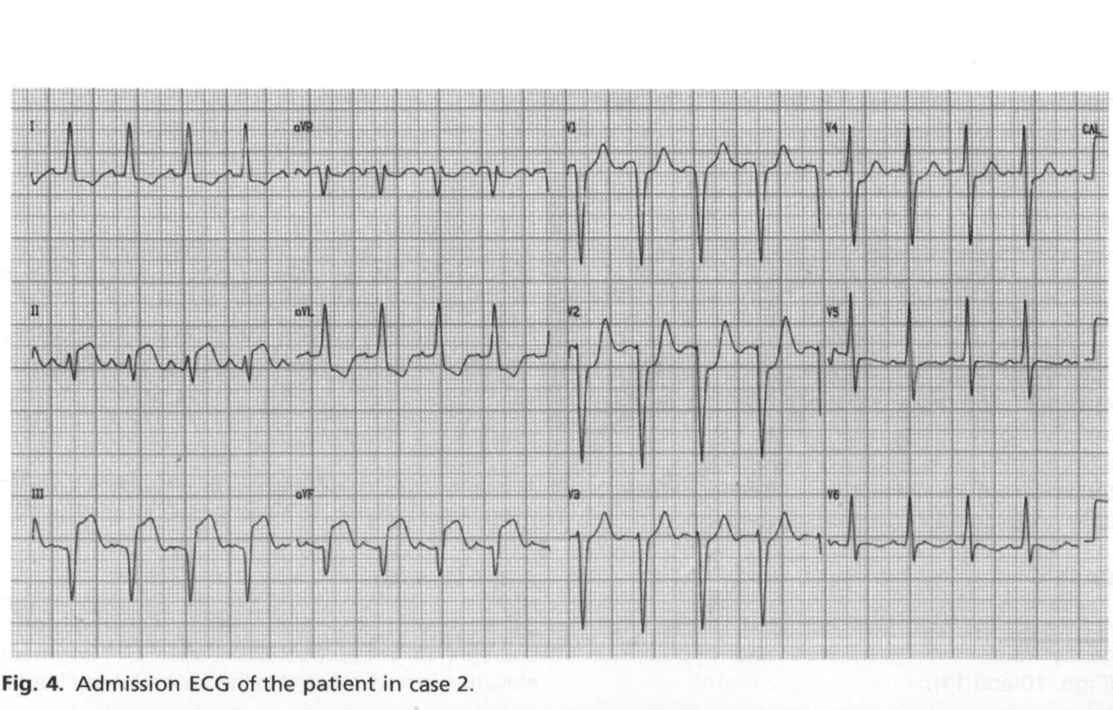

Fig. 4. Admission ECG of the patient in case 2.

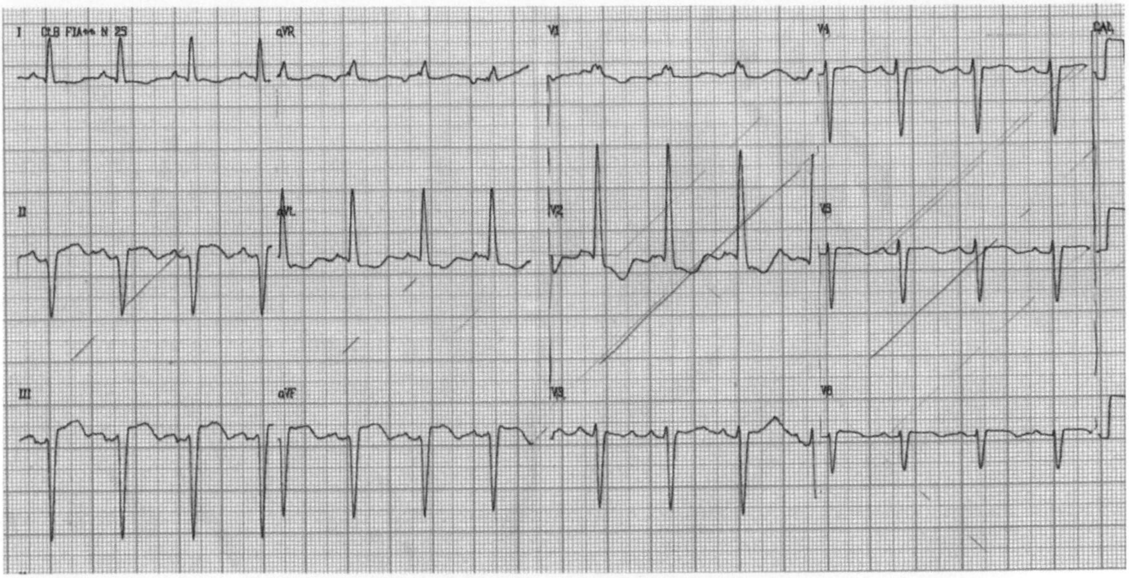

Fig. 5. ECG of the patient in case 2 performed during her second anginal episode.

Summary

The vectorcardiogram shows the lateral wall infarction pattern (white area) with injury vector pointed toward lead III. Patients with a pattern of inferior MI with ST elevation in lead II greater than lead III suggest occlusion of the left circumflex coronary artery.

CASE 6

A patient presented with the ECG pattern shown in **Fig. 13**. Please describe, interpret, and give the location of the occluded vessel.

1. ST-segment elevation in aVL and aVR.
2. ST-segment depression in inferior leads.
3. ST-segment elevation $\geq$2 mm from V1 to V4.

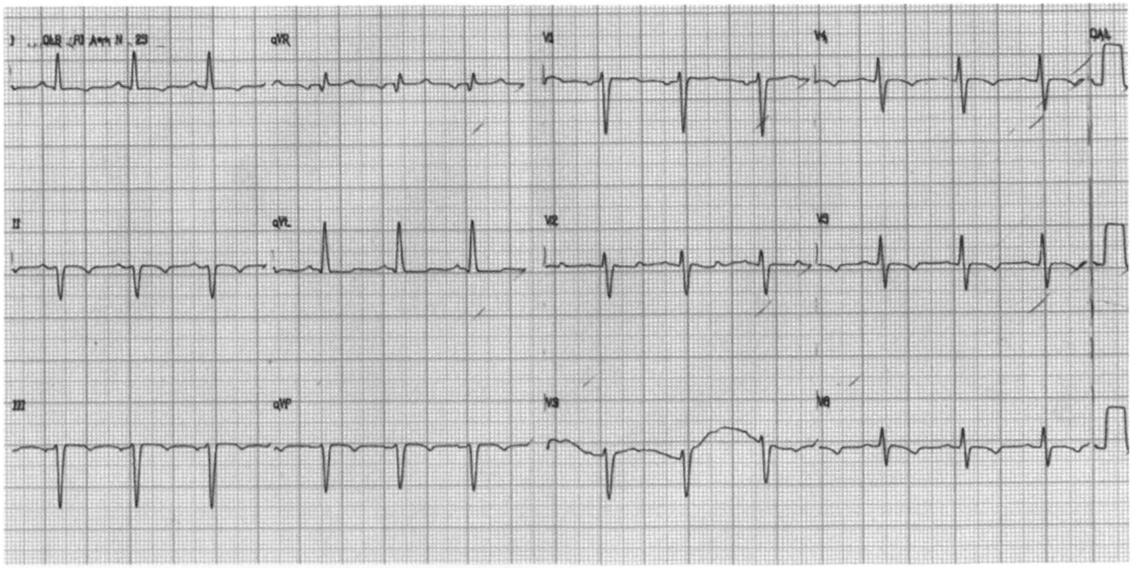

Fig. 6. ECG of the patient in case 2 recorded on day 3 after successful stenting of the LAD.

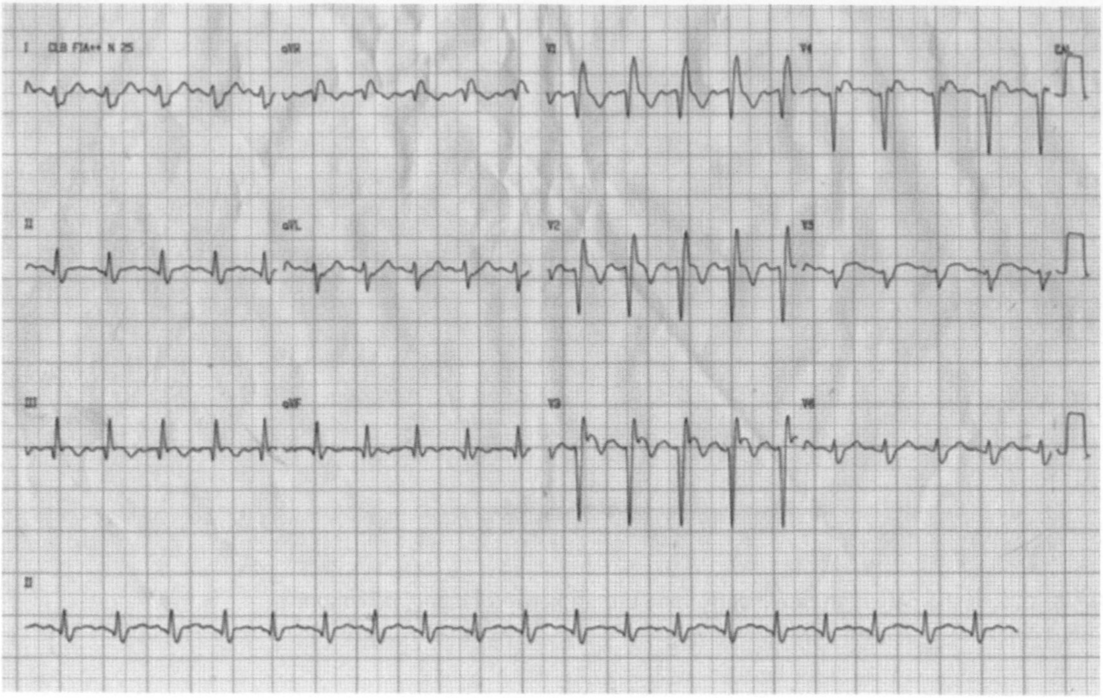

Fig. 7. Initial ECG performed in the patient in case 3 after 12 hours of precordial pain.

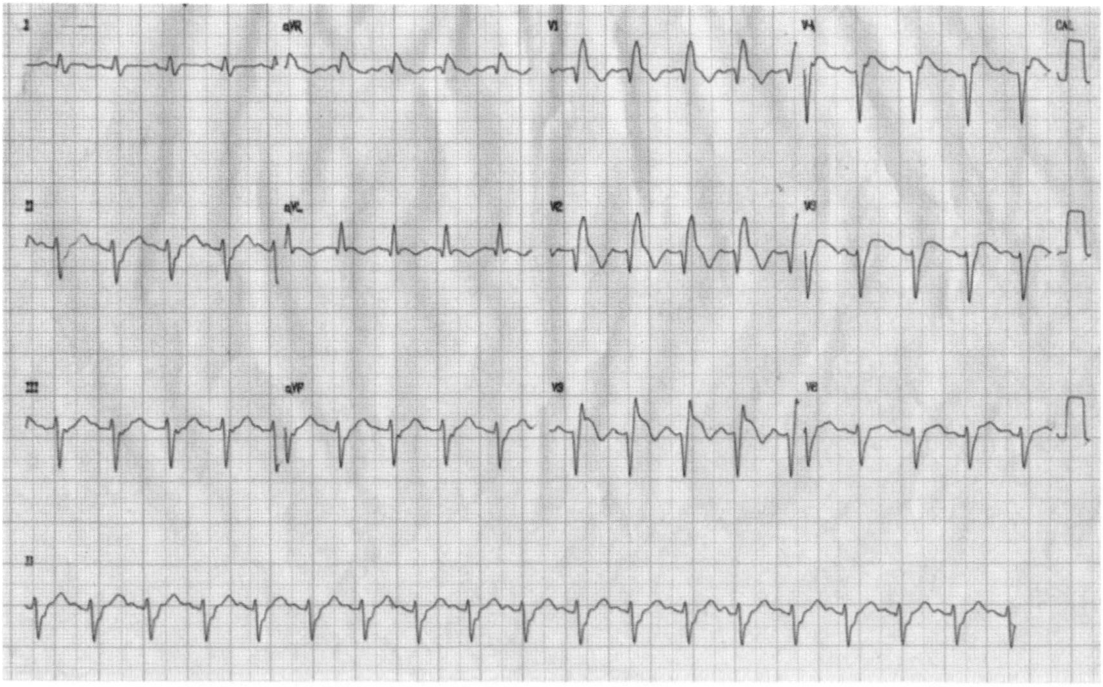

Fig. 8. ECG of the patient in case 3 taken on day 2.

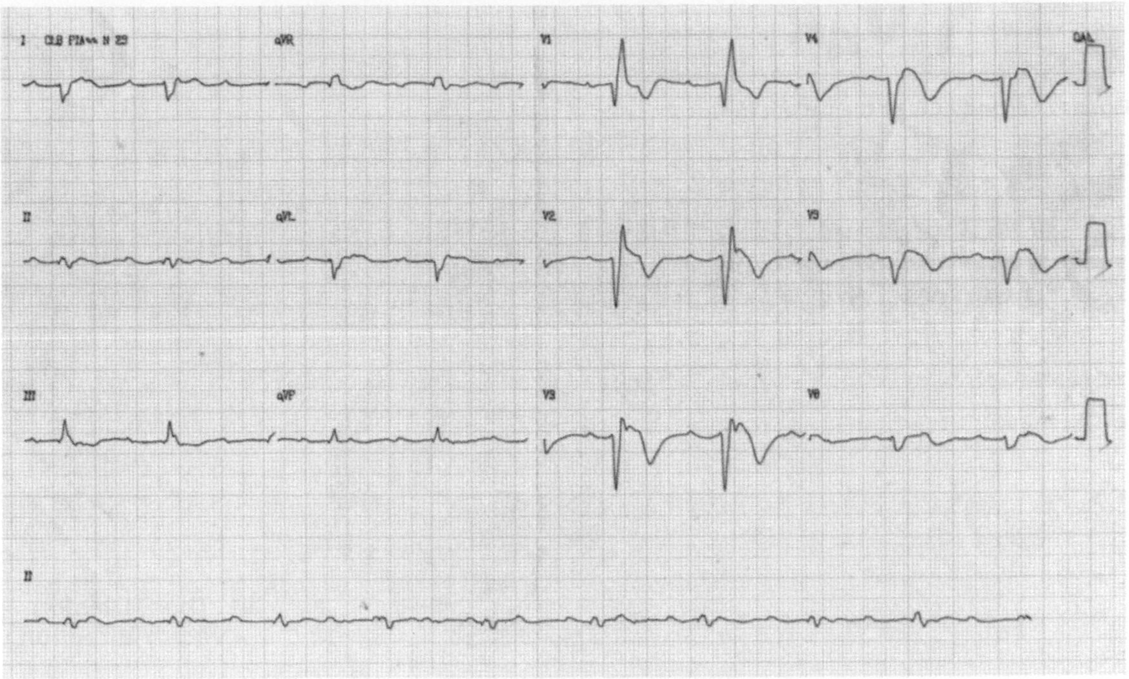

Fig. 9. A third ECG of the patient in case 3 was taken in the evening of day 2.

These ECG changes reflect occlusion of the LAD in a proximal location likely before the first septal and diagonal vessels.

CASE 7

A patient presented with the ECG shown in **Fig. 14**. Describe the abnormalities and location of occluded coronary vessel(s).

Summary

The patient had an inferior acute myocardial infarction: ST-segment elevation in II, III, and aVF, with ST elevation in lead III > lead II (right coronary occlusion pattern). Concomitantly, we observe ST depression in aVL and in leads V_4–V_6, suggestive of concomitant left anterior descending artery (LAD) stenosis or 3 vessel

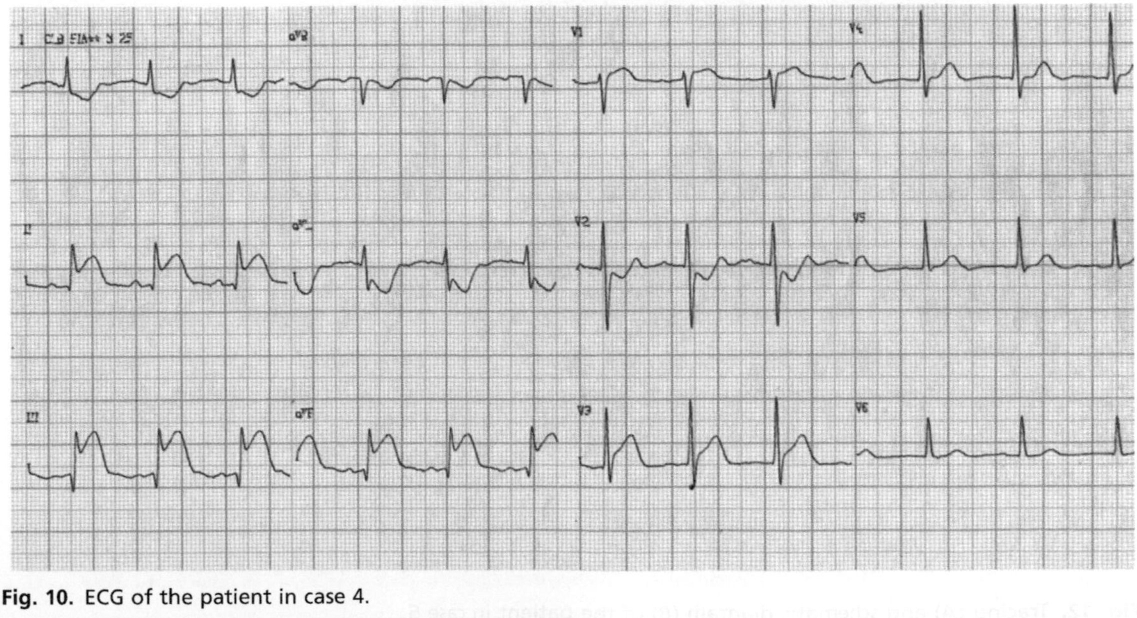

Fig. 10. ECG of the patient in case 4.

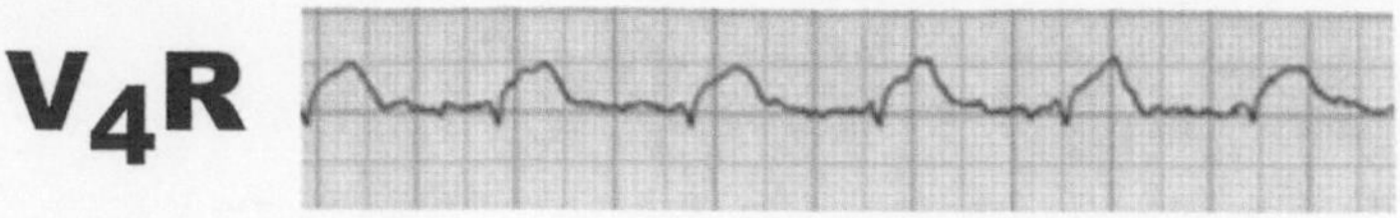

Fig. 11. Second ECG of the patient in case 4.

A

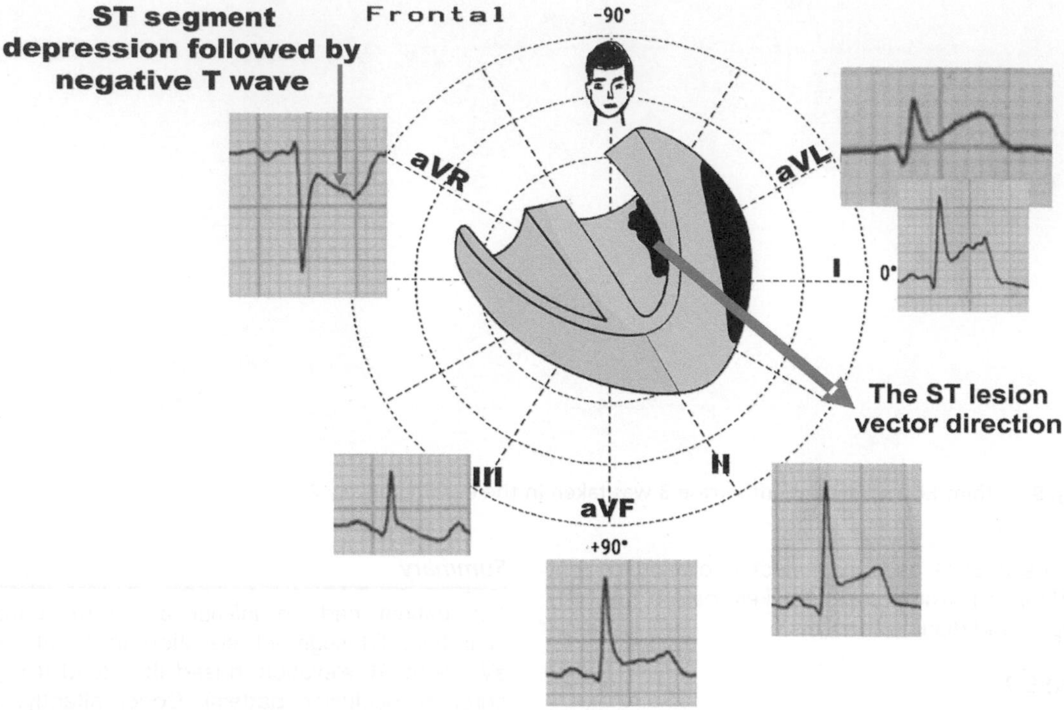

B

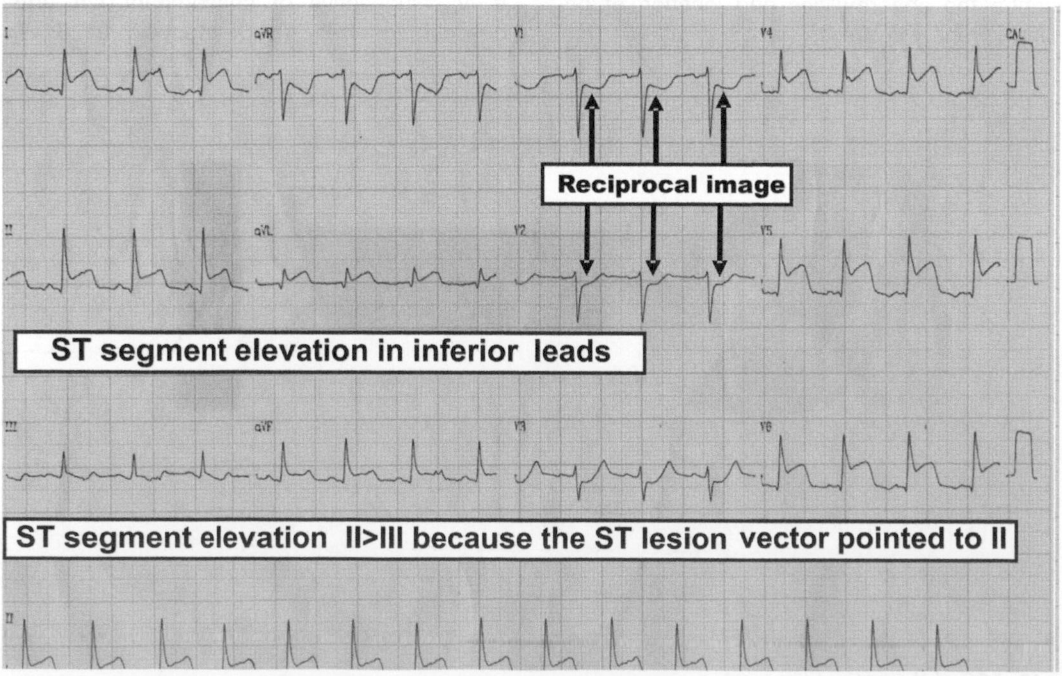

Fig. 12. Tracing (A) and schematic diagram (B) of the patient in case 5.

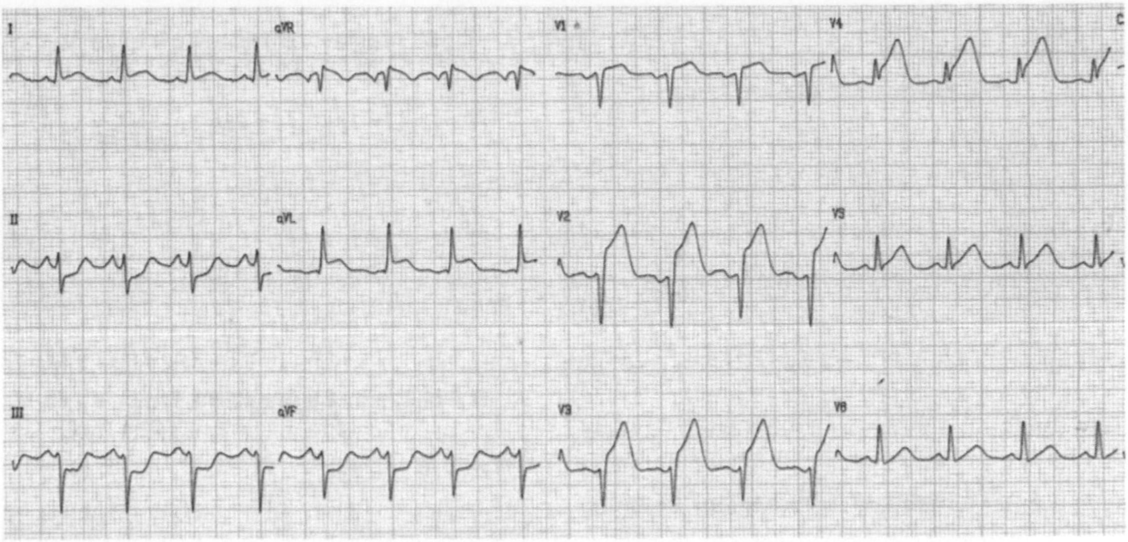

Fig. 13. ECG of the patient in case 6.

disease. Angiography showed complete occlusion of right coronary artery and critical occlusion of the LAD.

CASE 8

Diagnose the site of infarction and identify the occluded vessel from the ECG shown in **Fig. 15**. The injury vector first is directed anteriorly and leftward toward the ischemic zone over the left anterior wall (**Figs. 16** and **17**).

Discussion

In proximal occlusions of the LAD, the frontal plane vector is directed superiorly and to the left, yielding ST elevation in aVl and lead I with reciprocal depression in the inferior leads (see **Fig. 16**). The ST segment is flat in V_1, which suggests sparing of the first septal perforator and localizes the occlusion of the LAD to a site distal to the first septal perforator and proximal to the first diagonal branch of the LAD.

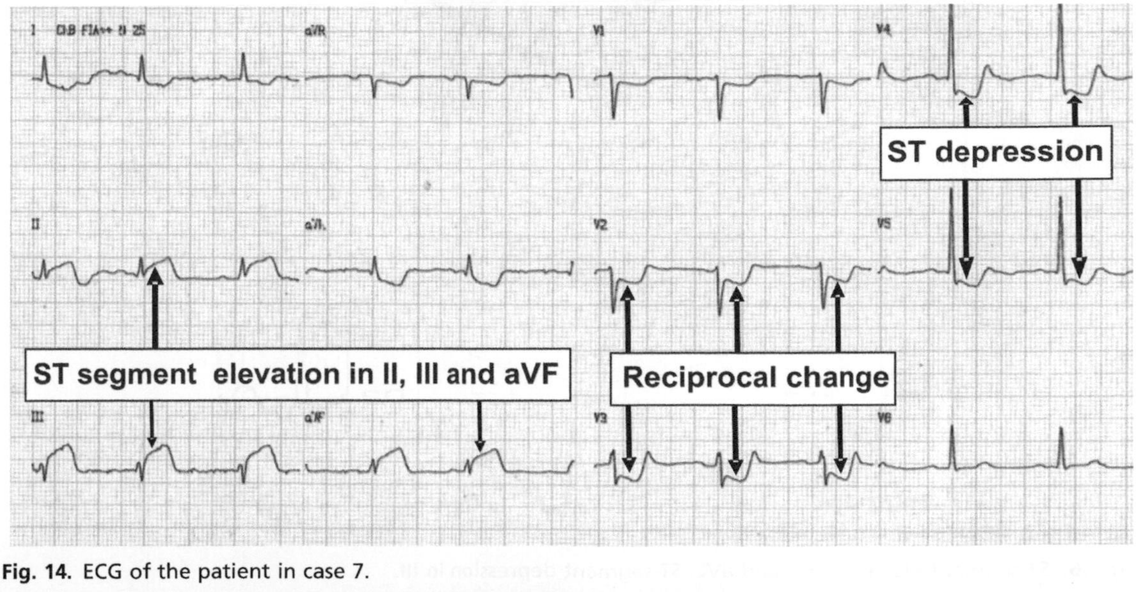

Fig. 14. ECG of the patient in case 7.

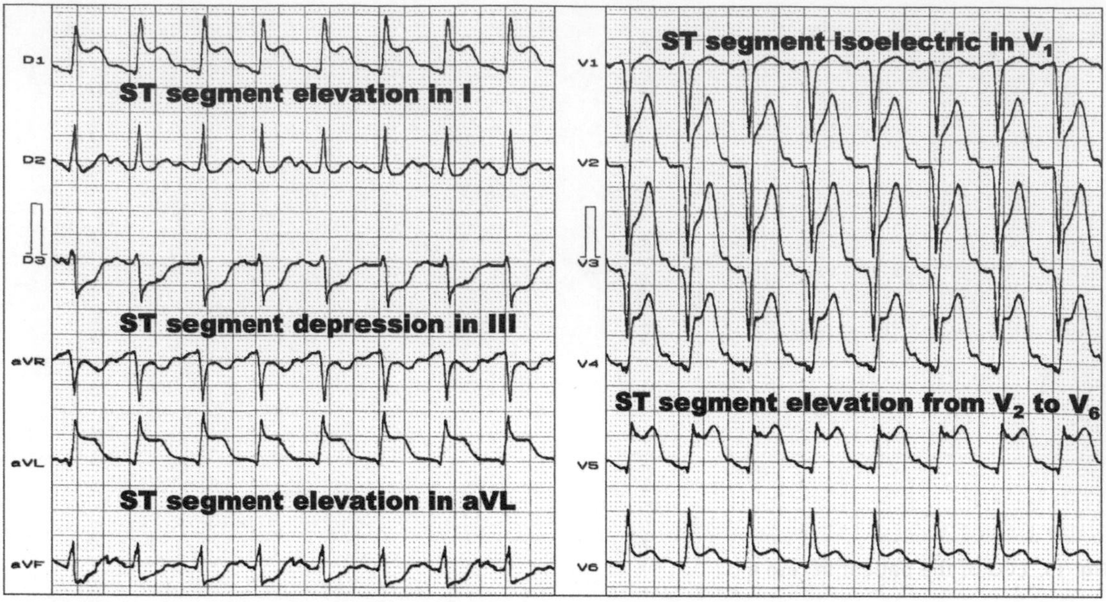

Fig. 15. ECG of the patient in case 8. Acute myocardial infarction caused by occlusion of LAD after the first septal perforator and before the first diagonal branch. Why this pattern? See **Fig. 16**.

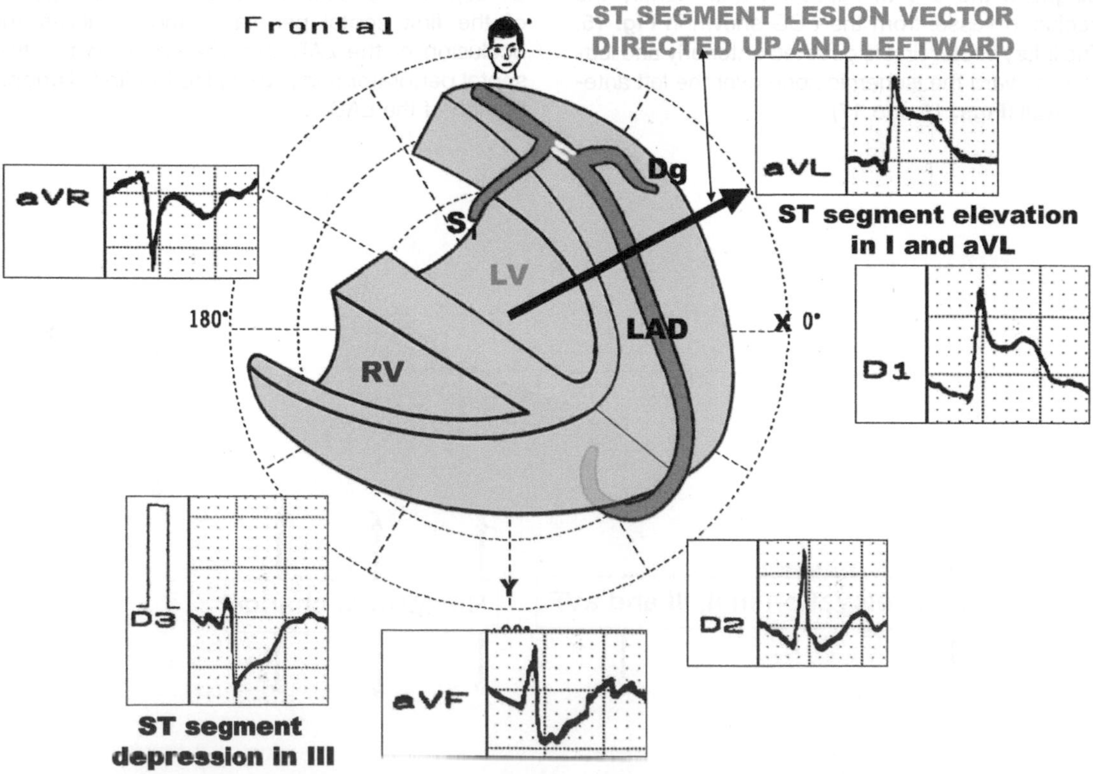

Fig. 16. ST-segment elevation in I and aVL. ST-segment depression in III.

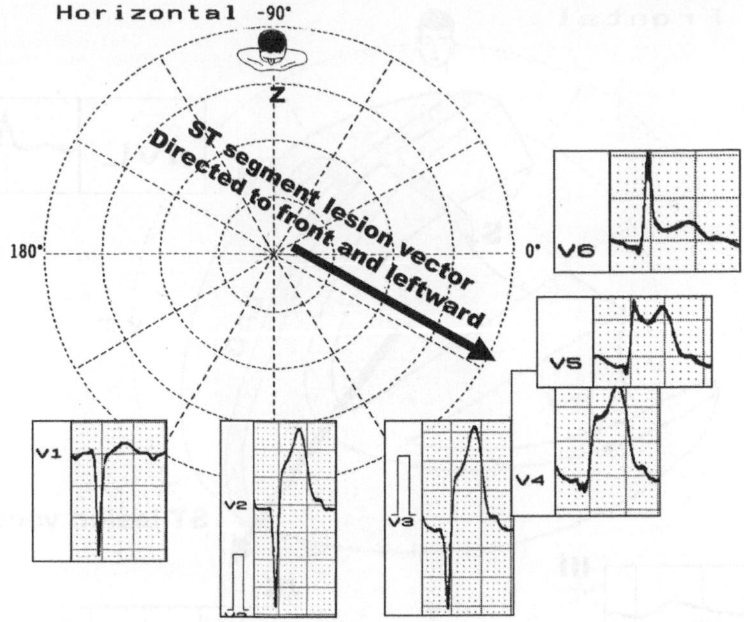

Fig. 17. ST-segment elevation from V_2 to V_6 and isoelectric in V_1.

CASE 9

Diagnose the site of infarction and explain the ECG pattern shown in **Fig. 18.**

Discussion

The ECG pattern reflects a more distal occlusion of the LAD (distal to the first septal perforator) and diagonal branches. In the frontal plane (**Fig. 19**), the injury vector points inferiorly reflecting ischemic damage to the inferior left ventricle. The horizontal plane injury vector is directed anteriorly and to the left (**Fig. 20**). The pattern reflects the "wrap around" feature of the LAD often supplying the inferior and anterior left ventricular myocardium.

Fig. 21 represents an overall summary of the injury vector dependent on the site of the LAD occlusion. In the frontal plane, a left main occlusion

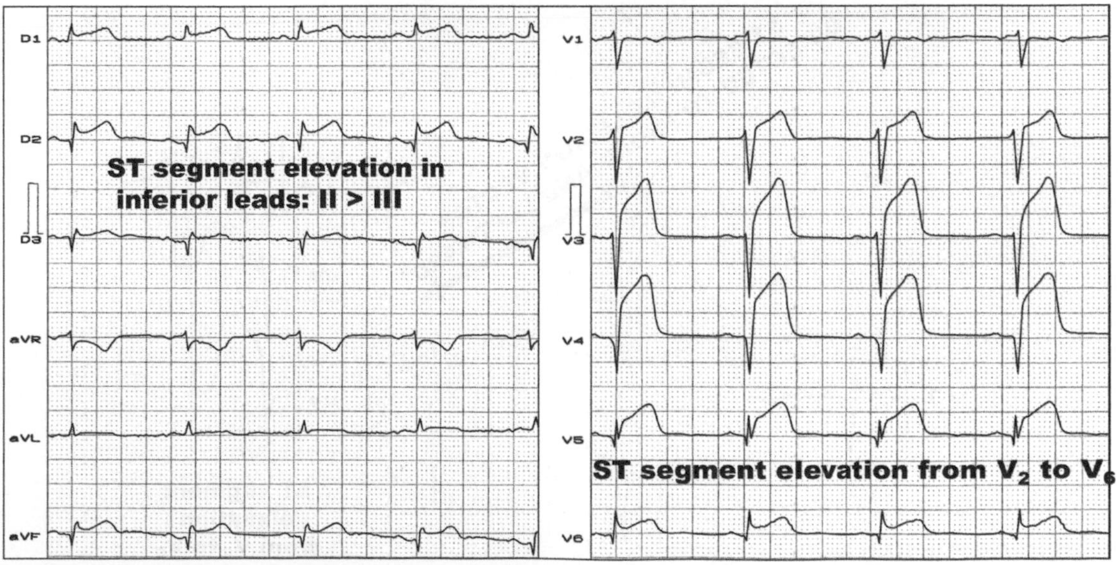

Fig. 18. ECG of patient in case 9. Why this pattern?

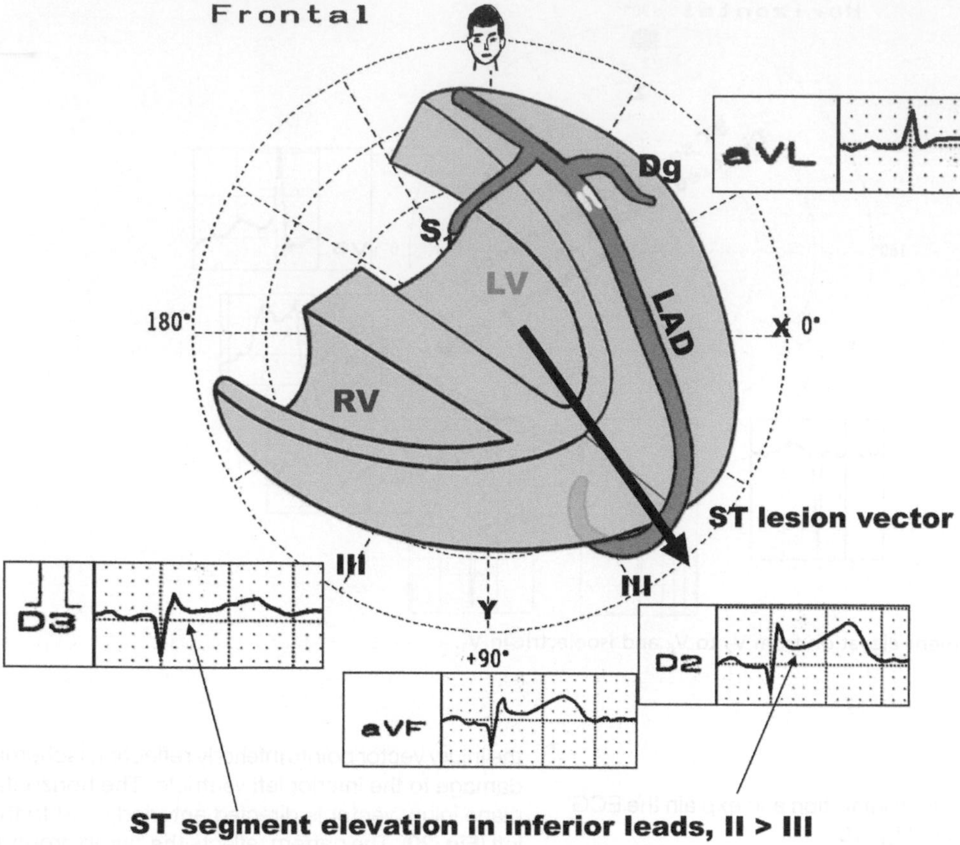

Fig. 19. In the frontal plane, the injury vector points inferiorly reflecting ischemic damage to the inferior left ventricle.

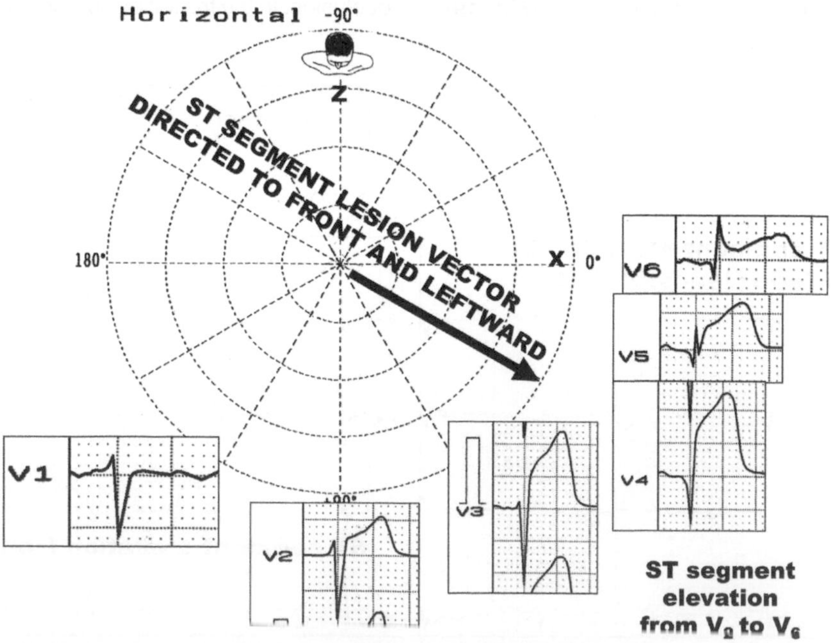

Fig. 20. The horizontal plane injury vector is directed anteriorly and to the left.

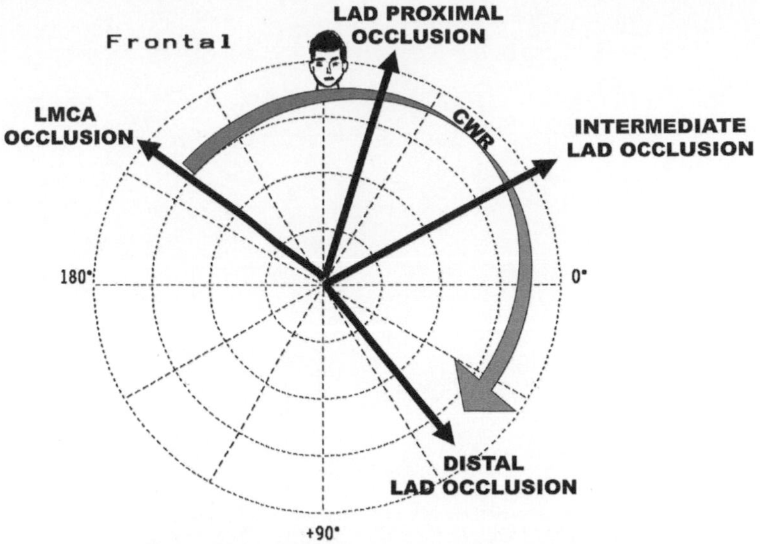

Fig. 21. Summary of ST lesion vector direction on FP. CWR, clockwise rotation.

is reflected by an injury vector pointing superiorly and rightward reflecting the ST elevation in aVr > than in V1 (see Case 2).

A proximal LAD occlusion is attended by an injury vector oriented superiorly and the left, yielding ST elevation in leads I and aVl and reciprocal changes in the inferior leads (see Case 8) as well as an anteriorly directed injury vector in the horizontal plane. More distal LAD occlusions may result in an injury vector directed inferiorly (ST elevation in the inferior leads) and anteriorly.

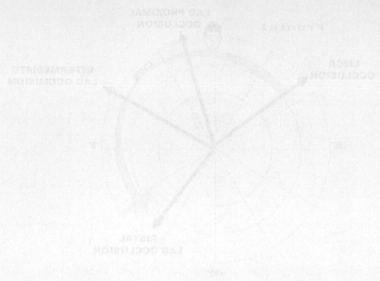

Supraventricular Tachycardia

Nitish Badhwar, MBBS

KEYWORDS

- Paroxysmal supraventricular tachycardia • Wolff-Parkinson-White syndrome
- Permanent reciprocal junctional tachycardia • Atrioventricular reentrant tachycardia

KEY POINTS

- Paroxysmal supraventricular tachycardia (PSVT) is frequently encountered in otherwise healthy patients without structural heart disease, and symptoms vary from palpitations and dyspnea to tachycardia-induced cardiomyopathy.
- The 3 most common causes of PSVT include atrioventricular nodal reentrant tachycardia (50%–60%), followed by atrioventricular reentrant tachycardia in patients with Wolff-Parkinson-White syndrome (25%–30%) and atrial tachycardia (10%).
- Rare causes of PSVT include focal junctional tachycardia, atriofascicular tachycardia, permanent reciprocating junctional tachycardia, and nodoventricular/nodofascicular tachycardia.
- Dagnostic maneuvers in challenging PSVT cases are described here.

Paroxysmal supraventricular tachycardia (PSVT) denotes a clinical syndrome characterized by a rapid tachycardia with an abrupt onset and termination. These arrhythmias are frequently encountered in otherwise healthy patients without structural heart disease, and symptoms vary from palpitations and dyspnea to tachycardia-induced cardiomyopathy. The 3 most common causes of PSVT include atrioventricular nodal reentrant tachycardia (AVNRT) (50%–60%), followed by atrioventricular reentrant tachycardia (AVRT) in patients with Wolff-Parkinson-White (WPW) syndrome (25%–30%) and atrial tachycardia (AT) (10%). Rare causes of PSVT include focal junctional tachycardia (JT), atriofascicular tachycardia, permanent reciprocating junctional tachycardia (PJRT), and nodoventricular/nodofascicular tachycardia (NVT/NFT). This section includes challenging PSVT cases that posed a diagnostic or therapeutic dilemma in the electrophysiology (EP) laboratory.

Surface electrocardiography offers some useful clues to the diagnosis of PSVT. Typical AVNRT is the most likely diagnosis if there is an A-on-V tachycardia that usually presents as pseudo R′ in V1 or terminal S wave in inferior leads. The most likely diagnosis of a short RP tachycardia is AVRT followed by atypical AVNRT and AT. The most likely diagnosis of a long RP tachycardia is AT followed by atypical AVNRT, and PJRT especially if it is incessant. If the tachycardia is associated with atrioventricular (AV) dissociation, the diagnosis of AVRT is excluded. If there are more atrial complexes than ventricular complexes, the most likely diagnosis is AT with AV block, although AVNRT with lower common pathway block is also possible. Narrow-complex SVT with ventriculoatrial (VA) block can be seen with AVNRT, JT and NFT/NVT.

Baseline findings in the EP laboratory that show lack of VA conduction despite the use of isoproterenol argue against AVRT as the SVT mechanism. SVT initiation dependent on a critical atrial-His (AH) interval favors AVNRT, although AT and AVRT are not completely excluded. Spontaneous termination of SVT with an atrial depolarization argue against AT as the mechanism, as does termination with VA block during ventricular pacing.

Cardiac Electrophysiology, University of California San Francisco, 500 Parnassus Avenue, MUE 431, San Francisco, CA 94143-1354, USA
E-mail address: badhwar@medicine.ucsf.edu

Card Electrophysiol Clin 4 (2012) 493–495
http://dx.doi.org/10.1016/j.ccep.2012.08.037
1877-9182/12/$ – see front matter

A septal VA interval of less than 70 milliseconds rules out orthodromic AVRT as the mechanism of SVT.[1] Short VA intervals are not typically seen in AT.

It is important from an ablation standpoint to confirm the participation of an accessory pathway (AP) in AVRT. The presence of any of 4 criteria can be used to establish this, which include (1) tachycardia termination obtained with a ventricular stimulus delivered during His refractoriness and without atrial depolarization, (2) delay in the next atrial depolarization when a ventricular stimulus is delivered during His refractoriness, (3) increase in VA interval with ipsilateral bundle branch block (BBB) during tachycardia,[2] and (4) an increase in His-ventricle (HV) interval results in an increase in His-atrial (HA) interval during tachycardia. It is important that in the case of AVNRT, the HA is fixed during tachycardia but may wobble at the initiation of tachycardia.

Differentiation of atypical AVNRT from orthodromic AVRT using a septal pathway can be a diagnostic dilemma that often requires different pacing maneuvers. Martinez-Alday and colleagues[3] measured the VA interval with differential pacing from the right ventricular apex (RVA) and right ventricular posterobasal region (RVB) during sinus rhythm. VA timing during RVA pacing was more than VA timing during RVB pacing (always >10 milliseconds) with posteroseptal AP conduction. VA timing during RVA pacing was less than or equal to VA timing during RVB pacing with normal AV nodal conduction. Para-Hisian pacing during sinus rhythm and para-Hisian entrainment during tachycardia has also been shown to have diagnostic value in differentiating AVNRT from orthodromic AVRT using a septal AP.[4,5] The number of beats required to capture the atrium with para-Hisian pacing during SVT has been used to differentiate AVRT (first beat) from AVNRT (>2 beats).[6] In another study, data from RVA pacing that leads to entrainment of tachycardia was used to differentiate atypical AVRT from septal AVNRT.[7] The investigators measured the VA interval and tachycardia cycle length (TCL) just before the initiation of right ventricular pacing, and the interval between the last pacing stimulus and the last entrained atrial depolarization (stimulus-atrial [SA] interval) and the post-pacing interval (PPI) at the RVA. Atypical AVNRT was associated with an SA-VA interval greater than 85 milliseconds and a PPI-TCL interval greater than 115 milliseconds. By contrast, orthodromic AVRT using a septal pathway was associated with an SA-VA interval of less than 85 milliseconds and a PPI-TCL interval of less than 115 milliseconds. Miller and colleagues[8] have shown that the change in HA intervals measured during SVT (HA_{svt}) as well as ventricular pacing at the same tachycardia rate (HA_{pace}) can be used to differentiate AVNRT from orthodromic AVRT using a septal AP. These investigators concluded that ΔHA ($HA_{pace} - HA_{svt}$) of more than -10 milliseconds reliably differentiates AVNRT ($\Delta HA > 0$ milliseconds) from orthodromic AVRT using a septal AP ($\Delta HA < -27$ milliseconds) without overlap. This technique is limited by technical problems in recording the retrograde His during ventricular pacing. Finally, delivery of late ventricular extra-stimulus (preferably from the RVA) at the time of His refractoriness during tachycardia is a very useful diagnostic maneuver. This maneuver is diagnostic of AVRT if it pulls in the A with the same activation sequence and resetting of tachycardia, pushes out the A or terminates tachycardia with VA block. It is important to deliver the late ventricular extra-stimuli from the RVB (because it is closer to the insertion site of accessory pathways) if the RVA extra-stimuli are ineffective.[9]

Differentiating AVNRT from JT can be a diagnostic dilemma in some cases where the SVT initiation occurs with atrial or ventricular overdrive pacing and is not dependent on a critical AH interval. The magnitude of the difference between the HA interval during tachycardia (HA_{tach}) and that seen during ventricular pacing (HA_{pace}) at the RVB may be useful for distinguishing these arrhythmias.[10] It has been shown that the insertion of a late premature atrial contraction (PAC) from coronary sinus ostium during SVT when the septal A is committed can advance or delay the subsequent His or terminate SVT in patients with AVNRT and not in those with JT.[11] Earlier PACs can potentially affect JT by slowing, accelerating, terminating, or having no effect on the tachycardia focus.[12] Response to atrial overdrive pacing (AOD) during SVT can also be used to differentiate AVNRT (A-H-A after termination of AOD) and JT (A-H-H-A after termination of AOD).[13]

Focal AT is an important differential diagnosis in long RP tachycardia. AT is the most likely mechanism when an atrial-atrial-ventricular, or A-A-V, response is seen on cessation of overdrive ventricular pacing during SVT that captures the atrium, especially when the atrial activation sequence during ventricular pacing is different to that during tachycardia.[14] Man and colleagues[15] found that AT or AVRT consistently showed an AH interval that was similar ($\Delta AH < 20$ milliseconds) to the AH interval with right atrial (RA) pacing at TCL in a patient with long RP tachycardia. Atypical AVNRT was always associated with a shorter AH interval ($\Delta AH > 20$ milliseconds) than the AH during RA pacing at TCL. Demonstration of VA linking is another diagnostic maneuver that differentiates AT from AVNRT or AVRT. AOD during SVT is performed from different sites in the atrium. The VA interval of the return beat after AOD will be similar to the VA interval during tachycardia, thus linking the ventricle and atrium and favoring a diagnosis of AVNRT or AVRT.[16]

The SVT section in this issue focuses on difficult cases of AVNRT, WPW with recurrent AVRT despite multiple ablations, nodofascicular SVT, and tachycardia-induced cardiomyopathy associated with double fire, PJRT, and AT. There is emphasis on the use of diagnostic maneuvers to make the appropriate diagnosis and on appropriate ablation strategy in patients with recurrent SVT.

REFERENCES

1. Knight BP, Ebinger M, Oral H, et al. Diagnostic value of tachycardia features and pacing maneuvers during paroxysmal supraventricular tachycardia. J Am Coll Cardiol 2000;36(2):574–82.
2. Kerr CR, Gallagher JJ, German LD. Changes in ventriculoatrial intervals with bundle branch block aberration during reciprocating tachycardia in patients with accessory atrioventricular pathways. Circulation 1982;66(1):196–201.
3. Martinez-Alday JD, Almendral J, Arenal A, et al. Identification of concealed posteroseptal Kent pathways by comparison of ventriculoatrial intervals from apical and posterobasal right ventricular sites. Circulation 1994;89(3):1060–7.
4. Hirao K, Otomo K, Wang X, et al. Para-Hisian pacing. A new method for differentiating retrograde conduction over an accessory AV pathway from conduction over the AV node. Circulation 1996; 94(5):1027–35.
5. Reddy VY, Jongnarangsin K, Albert CM, et al. Para-Hisian entrainment: a novel pacing maneuver to differentiate orthodromic atrioventricular reentrant tachycardia from atrioventricular nodal reentrant tachycardia. J Cardiovasc Electrophysiol 2003; 14(12):1321–8.
6. Viswanathan MN, Badhwar N, Lee BK, et al. His bundle pacing and entrainment: a single pacing maneuver to differentiate mechanisms of supraventricular tachycardias [abstract]. Heart Rhythm 2007;4(5):S77.
7. Michaud GF, Tada H, Chough S, et al. Differentiation of atypical atrioventricular node re-entrant tachycardia from orthodromic reciprocating tachycardia using a septal accessory pathway by the response to ventricular pacing. J Am Coll Cardiol 2001; 38(4):1163–7.
8. Miller JM, Rosenthal ME, Gottlieb CD, et al. Usefulness of the delta HA interval to accurately distinguish atrioventricular nodal reentry from orthodromic septal bypass tract tachycardias. Am J Cardiol 1991;68(10): 1037–44.
9. Matsushita G, Badhwar N, Collins KK, et al. Usefulness of a ventricular extrastimulus from the summit of the ventricular septum in diagnosis of septal accessory pathway in patients with supraventricular tachycardia. Am J Cardiol 2004;93:643–6.
10. Srivathsan K, Gami AS, Barrett R, et al. Differentiating atrioventricular nodal reentrant tachycardia from junctional tachycardia: novel application of the delta H-A interval. J Cardiovasc Electrophysiol 2008;19(1):1–6.
11. Viswanathan MN, Scheinman MM, Badhwar N. A new diagnostic maneuver to differentiate atrioventricular nodal reentrant tachycardia from junctional tachycardia: a difficult distinction [abstract]. Heart Rhythm 2007;4(5):S288.
12. Padanilam BJ, Manfredi JA, Steinberg LA, et al. Differentiating junctional tachycardia and atrioventricular node re-entry tachycardia based on response to atrial extrastimulus pacing. J Am Coll Cardiol 2008; 52(21):1711–7.
13. Fan R, Tardos JG, Almasry I, et al. Novel use of atrial overdrive pacing to rapidly differentiate junctional tachycardia from atrioventricular nodal reentrant tachycardia. Heart Rhythm 2011;8(6):840–4.
14. Knight BP, Zivin A, Souza J, et al. A technique for the rapid diagnosis of atrial tachycardia in the electrophysiology laboratory. J Am Coll Cardiol 1999; 33(3):775–81.
15. Man KC, Niebauer M, Daoud E, et al. Comparison of atrial-His intervals during tachycardia and atrial pacing in patients with long RP tachycardia. J Cardiovasc Electrophysiol 1995;6(9):700–10.
16. Sarkozy A, Richter S, Chierchia G-B, et al. A novel pacing manoeuvre to diagnose atrial tachycardia. Europace 2008;10(4):459–66.

Para-Hisian Atrial Tachycardia

Lea El Hage, MD, Nitish Badhwar, MBBS*

KEYWORDS

• Para-Hisian atrial tachycardia • Catheter ablation • Atrioventricular block

KEY POINTS

- Incessant supraventricular tachycardia that presented with short RP and long RP tachycardia at the same cycle length.
- Presence of distinctive P wave morphology.
- Suggested mechanism was a cyclic adenosine monophosphate–dependent triggered activity based on response to adenosine.
- Mapped and successfully ablated at right para-Hisian region without atrioventricular block or PR prolongation.

CLINICAL PRESENTATION

A 77-year-old man with a history of coronary artery disease, status post coronary artery bypass graft, presented with a 5-month history of palpitation, lightheadedness, and dizziness. No episodes of syncope were noted. The patient failed initial treatment with β-blockers and calcium-channel blockers. Holter monitoring revealed persistent narrow complex tachycardia at a rate of 150 to 160 beats/min. He was scheduled for electrophysiology study and possible ablation.

ELECTROPHYSIOLOGY STUDY

Multipolar electrode catheters were positioned in the high right atrium, right ventricular apex, His bundle region, and coronary sinus via percutaneous introduction from the right femoral and internal jugular veins. Bipolar and unipolar electrograms were displayed and stored using a digital recording system (EP MedSystems, West Berlin, NJ). The CARTO system (Biosense Webster, Diamond Bar, CA) was used for 3-dimensional electroanatomic mapping. The patient's sinus rhythm electrocardiogram (ECG) is shown in **Fig. 1**.

The patient was noted to have incessant supraventricular tachycardia (SVT) during electrophysiology study with a cycle length (CL) of 527 milliseconds. A short RP and long RP tachycardia at the same CL were noted (**Fig. 2**). Adenosine administration resulted in conversion of the short RP tachycardia to long RP tachycardia, and eventual termination of the tachycardia (**Fig. 3**).

QUESTION: WHAT IS THE DIAGNOSIS?

The change from short RP to long RP tachycardia without change in the CL argues against atrioventricular (AV) reentry tachycardia using an accessory pathway and AV nodal reentry tachycardia, and makes atrial tachycardia (AT) the most likely diagnosis. The change from short RP SVT to long RP SVT is due to block in slow pathway conduction that is sensitive to low-dose adenosine; this suggests the presence of dual AV-node physiology in this patient. The diagnosis of AT was also supported by the dissociation of the ventricular signal from SVT during ventricular overdrive pacing and lack of ventriculoatrial linking shown by introduction of

Section of Electrophysiology, Division of Cardiology, University of California San Francisco, San Francisco, CA, USA
* Corresponding author. Cardiac Electrophysiology, University of California San Francisco, 500 Parnassus Avenue, MUE 431, San Francisco, CA 94143-1354, USA.
E-mail address: badhwar@medicine.ucsf.edu

Card Electrophysiol Clin 4 (2012) 497–502
http://dx.doi.org/10.1016/j.ccep.2012.08.022
1877-9182/12/$ – see front matter

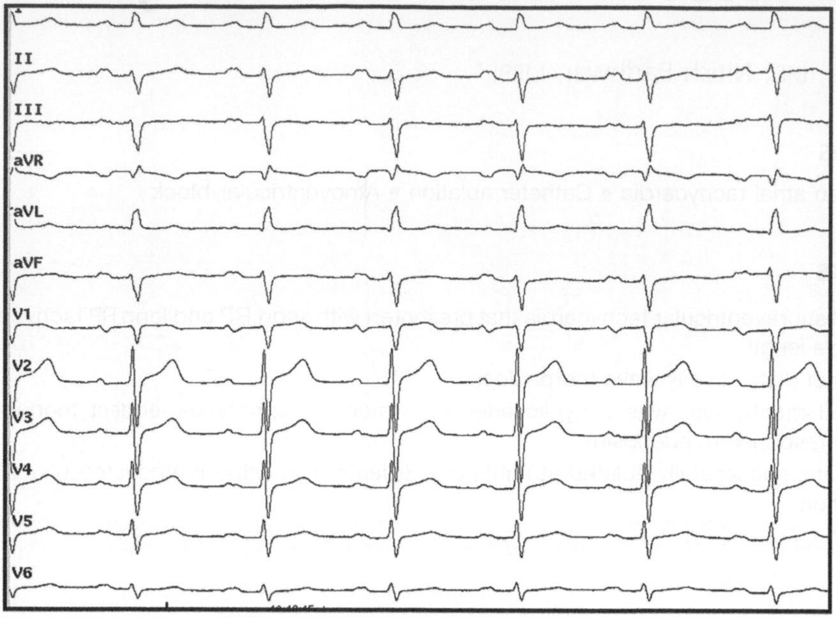

Fig. 1. Twelve-lead electrocardiogram (ECG) during sinus rhythm.

premature ventricular contractions, premature atrial contractions, and atrial overdrive pacing during SVT. Evaluation of the P-wave morphology reveals shorter P-wave duration during tachycardia in comparison with sinus rhythm, suggesting septal origin. Positive P waves in leads I and aVL, and biphasic P waves with terminal negative in V_1 indicated a right atrial focus, while negative P waves in II, III, and aVF indicated an inferior atrial location. Intracardiac recording confirmed that the earliest atrial electrogram (A) was at proximal His.

The CARTO mapping system was suggestive of a focal mechanism, with earliest atrial activation at His region supporting a para-Hisian focal AT (**Fig. 4**). The A signal was fractionated at this site and preceded the P wave by 39 milliseconds. Termination with adenosine is suggestive of triggered activity. A high-resolution map of the His cloud and AT focus was obtained, which revealed that the earliest site of activation was slightly superior and posterior to the His cloud. Low-energy radiofrequency (RF) applied to this site led to termination of SVT within 3 seconds of RF ablation (**Fig. 5**). The patient had no inducible tachycardia after ablation despite aggressive atrial extrastimuli on and off isoproterenol.

DISCUSSION

Focal ATs mainly originate from the crista terminalis, AV annuli, pulmonary vein ostia, coronary sinus ostium/musculature, and triangle of Koch.[1,2] The triangle of Koch is formed by the tendon of Todaro, attachment of the septal leaflet of the tricuspid valve, and the orifice of the coronary sinus. A para-Hisian location is considered when either a His deflection is observed at the site of earliest atrial activation during tachycardia or successful ablation along the tricuspid annulus is within 1 cm of the site recording the potential of the His bundle.[3] AT originating from the para-Hisian area are suggested to be a subset of "annular" (tricuspid) ATs owing to their similar properties, being differentiated only by the proximity of the His bundle.[4,5]

In general, adenosine is capable of differentiating between macro-reentrant and focal AT.[2] It terminates triggered focal AT and suppresses focal AT caused by enhanced automaticity, and has no effect on macro-reentrant AT (with the exception of AT involving partially depolarized tissue). Adenosine has been shown to inhibit the L-type calcium current ($I_{ca(L)}$) as well as the transient inward current (I_{Ti}), resulting in a decrease in the intracellular cyclic adenosine monophosphate (cAMP). Termination of the AT with adenosine is suggestive of a cAMP-dependent triggered activity as the mechanism of the tachycardia.

Several algorithms have described localization of the focal AT site by analysis of the P waves during tachycardia. P-wave morphology in leads aVL and V_1 can be used to differentiate between

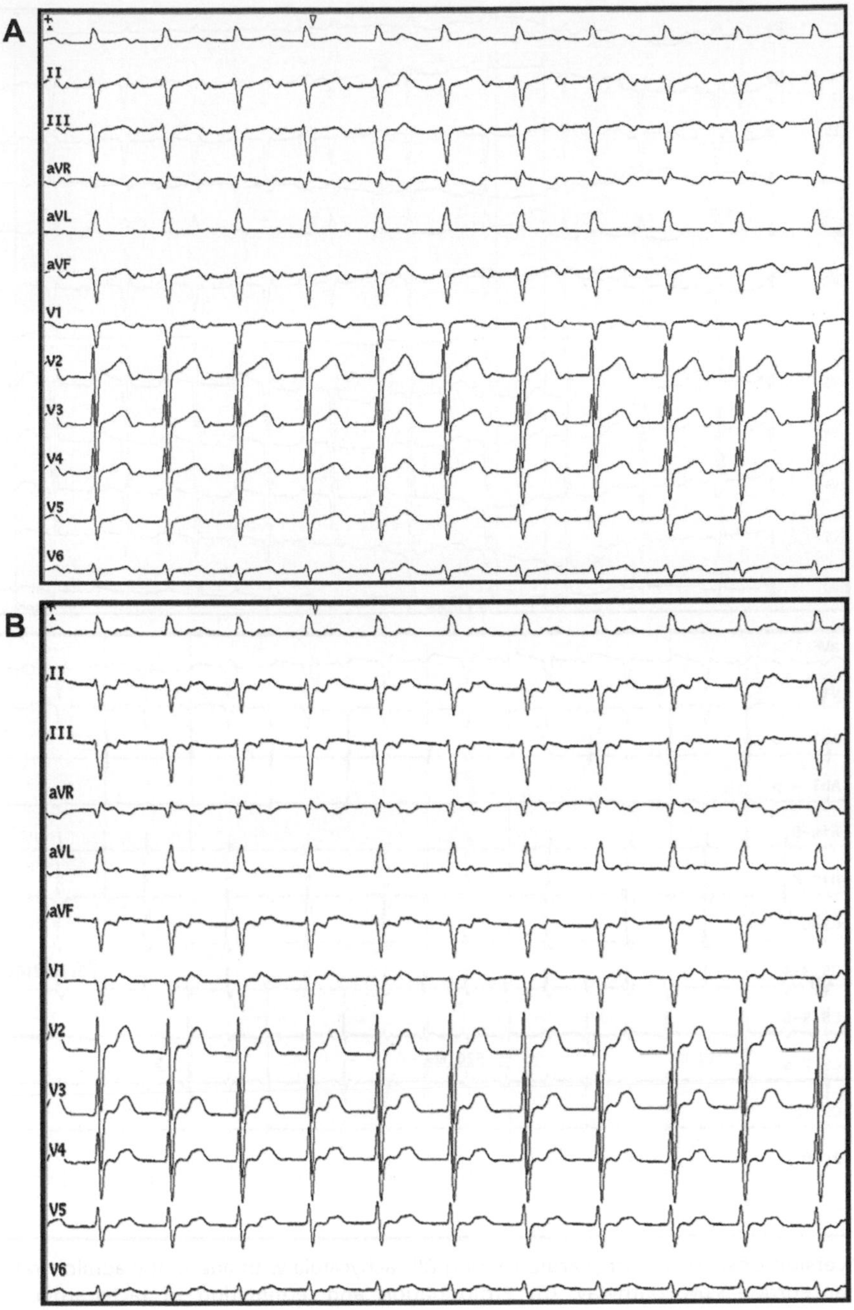

Fig. 2. (*A*) Twelve-lead ECG showing narrow complex long RP tachycardia. (*B*) Twelve-lead ECG showing narrow complex short RP tachycardia at the same cycle length as in *A*.

a left and right AT focus. A positive or biphasic P wave in lead aVL is predictive of a right atrial focus.[6] Negative or positive-negative biphasic P waves in V_1 are predictive of a right AT origin, whereas positive or negative-positive biphasic P waves in V_1 predict a left atrial origin.[7] Evaluation of P-wave morphology in leads II, III, and aVF can determine a superior versus inferior AT focus. Analysis of the P-wave morphology in this patient revealed an inferior right atrial focus. Findings indicative of para-Hisian AT on the ECG include narrowing of the P wave during SVT compared with sinus rhythm, and biphasic P waves in V_1 with early precordial transition.[4]

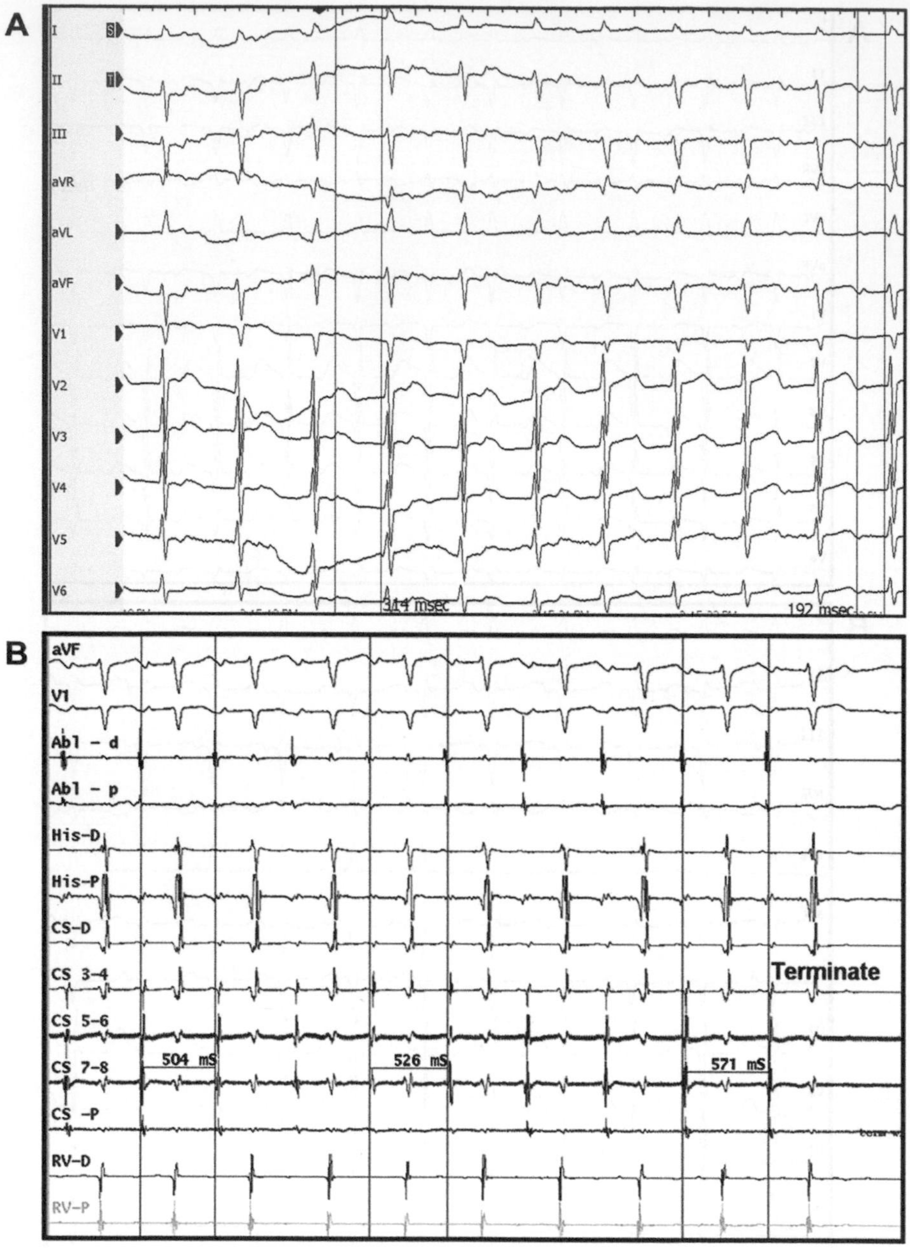

Fig. 3. (*A*) Conversion of short RP tachycardia to long RP tachycardia with adenosine administration, because of block in the antegrade slow pathway. (*B*) Prolongation and termination of tachycardia with adenosine administration.

ATs arising from the para-Hisian area at the apex of the triangle of Koch can be challenging to ablate because of their proximity to the AV node.[8] Even with careful attention, complete AV block can occur. Despite this increased risk, catheter ablation of para-Hisian AT has been shown to be effective.[4] Para-Hisian AT ablation can be also be mapped and ablated in the noncoronary cusp (NCC) of the aortic valve.[9] The specialized conduction system has been shown to be around the aortic root and AV canal in early embryonic stages that regress with age.[10] Because of the proximity of the NCC to the AV node, ablation in the NCC has been shown to cure para-Hisian AT with a decreased risk of AV block.[9]

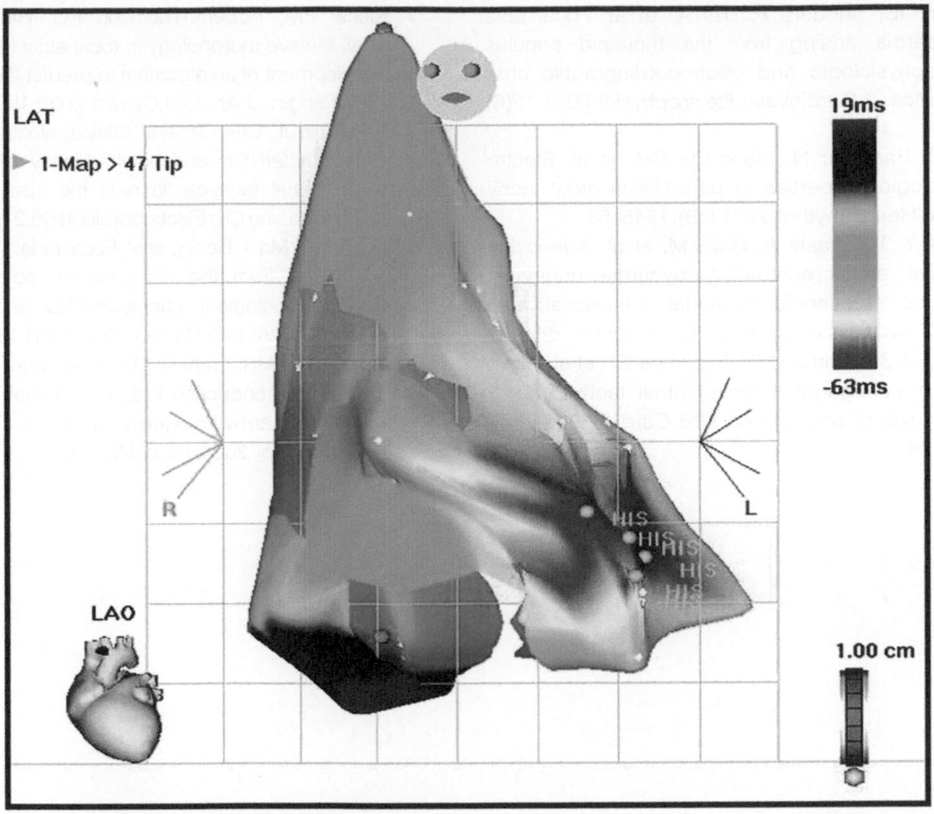

Fig. 4. Three-dimensional CARTO activation map shows focal activation of the atrial tachycardia from the para-Hisian region. The yellow dots signify points with His signal.

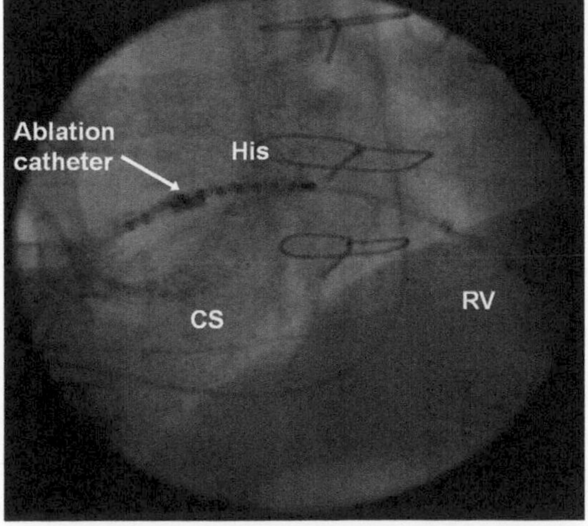

Fig. 5. Fluoroscopy showing site of successful ablation of the para-Hisian tachycardia. CS, coronary sinus; RV, right ventricle.

SUMMARY

Para-Hisian ATs can be classified as a subgroup of annular AT, owing to their similar location and properties. These ATs are associated with distinctive P-wave morphology. This report describes a case of para-Hisian AT associated with short RP and long RP tachycardias at the same CL. The response to adenosine suggested a cAMP-dependent triggered activity as the mechanism. Right atrial catheter ablation was successful, without atrioventricular block or prolongation of PR interval.

REFERENCES

1. Iwai S, Badhwar N, Stambler BS, et al. Para-Hisian atrial tachycardia: distinct entity or subset of annular atrial tachycardia? Circulation 2005;112(17):U811.
2. Iwai S, Markowitz SM, Stein KM, et al. Response to adenosine differentiates focal from macroreentrant atrial tachycardia: validation using three-dimensional electroanatomic mapping. Circulation 2002;106(22):2793–9.

3. Morton JB, Sanders P, Das A, et al. Focal atrial tachycardia arising from the tricuspid annulus: electrophysiologic and electrocardiographic characteristics. J Cardiovasc Electrophysiol 2001;12(6): 653–9.
4. Iwai S, Badhwar N, Markowitz SM, et al. Electrophysiologic properties of para-Hisian atrial tachycardia. Heart Rhythm 2011;8(8):1245–53.
5. Iesaka Y, Takahashi A, Goya M, et al. Adenosine-sensitive atrial reentrant tachycardia originating from the atrioventricular nodal transitional area. J Cardiovasc Electrophysiol 1997;8(8):854–64.
6. Tang CW, Scheinman MM, Van Hare GF, et al. Use of P wave configuration during atrial tachycardia to predict site of origin. J Am Coll Cardiol 1995;26(5): 1315–24.
7. Kistler PM, Roberts-Thomson KC, Haqqani HM, et al. P-wave morphology in focal atrial tachycardia: development of an algorithm to predict the anatomic site of origin. J Am Coll Cardiol 2006;48(5):1010–7.
8. Lai LP, Lin JL, Chen TF, et al. Clinical, electrophysiological characteristics, and radiofrequency catheter ablation of atrial tachycardia near the apex of Koch's triangle. Pacing Clin Electrophysiol 1998;21(2):367–74.
9. Ouyang F, Ma J, Ho SY, et al. Focal atrial tachycardia originating from the non-coronary aortic sinus—electrophysiological characteristics and catheter ablation. J Am Coll Cardiol 2006;48(1):122–31.
10. Jongbloed MR, Schalij MJ, Poelmann RE, et al. Embryonic conduction tissue: a spatial correlation with adult arrhythmogenic areas. J Cardiovasc Electrophysiol 2004;15(3):349–55.

Incessant Long RP Tachycardia

Marwan Refaat, MD[a], Nitish Badhwar, MBBS[a,b,*]

KEYWORDS

• Catheter ablation • Atrial tachycardia • Coronary sinus

KEY POINTS

- Incessant supraventricular tachycardia (SVT) can lead to systolic heart failure.
- Long RP SVT with negative P waves in the inferior leads can be caused by atrial tachycardia from the coronary sinus, atypical atrioventricular nodal reentrant tachycardia (AVNRT), and permanent reciprocating junctional tachycardia (PJRT) using a decremental accessory pathway.
- Spontaneous atrioventricular block during SVT ruled out PJRT and lack of ventriculoatrial linking ruled out AVNRT.
- P-wave analysis and 3-dimensional electroanatomic mapping localized the origin to the proximal coronary sinus, where catheter ablation was curative for SVT.

CLINICAL PRESENTATION

A 68-year-old woman had palpitations and dyspnea occurring on a daily basis for several months. She presented with increasing dyspnea, abdominal girth, and peripheral edema, and was found to be in decompensated systolic congestive heart failure. She was noted to have incessant episodes of supraventricular tachycardia (SVT) that was a long RP tachycardia (**Fig. 1**). Coronary angiography did not show significant coronary artery disease. She continued to have episodes of SVT despite treatment with β-blockers. She was referred for electrophysiology study and ablation.

ELECTROPHYSIOLOGY STUDY

Multipolar electrode catheters were introduced percutaneously from the right femoral and internal jugular veins and positioned into the high right atrium (HRA), right ventricular apex (RVA), His-bundle region, and coronary sinus (CS). Bipolar electrograms (30–500 Hz) and unipolar electrograms (0.5–500 Hz) were displayed and stored using a digital recording system (EP Med-Systems, West Berlin, NJ). Three-dimensional electroanatomic mapping was performed with Ensite NavX (St Jude Medical, St Paul, MN).

At baseline, the patient was in SVT with a tachycardia cycle length of 430 milliseconds (see **Fig. 1**) that would terminate with premature atrial contractions (PACs) and reinitiate with PACs (**Fig. 2**). Baseline atrial-His (AH) and His-ventricular (HV) intervals were within normal limits. No ventriculoatrial (VA) conduction was observed with or without isoproterenol infusion. Sustained long RP tachycardia was reliably induced, with earliest atrial activation in the proximal CS.

The diagnosis of atrial tachycardia (AT) was confirmed using the following criteria. (1) Absence of VA conduction at baseline, and VA dissociation during right ventricular pacing during SVT. Spontaneous atrioventricular block during SVT (see **Fig. 2**) ruled out PJRT and limited the differential diagnosis to AVNRT and AT. (2) Lack of critical AH interval required for SVT initiation. (3) No VA linking during

[a] Cardiac Electrophysiology Section, Cardiology Division, University of California, San Francisco, San Francisco, CA, USA; [b] Cardiac Electrophysiology, University of California San Francisco, 500 Parnassus Avenue, MUE 431, San Francisco, CA 94143-1354, USA
* Corresponding author.
E-mail address: badhwar@medicine.ucsf.edu

Card Electrophysiol Clin 4 (2012) 503–507
http://dx.doi.org/10.1016/j.ccep.2012.08.038

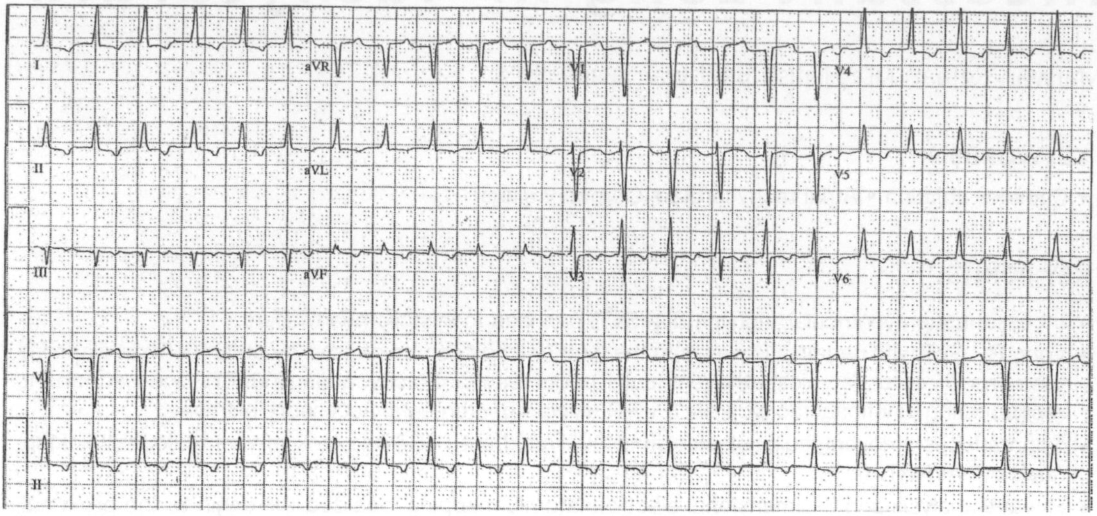

Fig. 1. Long RP supraventricular tachycardia (SVT) with negative P waves in the inferior leads.

SVT. Overdrive atrial pacing from the lateral right atrium showed VA interval of 180 milliseconds in the return beat (**Fig. 3**A) while the VA on the return beat after atrial overdrive pacing from the proximal CS was 120 milliseconds (see **Fig. 3**B). Hence, the difference of VA coupling interval was 60 milliseconds, which favors a diagnosis of AT.

QUESTION: WHERE IS THE SITE OF ORIGIN OF THE FOCAL ATRIAL TACHYCARDIA?

During tachycardia, the earliest atrial activation was noted in the proximal CS. Analysis of P-wave morphology during tachycardia revealed narrower P waves than the P waves during sinus rhythm, suggesting septal origin of the AT. An isoelectric/positive P wave was seen in lead V1. The P wave in lead aVL was difficult to visualize because of its inscription in the preceding T wave. The P wave was negative in the inferior leads, with P wave in lead II being more negative than P wave in lead III and lead aVF.

A 7F closed-irrigation ablation catheter with a 4-mm tip (Boston Scientific, Natick, MA) was advanced into the right atrium for mapping and ablation. The earliest bipolar electrogram (relative to P-wave onset) associated with a negative unipolar deflection was considered to be the site of AT origin. After detailed mapping of the right atrium, the site of AT origin was localized to the roof of the CS ostium (**Fig. 4**). This region was also characterized by a fractionated atrial electrogram that preceded the P wave during tachycardia by 60 milliseconds (**Fig. 5**). Termination of the tachycardia was

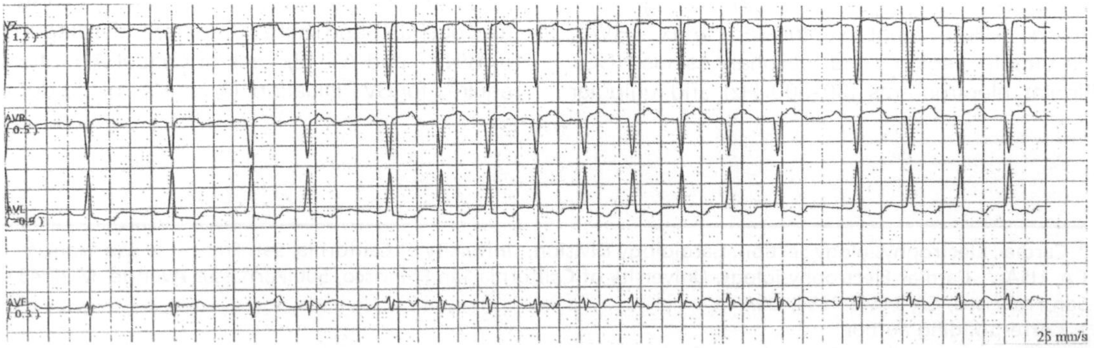

Fig. 2. Spontaneous atrioventricular block during supraventricular tachycardia (SVT) rules out atrioventricular reentrant tachycardia as the mechanism.

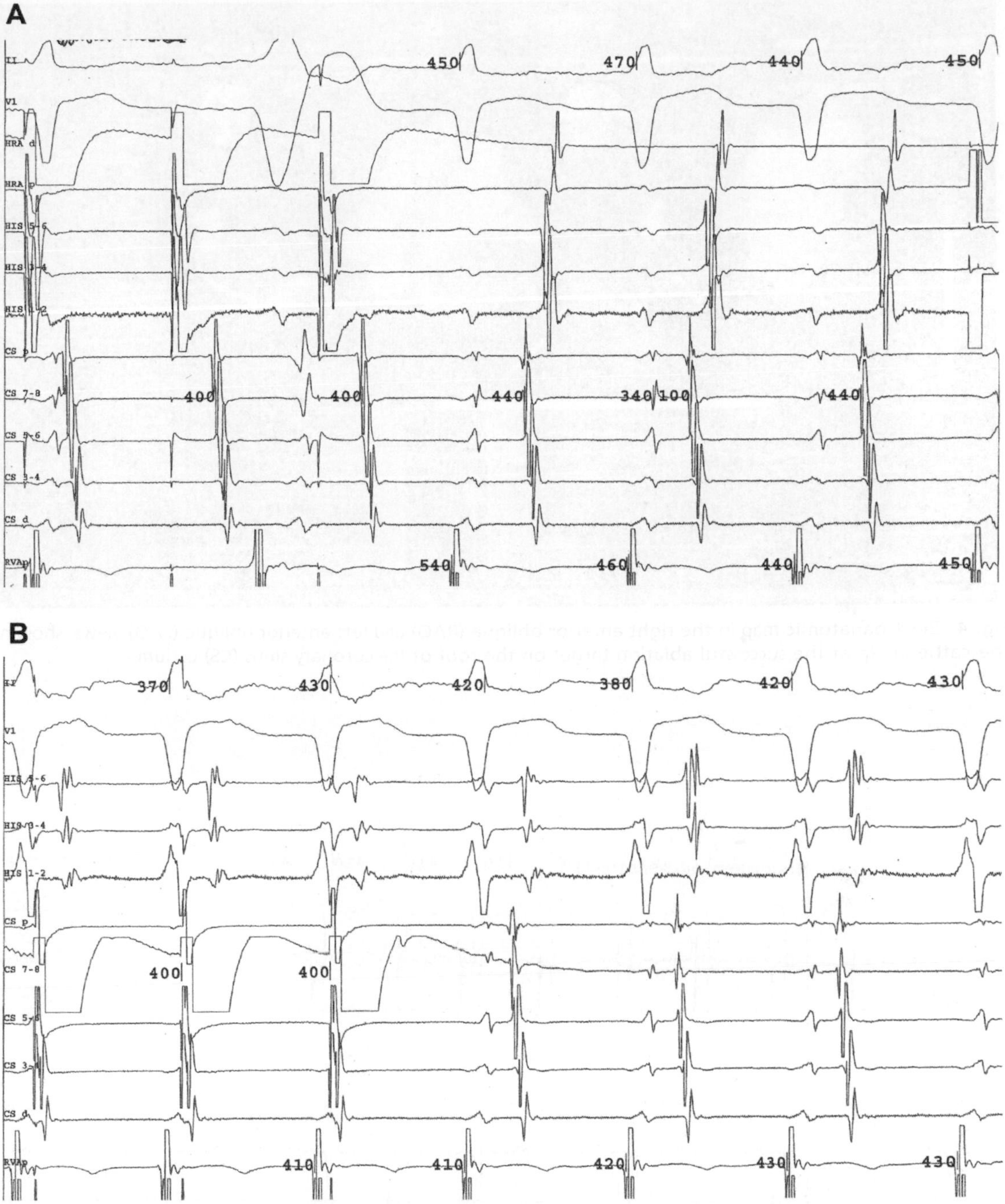

Fig. 3. Atrial overdrive pacing during tachycardia from the lateral right atrium (*A*) and CS ostium (*B*) shows variable ventriculoatrial interval of the return beat after pacing. This finding favors atrial tachycardia over atrioventricular nodal reentrant tachycardia as the mechanism of the SVT. HIS, His-bundle recordings; CS, coronary sinus recordings; RVA, right ventricular recordings.

observed after 2.6 seconds of radiofrequency ablation applied to the roof of the CS ostium (see **Fig. 5**). Tachycardia was not inducible after ablation at this site despite the use of isoproterenol up to 2 μg/min and aggressive atrial pacing with programmed atrial extra-stimuli. The patient has been symptom-free and off medications with normalization of left ventricular ejection fraction for more than 1 year.

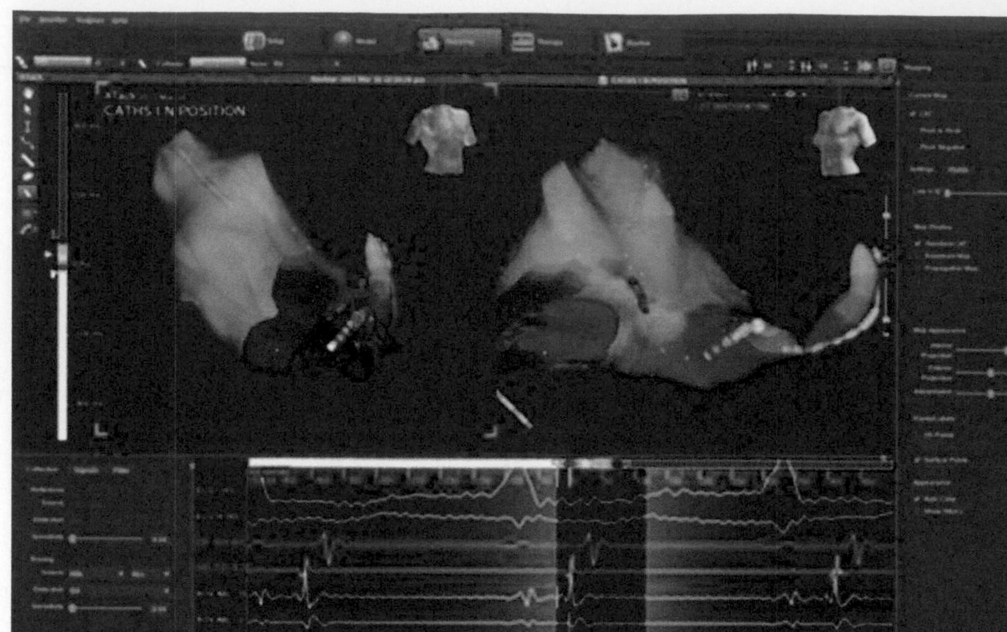

Fig. 4. Electroanatomic map in the right anterior oblique (RAO) and left anterior oblique (LAO) views, showing the catheter tip at the successful ablation target on the roof of the coronary sinus (CS) ostium.

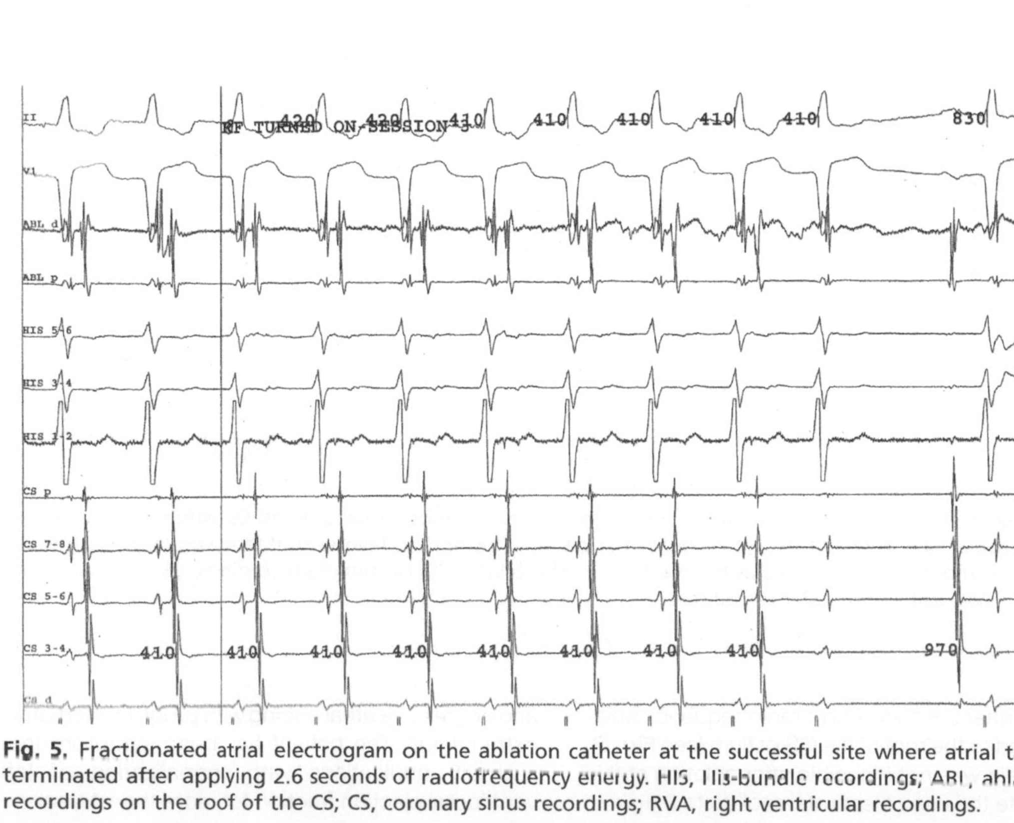

Fig. 5. Fractionated atrial electrogram on the ablation catheter at the successful site where atrial tachycardia terminated after applying 2.6 seconds of radiofrequency energy. HIS, His-bundle recordings; ABL, ablator signal recordings on the roof of the CS; CS, coronary sinus recordings; RVA, right ventricular recordings.

DISCUSSION

Focal ATs are uncommon causes of SVTs in adults, accounting for 5% to 10% of the cases. Focal ATs usually occur along the crista terminalis in the right atrium and near the pulmonary veins in the left atrium. Less frequently they can arise from the aortic cusps, CS ostium and musculature, the para-Hisian region, the appendages, or along the tricuspid or mitral annulus.[1] This case illustrates an AT originating from the roof of the CS ostium that was incessant, leading to tachycardia-induced cardiomyopathy.

Analysis of P-wave morphology during SVT and/or ectopic atrial impulses is useful in localizing the site of focal ATs. Several P-wave algorithms have been developed to help determine the site of origin of focal AT.[1,2] In a recent algorithm, Kistler and colleagues[1,3] reported P-wave morphology during SVT that was biphasic with terminal positive in lead V1, positive in lead aVL, and deep negative in the inferior leads, favoring CS ostial AT. The present case had a negative P wave in the inferior leads with a P wave in lead II more negative than lead III, which favors AT focus in the proximal CS rather than in the right posterior septal region. This focus was confirmed by the use of 3-dimensional mapping, which showed the site of earliest atrial activation with reference to the surface P wave to be at the roof of the CS ostium. Catheter ablation at this site terminated the AT.

Atrial pacing maneuvers are helpful in the diagnosis of AT by pacing in the atrium at a rate faster than the tachycardia rate at 2 different sites. If the VA interval of the return cycle length is within 10 milliseconds of the VA interval during the tachycardia, there is "VA linking," and AVNRT or AVRT is the most likely diagnosis. If the VA interval is variable, AT is most likely.[4]

SUMMARY

This case illustrates an uncommon cause of incessant long RP tachycardia leading to symptoms of heart failure. The SVT showed negative P wave in the inferior leads. The SVT was proved to be AT based on dissociation of the ventricle from SVT and the lack of VA linking. P-wave morphology during SVT suggested inferior septal origin and negative P wave in lead II that was more prominent than P wave in lead III, favoring CS origin of AT. The 3-dimensional mapping helped localize the exact site on the roof of CS ostium, where successful catheter ablation was performed.

REFERENCES

1. Kistler PM, Roberts-Thomson KC, Haqqani HM, et al. P-wave morphology in focal atrial tachycardia: development of an algorithm to predict the anatomic site of origin. J Am Coll Cardiol 2006;48(5):1010–7.
2. Tang CW, Scheinman MM, Van Hare GF, et al. Use of P wave configuration during atrial tachycardia to predict site of origin. J Am Coll Cardiol 1995;26(5):1315–24.
3. Kistler PM, Fynn SP, Haqqani HM, et al. Focal atrial tachycardia from the ostium of the coronary sinus: electrocardiographic and electrophysiological characterization and radiofrequency ablation. J Am Coll Cardiol 2005;45:1488–93.
4. Sarkozy A, Richter S, Chierchia G-B, et al. A novel pacing manoeuvre to diagnose atrial tachycardia. Europace 2008;10(4):459–66.

Atrial Refractory Stimulation to Identify the Optimal Slow-Pathway Ablation Site for Treatment of Atypical Atrioventricular Nodal Reentrant Tachycardia

Russell R. Heath, MD, Duy Thai Nguyen, MD, Royce L. Bargas, DO, William H. Sauer, MD*

KEYWORDS

- Atrioventricular nodal reentrant tachycardia • Slow-pathway potential • Catheter ablation
- Supraventricular tachycardia

KEY POINTS

- Atypical atrioventricular nodal reentrant tachycardia (AVNRT) provides a unique opportunity to localize the slow pathway in ways not possible with the typical form of AVNRT.
- Atrial refractory stimulation during atypical AVNRT in the region of the slow pathway will advance the subsequent A and V if stimulation captures the slow pathway, thus providing localization of the slow pathway.
- Using alternative methods to localize the slow pathway during atypical AVNRT can reduce the chance of heart block by guiding ablation more distant from the compact AV node.

CASE PRESENTATION

A 52-year-old man with a history of ablation for the treatment of atrial fibrillation and typical AVNRT presented with complaints of persistent palpitations. An event monitor demonstrated a regular tachycardia with a right bundle branch block identical to his QRS complex during sinus rhythm. The patient was then referred for electrophysiology study and ablation of tachycardia.

QUESTION

In atypical AVNRT, what methods can be used to localize the slow pathway?

ELECTROPHYSIOLOGY STUDY

Anterograde dual AV nodal physiology was demonstrated with atrial extra-stimuli. Retrograde VA conduction was concentric and decremental. Para-Hisian pacing, as well as apical and basal ventricular pacing, were consistent with a nodal response without evidence of accessory pathway conduction. A supraventricular tachycardia (SVT) with a cycle length of 480 milliseconds was induced. Resetting of the tachycardia with ventricular pacing resulted in a V-A-H-V response with a postpacing interval minus the tachycardia cycle length of greater than 115 milliseconds. Using CARTO (Biosense Webster, Diamond Bar, CA)

Conflicts of interest: None pertaining to this article.
Section of Cardiac Electrophysiology, Division of Cardiology, University of Colorado School of Medicine, 12401 E 17th Avenue, B-136, Aurora, CO 80045, USA
* Corresponding author.
E-mail address: william.sauer@ucdenver.edu

Card Electrophysiol Clin 4 (2012) 509–512
http://dx.doi.org/10.1016/j.ccep.2012.08.028
1877-9182/12/$ – see front matter

3-dimensional electroanatomic mapping, the earliest atrial activation during tachycardia was mapped to the base of the coronary sinus (**Fig. 1**). At the earliest point a distinct near-field electrogram was identified to precede the atrial electrogram. During tachycardia, atrial stimulation was delivered during atrial refractoriness in an attempt to capture the slow pathway. Atrial stimulation was delivered in and around the posterior, inferior, and anterior aspects of the coronary sinus. With pacing during atrial refractoriness, delivered at the earliest site at the inferior and posterior aspect of the coronary sinus, and at the location of the near-field potential, stimulation advanced the subsequent atrial and ventricular activation (**Fig. 2**). Pacing at this site with shorter atrial to stimulation intervals terminated the tachycardia. Radiofrequency ablation at this site performed during tachycardia resulted in termination of the arrhythmia and subsequent accelerated junctional rhythm with intact AV and VA conduction (**Fig. 3**). Following ablation, there was no evidence of anterograde or retrograde slow-pathway conduction with and without isoproterenol infusion.

DISCUSSION

This case supports the theory that there are insulated conducting fibers that provide the inferior input to the AV node.[1] The use of atrial stimulation to identify the effective site for ablation of the AV nodal slow pathway for the treatment of typical AVNRT has been previously described.[2,3] This case illustrates a useful technique for identifying the location of the slow AV nodal pathway during the uncommon form of AVNRT. Atrial refractory stimulation delivered during atypical AVNRT could reduce the risk of heart block by localizing a suitable ablation site remote from the AV node, as was the case in this patient. Further investigation is needed for evaluating this maneuver in other forms of AVNRT.

CLINICAL COURSE

Following ablation the patient's HV interval was unchanged. After an 18-month follow-up there has been no recurrence of SVT or atrial fibrillation.

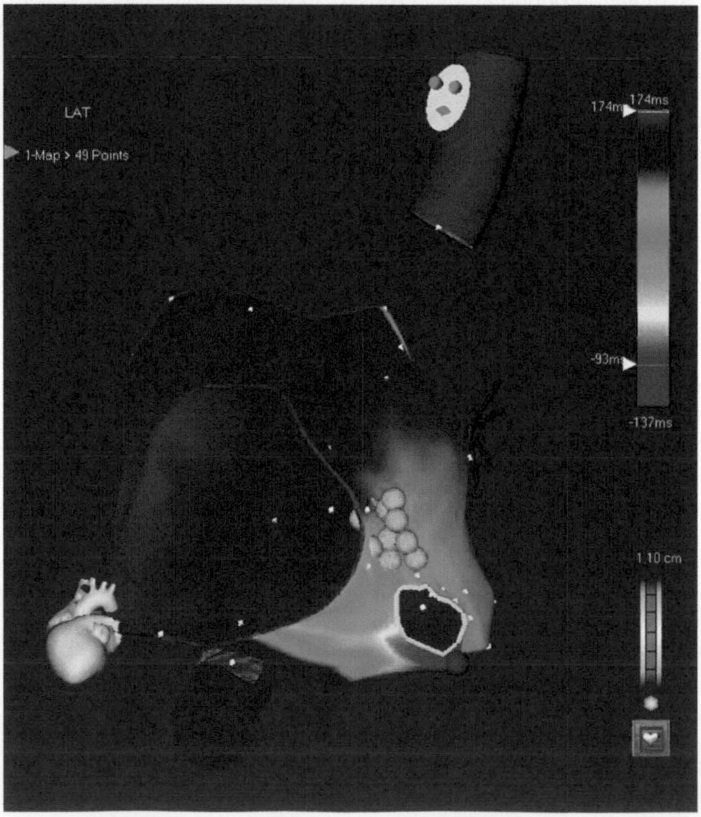

Fig. 1. Three-dimensional map of the earliest retrograde atrial activation during atypical atrioventricular nodal reentrant tachycardia (AVNRT). The red area represents the earliest site of activation and the red circle represents the area in which successful ablation was performed.

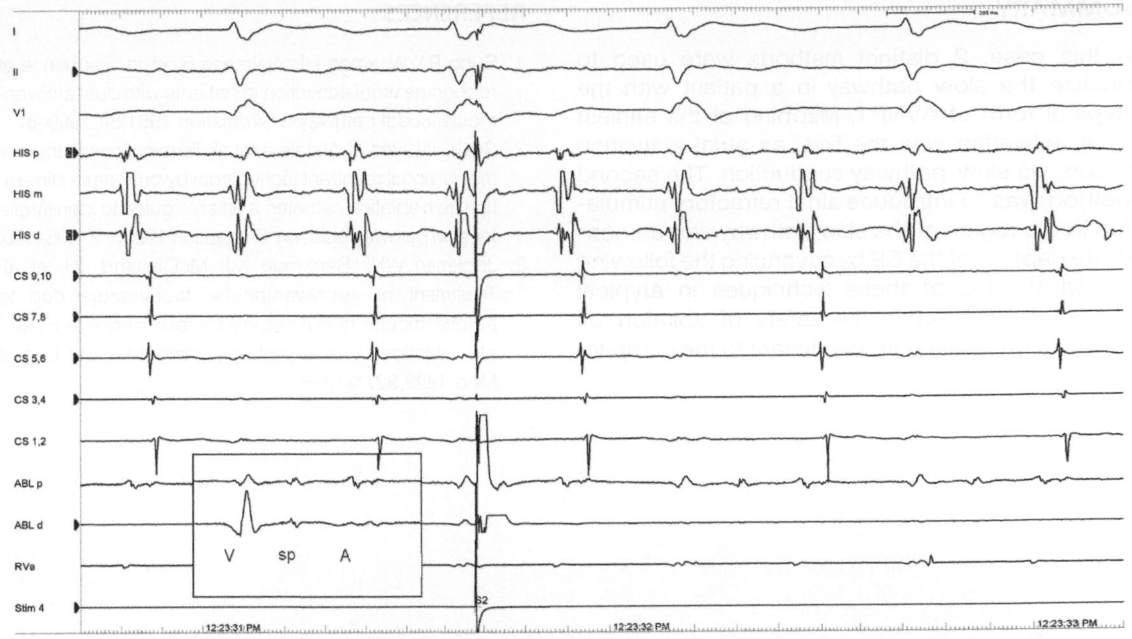

Fig. 2. Slow-pathway capture during AVNRT advances subsequent ventricular and atrial activation. Shown are surface leads I, II, and V1 as well as intracardiac electrograms from the proximal, mid, and distal His bundle, the decapolar catheter in the coronary sinus, the right ventricular catheter (which has been minimally gained), and the ablation catheter, which is positioned at the site of the earliest atrial activation. Because of a pacing artifact on the distal ablator, the EGMs are not discernible. The EGM before pacing is displayed in the inset box at the lower left of the figure.

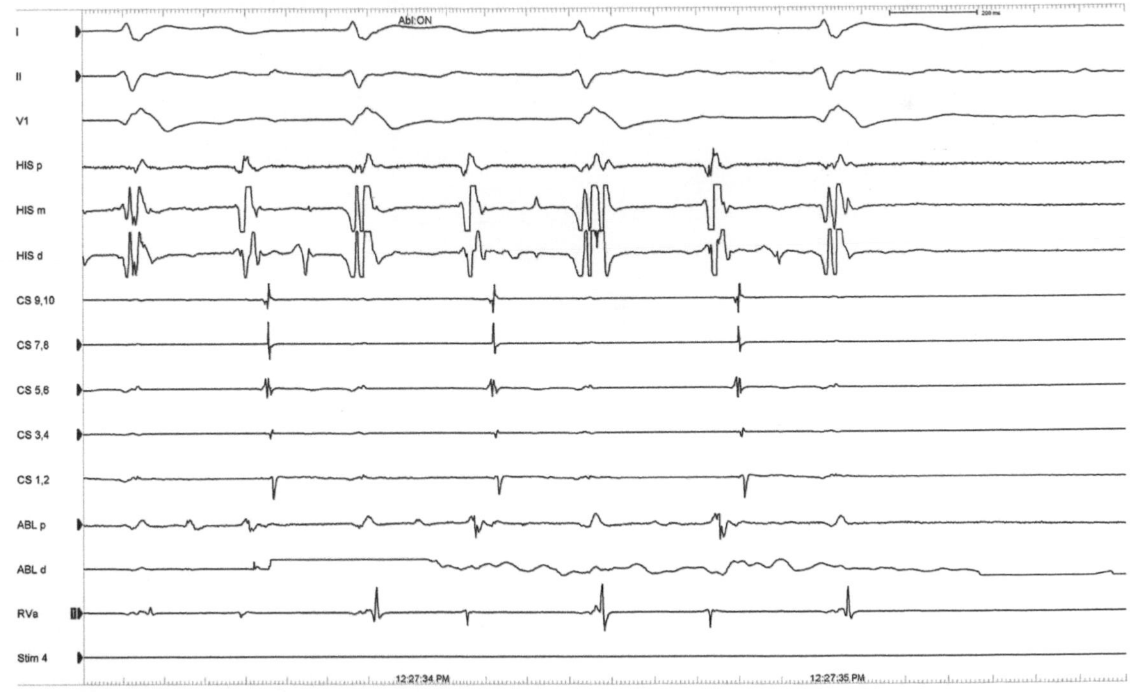

Fig. 3. Ablation at the earliest site of atrial activation and where the slow-pathway potential was identified results in termination of tachycardia without residual slow-pathway conduction. Shown are surface leads I, II, and V1 as well as intracardiac electrograms from the proximal, mid, and distal His bundle, The decapolar catheter in the coronary sinus, the right ventricular catheter, and the ablation catheter, which is positioned at the site of the earliest atrial activation.

SUMMARY

In this case, 2 distinct methods were used to localize the slow pathway in a patient with the atypical form of AVNRT. Mapping of the earliest atrial activation was the first, as atrial activation occurs via slow-pathway conduction. The second method was to introduce atrial refractory stimulation in the region of the slow pathway and demonstrate capture of the SP by advancing the following A and V. Use of these techniques in atypical AVNRT may improve the safety of ablation by localizing the slow pathway distant to the compact AV node.

REFERENCES

1. Sung RJ, Waxman HL, Saksena S, et al. Sequence of retrograde atrial activation in patients with dual atrioventricular nodal pathways. Circulation 1981;64:1059–67.
2. Sra J, Jazayeri M, Natale A, et al. Termination of atrioventricular nodal reentrant tachycardia by premature stimulation from ablation catheter: a reliable guide to identify site for slow pathway ablation. Circulation 1995;91:1095–100.
3. Jackman WM, Beckman KJ, McClelland JH, et al. Treatment of supraventricular tachycardia due to atrioventricular nodal reentry by radiofrequency catheter ablation of slow-pathway conduction. N Engl J Med 1992;327:313–8.

A Regularly Irregular Tachycardia in a Patient with New Cardiomyopathy

Duy Thai Nguyen, MD*, Russell R. Heath, MD,
William H. Sauer, MD

KEYWORDS

• Catheter ablation • Junctional tachycardia • Atrioventricular nodal reentrant tachycardia
• Double-fire • Dual AV node physiology

KEY POINTS

- A regularly irregular tachycardia should not be mistaken for atrial fibrillation.
- The differential diagnosis for an A-on-V tachycardia includes atrioventricular nodal reentrant tachycardia (AVNRT) and junctional tachycardia (JT).
- Late-coupled atrial premature beats during supraventricular tachycardia can differentiate between AVNRT and JT.
- Cryoablation should be considered when ablating near the His bundle, when radiofrequency ablation of the typical slow-pathway region is unsuccessful.
- In the setting of a new cardiomyopathy of unknown etiology, an abnormal tachycardia should be treated to ascertain whether the cardiomyopathy could be reversed.

CLINICAL HISTORY

A 26-year-old man, with no significant medical history, presented with frequent palpitations since childhood. He had 3 previous catheter ablations performed for supraventricular tachycardia (SVT) that were unsuccessful. He was referred because of persistent symptoms despite multiple medications. His presenting electrocardiogram showed a regularly irregular atrial rhythm (**Fig. 1**), and he had an echocardiogram demonstrating moderately decreased left ventricular dysfunction.

ELECTROPHYSIOLOGY STUDY

Multipolar catheters were placed in the right atrium, His-bundle region, right ventricle (RV), and coronary sinus. At baseline, the patient was in normal sinus rhythm with normal atrial-His (AH) and a prolonged His-ventricular (HV) interval of 60 milliseconds, thought to be due to his prior ablations.

Ventricular pacing at baseline demonstrated complete ventriculoatrial (VA) dissociation. SVT was consistently induced with burst atrial pacing on high doses of isoproterenol. Atrial activation during SVT was concentric, and the septal VA time was less than 70 milliseconds, thus excluding atrioventricular (AV) reentrant tachycardia. Ventricular overdrive pacing resulted in a V-A-H-V response, thus ruling out atrial tachycardia. Atrial burst pacing initiated the tachycardia with simultaneous A and V activation (**Fig. 2**), thus narrowing the differential diagnosis to typical AV nodal reentrant tachycardia (AVNRT) with double-response or focal junctional tachycardia (JT). Attempts to atrial-overdrive pace the tachycardia consistently

Disclosures: None.
Cardiac Electrophysiology, Division of Cardiology, University of Colorado, Denver, Anschutz Medical Campus, 12401 East 17th Avenue, B-132, Aurora, CO 80045, USA
* Corresponding author.
E-mail address: duy.t.nguyen@ucdenver.edu

Card Electrophysiol Clin 4 (2012) 513–516
http://dx.doi.org/10.1016/j.ccep.2012.08.033
1877-9182/12/$ – see front matter

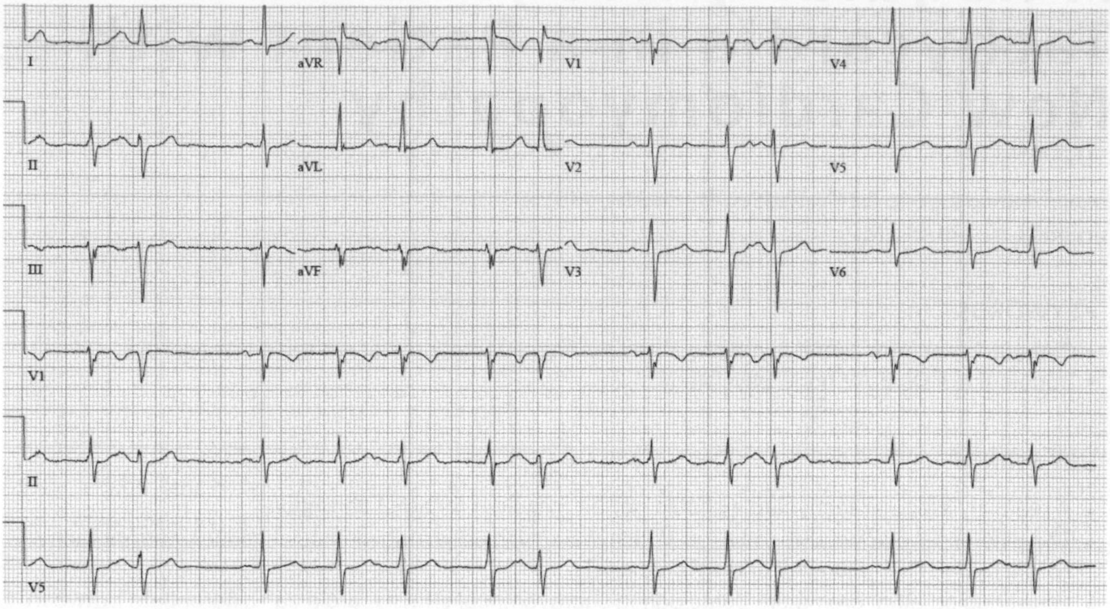

Fig. 1. Twelve-lead electrocardiogram of a regularly irregular atrial rhythm.

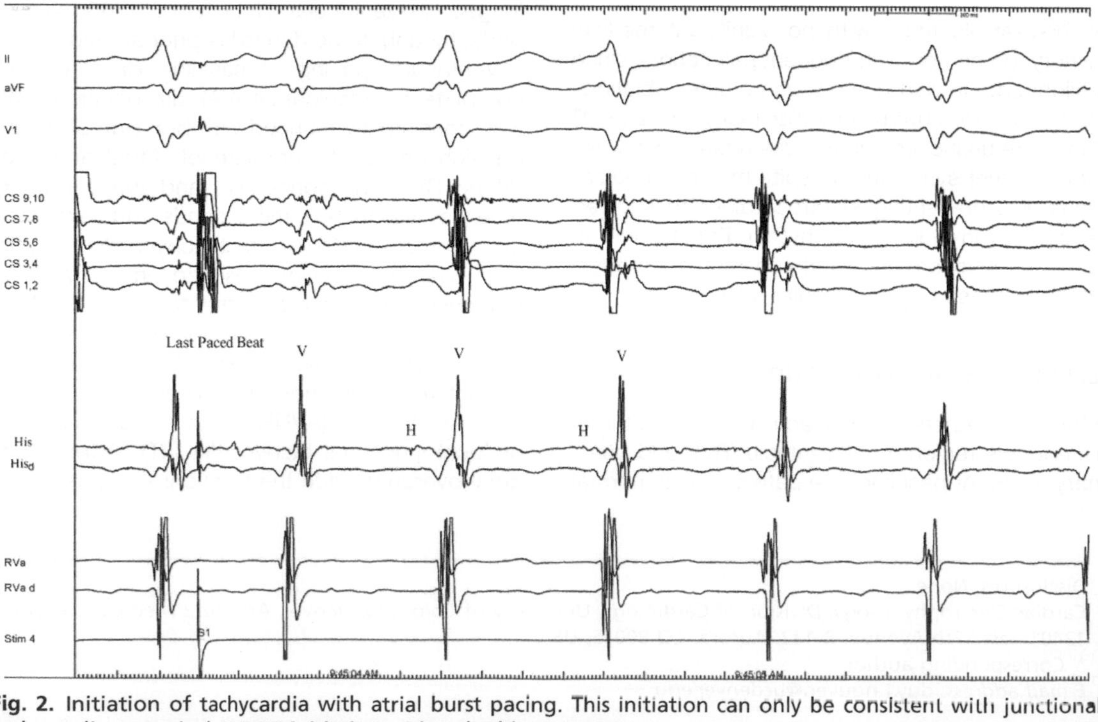

Fig. 2. Initiation of tachycardia with atrial burst pacing. This initiation can only be consistent with junctional tachycardia or typical AVNRT initiating with a double response.

terminated the tachycardia each time. During SVT, late-coupled atrial premature beats (APBs) were introduced, when the septal atrial activation (atrial signal on the His recording) was committed (**Fig. 3**).

QUESTION

What is the most likely mechanism of the tachycardia?

DISCUSSION

In this case, the lack of VA conduction would appear to make AVNRT much less likely. Initiation with atrial burst pacing in the setting of A-on-V tachycardia would favor JT; otherwise, the alternative explanation for **Fig. 2** is a double-fire from the last atrial paced beat causing typical AVNRT. Differentiation between AVNRT and JT remains a challenge given their similar characteristics, but is an important distinction because the approach to ablation and the site of ablation may differ. Srivathsan and colleagues[1] examined the difference between the AH interval in tachycardia and the AH interval during ventricular pacing at the basal RV, and found that the magnitude of this difference may be useful in distinguishing these arrhythmias; however, this maneuver was not possible in this case.

An alternative method to differentiate AVNRT from JT would be to insert a late APB from the slow AV nodal pathway region, during tachycardia when the septal atrial electrogram (A) was committed; this late APB could advance or delay the subsequent His or terminate tachycardia in patients with AVNRT, but not in patients with JT.[2] Late APBs, before the septal A is committed, can potentially affect JT or AVNRT by advancing the subsequent His and ventricular electrogram. However, termination of tachycardia or delay of the next His should be absolutely diagnostic in differentiating AVNRT (reentrant mechanism with a slow decremental limb) from JT (focal origin with triggered or automatic mechanism).[3] The exclusion of junctional tachycardia therefore confirms the diagnosis of AVNRT, and the initiation of the tachycardia is therefore one of double-fire. This feature further explained the patient's presenting electrocardiogram of a regularly irregular tachycardia attributable to a 2-for-1 response.

CLINICAL COURSE

In this case, delay of the next His during SVT with a late APB was diagnostic for AVNRT, because JT would not have been delayed by a late APB.

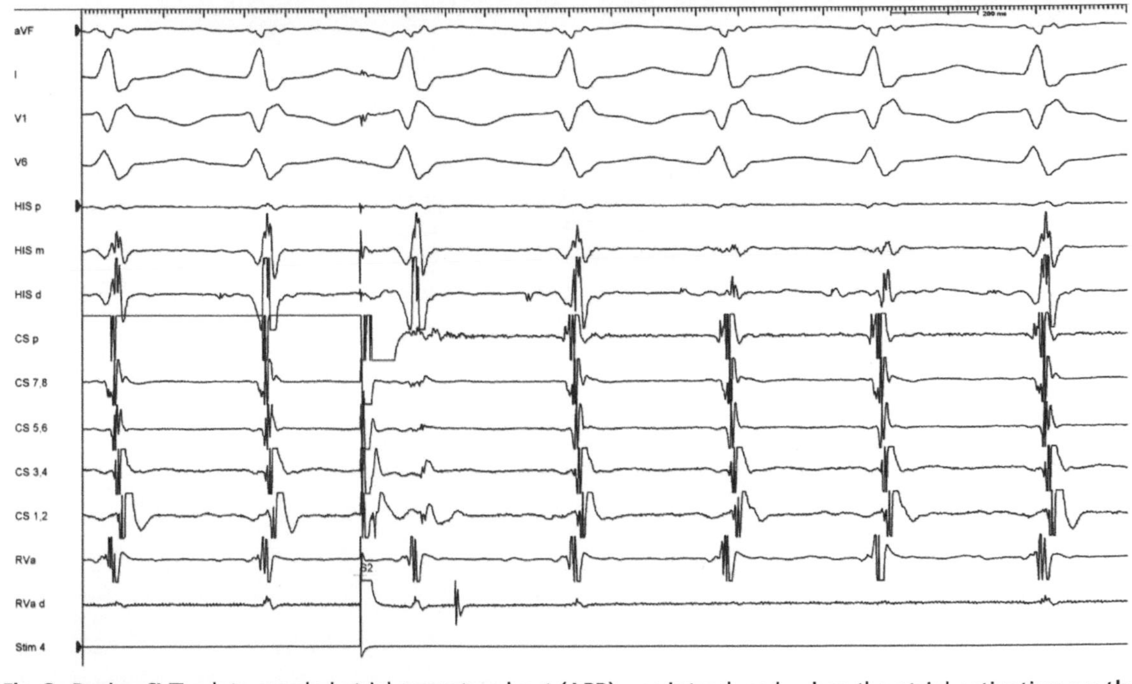

Fig. 3. During SVT, a late-coupled atrial premature beat (APB) was introduced, when the atrial activation on the His recording was committed. The APB delayed the following His and V signal, thus ruling in AVNRT, because it had to have entered the slow pathway to cause the delay. JT would not have been affected by the late APB. CS d, distal coronary sinus; CS p, proximal coronary sinus; H, His electrogram; His d, distal His; His m, mid His; His p, proximal His; HRA d, distal high right atrium; HRA p, proximal high right atrium; RVA d, distal right ventricular apex; RVA p, proximal right ventricular apex.

Ablation in the slow-pathway region resulted in junctional beats, but the same tachycardia remained inducible. Despite ablation in the coronary sinus and throughout the slow-pathway region, the tachycardia persisted. Finally, cryoablation was used while ablating above the roof of the coronary sinus with a His signal on the proximal pole but not on the distal pole of the cryoablation catheter. PR and HV intervals remained stable, and no atrioventricular block was observed. At the conclusion of several cryoablation freezes, SVT could no longer be induced. The patient has remained symptom-free during follow-up of 1 year, and his cardiomyopathy has resolved. His cardiomyopathy was presumed to be secondary to the regularly irregularly tachycardia caused by a 2-for-1 response from dual AV node physiology. After successful ablation of the patient's slow pathway this could no longer be sustained, and his cardiomyopathy improved.

SUMMARY

A regularly irregular tachycardia should not be mistaken for atrial fibrillation. The differential diagnosis for an A-on-V tachycardia includes AVNRT and JT. Late-coupled APBs during SVT can differentiate between AVNRT and JT. Cryoablation should be considered when ablating near the His bundle, when radiofrequency ablation of the typical slow-pathway region is unsuccessful. In the setting of a new cardiomyopathy of unknown etiology, an abnormal tachycardia should be treated to ascertain whether the cardiomyopathy could be reversed.

REFERENCES

1. Srivathsan K, Gami AS, Barrett R, et al. Differentiating atrioventricular nodal reentrant tachycardia from junctional tachycardia: novel application of the delta H-A interval. J Cardiovasc Electrophysiol 2008;19:1–6.
2. Hamdan MH, Badhwar N, Scheinman MM. Role of invasive electrophysiologic testing in the evaluation and management of adult patients with focal junctional tachycardia. Card Electrophysiol Rev 2002;6:431–5.
3. Viswanathan MN, Scheinman M, Badhwar N. A new diagnostic maneuver to differentiate atrioventricular nodal reentrant tachycardia from junctional tachycardia: a difficult distinction. Heart Rhythm 2007;4:S288 [abstract].

Incessant Supraventricular Tachycardia in a Patient with Cardiomyopathy

David F. Katz, MD, William H. Sauer, MD,
Duy Thai Nguyen, MD*

KEYWORDS

- Permanent junctional reciprocating tachycardia • Atrioventricular reentrant tachycardia
- Ventricular premature depolarization • Posteroseptal pathway ablation

KEY POINTS

- The differential diagnosis for a long RP supraventricular tachycardia includes atrial tachycardia, atypical atrioventricular nodal reentrant tachycardia, and atrioventricular reentrant tachycardia with a slowly conducting retrograde accessory pathway (AP), as seen in permanent junctional reciprocating tachycardia (PJRT).
- The combination of incessant tachycardia, a stable tachycardia cycle length, and a typical electrocardiogram P-wave morphology are highly suggestive of PJRT.
- Delay of atrial depolarization following delivery of a His-refractory ventricular premature depolarization during tachycardia demonstrates participation of a decremental AP.
- In a patient with cardiomyopathy of unknown etiology, incessant long RP tachycardia should raise concern for PJRT, ablation of which may result in improvement of the left ventricular ejection fraction.

CLINICAL HISTORY

A 30-year-old man presented to the emergency room with shortness of breath and hypotension. He was intubated and placed on vasopressors. An echocardiogram showed a dilated cardiomyopathy with severely depressed left ventricular (LV) ejection fraction. It was also noted that he was in incessant supraventricular tachycardia (SVT). Intravenous adenosine terminated the tachycardia multiple times, but it would immediately reinitiate. Amiodarone and procainamide were also used, but had minimal effect. Electrophysiology (EP) consultation was requested.

ELECTROPHYSIOLOGY STUDY AND ABLATION

The tachycardia was thought to contribute to the patient's cardiomyopathy and continued vasopressor requirement, resulting in referral for an EP study. Multipolar catheters were placed in the right atrium (RA), His-bundle region, right ventricle, and coronary sinus (CS). At baseline, the patient was in a long RP supraventricular tachycardia with a tachycardia cycle length (TCL) of 580 milliseconds (**Fig. 1**). Atrial activation was seen earliest on the proximal CS poles, and proceeded in a posterior to anterior direction along the His catheter (**Fig. 2**A) corresponding to the P-wave morphology seen on the surface electrocardiogram (ECG).

Attempts at entraining the tachycardia from the ventricle repeatedly resulted in termination of the tachycardia without exciting the atrium, ruling out atrial tachycardia (data not shown). Delivery of a relatively late-coupled, His-synchronous ventricular premature depolarization (VPD) from the right ventricular apex failed to alter the timing of the

Disclosures: None.
Cardiac Electrophysiology, Cardiology Division, University of Colorado Denver, Anschutz Medical Campus, 12401 East 17th Avenue, B-132, Aurora, CO 80045, USA
* Corresponding author.
E-mail address: duy.t.nguyen@ucdenver.edu

Card Electrophysiol Clin 4 (2012) 517–520
http://dx.doi.org/10.1016/j.ccep.2012.08.024

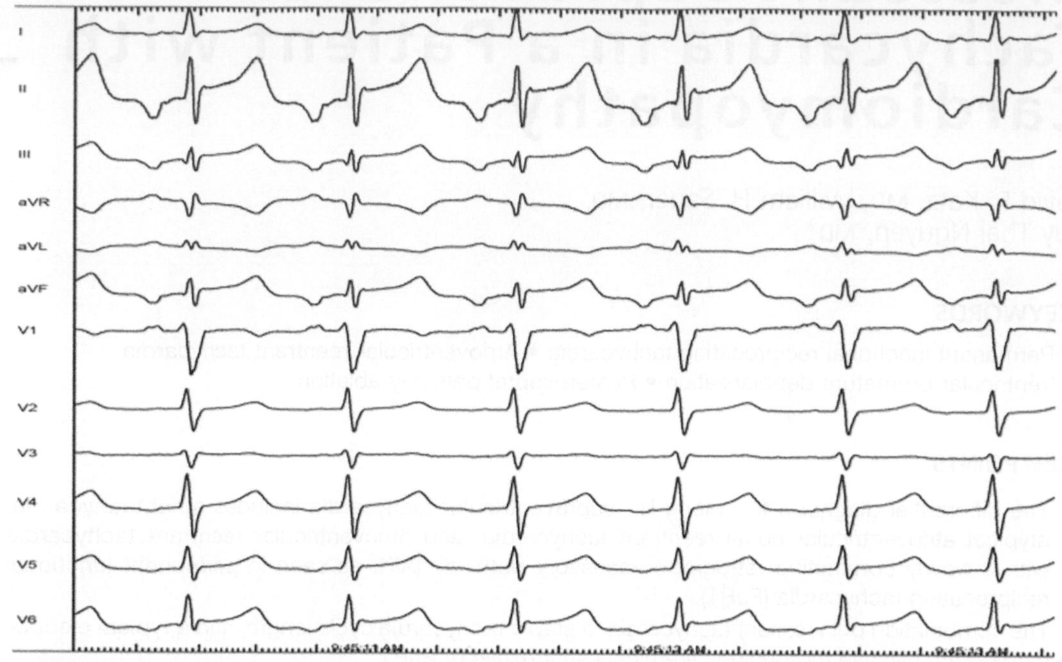

Fig. 1. Twelve-lead electrocardiogram of a narrow-complex tachycardia with long RP intervals.

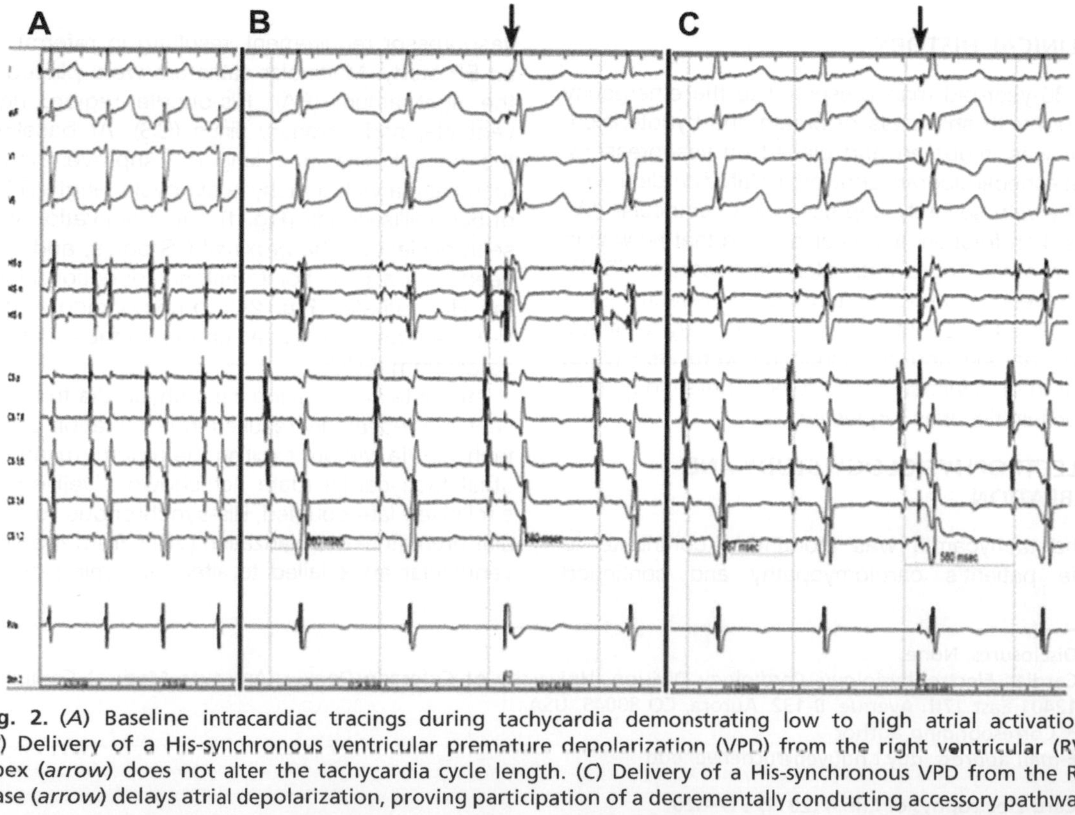

Fig. 2. (*A*) Baseline intracardiac tracings during tachycardia demonstrating low to high atrial activation. (*B*) Delivery of a His-synchronous ventricular premature depolarization (VPD) from the right ventricular (RV) apex (*arrow*) does not alter the tachycardia cycle length. (*C*) Delivery of a His-synchronous VPD from the RV base (*arrow*) delays atrial depolarization, proving participation of a decrementally conducting accessory pathway.

following atrial electrogram (**Fig. 2**B). When the His-synchronous VPD was delivered 10 milliseconds earlier and from the basal right ventricle, the next atrial electrogram was delayed by 15 milliseconds relative to the TCL, and the tachycardia was reset (**Fig. 2**C).

The site of earliest atrial activation during tachycardia was identified on the posterior right atrial septum adjacent to the CS ostium (**Fig. 3**). Ablation at this site (4 mm nonirrigated catheter) resulted in termination of the tachycardia within 3 seconds (**Fig. 4**). No further tachycardia was inducible. The patient remained stable without tachycardia recurrence; his vasopressors were weaned off, and he was extubated. A follow-up echocardiogram on discharge showed improvement in the LV ejection fraction.

QUESTION

How do His-synchronous VPDs provide diagnostic clarity in this case?

DISCUSSION

Many characteristics of the case presented here are typical of persistent/permanent junctional reciprocating tachycardia (PJRT), including the history of incessant tachycardia, the P-wave morphology observed on the ECG, and the tachycardia-induced cardiomyopathy. In fact, PJRT should always be suspected when the combination of incessant long RP tachycardia (>12 h/d) and the common PJRT P-wave appearance (deeply inverted in leads II, III), is observed.[1] Cardiomyopathy is seen in as many as 28% of patients diagnosed with PJRT and, in both the pediatric and adult literature, has been reported to resolve after therapy is provided.[2,3]

While clinical history and surface ECG may suggest a diagnosis of PJRT, invasive EP study allows both definitive diagnosis and ablation of the arrhythmia. Para-Hisian pacing during sinus rhythm may suggest the presence of an accessory pathway (AP), but does not demonstrate participation of an AP in tachycardia. This procedure could not be performed in this patient because he was in incessant tachycardia. Entrainment maneuvers during tachycardia can be helpful, particularly for differentiating atrial tachycardia from reentrant rhythms based on the activation sequence seen when pacing is ceased. Atrial tachycardia should demonstrate a V-A-A-V response; atypical atrioventricular nodal reentrant tachycardia (AVNRT) may yield a V-A-V response or a pseudo–V-A-A-V response, depending on the length of the paced V-A interval. PJRT, which is an orthodromic atrioventricular reentrant tachycardia (AVRT) using a concealed, decrementally conducting AP, should also demonstrate a V-A-V response to pacing. Entrainment is therefore useful for limiting the differential, although the response to pacing alone is not always diagnostic.[4] Comparison of the stim-to-atrial time with the V-A time during tachycardia, and comparison of the postpacing interval (PPI) with the TCL both can help differentiate between atypical AVNRT and PJRT.[5] However, this technique has not been validated in AVRT with decremental AP. In this case attempts at entrainment terminated the tachycardia, thus precluding evaluation of the response to pacing and measurement of the PPI.

Ultimately, delivery of a His-synchronous VPD confirmed definitively the diagnosis of PJRT in

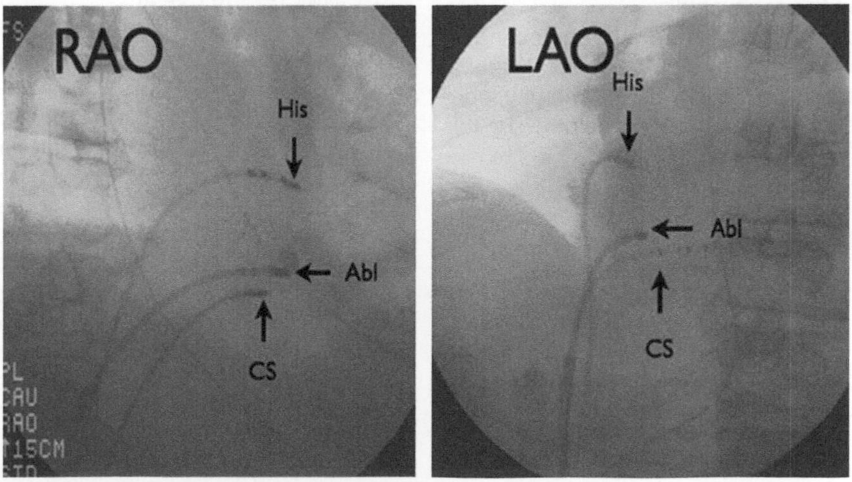

Fig. 3. Right anterior oblique (RAO) and left anterior oblique (LAO) projections demonstrating the site of successful ablation. Arrows indicate: Abl, ablation catheter; CS, coronary sinus catheter; His, His-bundle catheter.

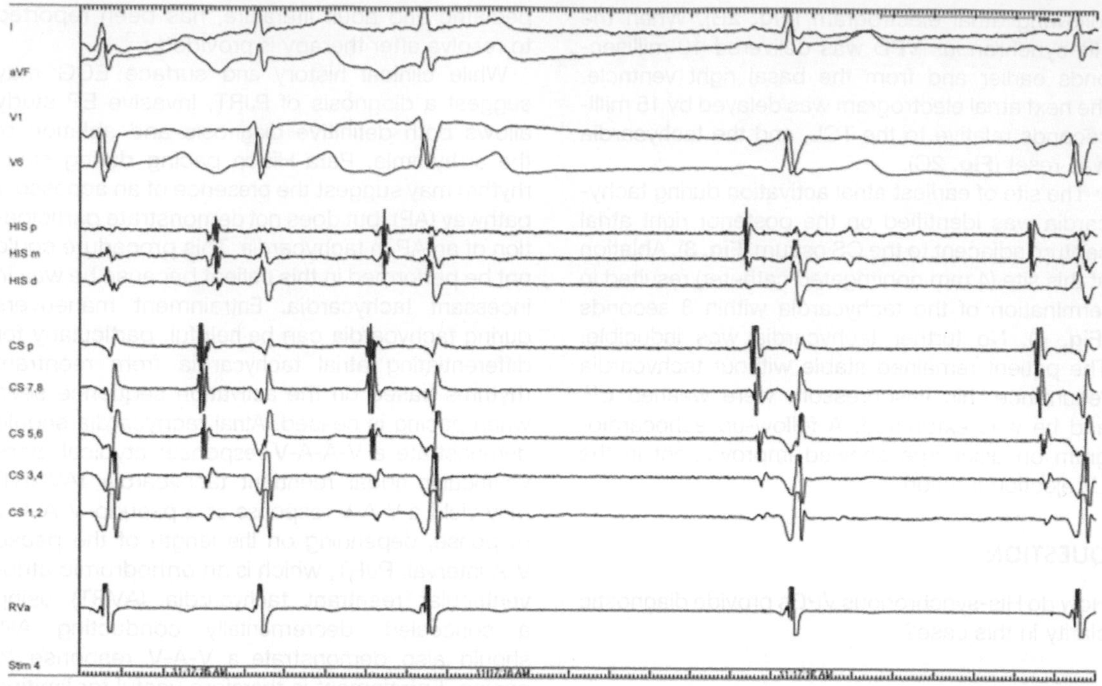

Fig. 4. Ablation on the posterior right atrial septum, adjacent the coronary sinus ostium, terminates tachycardia.

this patient. When a VPD was delivered at the right ventricular apex, there was no effect on the TCL, rendering the maneuver nondiagnostic. This situation is likely to occur because the relatively late-coupled VPD was given at site remote from the AP and so did not come about early enough to affect pathway conduction. When the His-synchronous VPD was delivered at the right ventricular base[6] at a slightly shorter coupling interval, the subsequent atrial depolarization was delayed and the tachycardia was reset, proving that a retrograde, decrementally conducting AP participated in the tachycardia.

Although the majority of APs participating in PJRT are located in the posteroseptal region of the right atrium,[1] a variety of AP pathway locations has been observed to participate in this tachycardia.[7]

SUMMARY

The key features of this case are the incessant nature of the long RP SVT, the ECG findings characteristic of PJRT, and utility of appropriately timed and spaced VPDs in making the diagnosis of PJRT. An understanding of the patient's clinical scenario and recognition that his cardiomyopathy was a result of his incessant tachycardia resulted in delivery of timely invasive care and the patient's recovery from critical illness.

REFERENCES

1. Zipes D, Jalife J. Cardiac electrophysiology from cell to bedside. 5th edition. Philadelphia: Saunders Elsevier; 2009. p. 942.
2. Vaksmann G, D'Hoinne C, Lucet V, et al. Permanent junctional reciprocating tachycardia in children: a multicentre study on clinical profile and outcome. Heart 2006;92:101–4.
3. Cruz FE, Cheriex EC, Smeets JL, et al. Reversibility of tachycardia-induced cardiomyopathy after cure of incessant supraventricular tachycardia. J Am Coll Cardiol 1990;16:739–44.
4. Knight BP, Zivin A, Souza J, et al. A technique for the rapid diagnosis of atrial tachycardia in the electrophysiology laboratory. J Am Coll Cardiol 1999;33:775–81.
5. Michaud G, Tada H, Chough S, et al. Differentiation of atypical atrioventricular node re-entrant tachycardia from orthodromic reciprocating tachycardia using a septal accessory pathway by the response to ventricular pacing. J Am Coll Cardiol 2001;38:1163–7.
6. Matsushita G, Badhwar N, Collins KK, et al. Usefulness of a ventricular extrastimulus from the summit of the ventricular septum in diagnosis of septal accessory pathway in patients with supraventricular tachycardia. Am J Cardiol 2004;93:643–6.
7. Ticho BS, Saul JP, Hulse JE, et al. Variable location of accessory pathways associated with the permanent form of junctional reciprocating tachycardia and confirmation with radiofrequency ablation. Am J Cardiol 1992;70:1559–64.

Recurrent Tachycardia in a Patient with Left Lateral Wolff-Parkinson-White Syndrome

Raphael K. Sung, MD, Nitish Badhwar, MBBS*

KEYWORDS

• Catheter ablation • Accessory pathway • Atrioventricular reentrant tachycardia

KEY POINTS

- Lateral pathways may have a slant, with ventricular and atrial insertion sites that are remote from each other, resulting in difficult or ineffective ablation of the accessory pathway (AP).
- When pacing at 2 different ventricular sites to activate the accessory pathway from opposite directions, a significant change in local ventriculoatrial (VA) timing at the site of the earliest atrial activation indicates the presence of a slanted AP.
- The ventricular activation wavefront causing the longer local VA timing is traveling in the opposite direction to the retrograde accessory pathway conduction.
- Ventricular pacing that causes ventricular activation in the opposite direction to AP conduction may be used to separate out local VA signal, to better assess for AP potential and extrapolate the ventricular insertion of the AP.

CLINICAL HISTORY

A 65-year-old man was admitted for his fourth electrophysiology study (EPS) for symptoms of palpitations and recurrent supraventricular tachycardia. His first EPS demonstrated Wolff-Parkinson-White syndrome, with successful ablation of antegrade and retrograde conduction over the left lateral accessory pathway (AP). He had recurrence of tachycardia following ablation that was consistent with atrioventricular reentrant tachycardia (AVRT) using the AP as the retrograde limb. The patient's second EPS was complicated by tamponade during ablation, and the third study was again unsuccessful, with recurrence of orthodromic AVRT following ablation. The patient continued to have tachycardia despite flecainide and β-blockers, and was admitted for another EPS. Physical examination was within normal limits and the echocardiogram showed normal left ventricular function. A 12-lead electrocardiogram (ECG) demonstrated sinus rhythm with normal intervals and QRS morphology and axis. There was no evidence of preexcitation.

ELECTROPHYSIOLOGY STUDY

A duodecapolar catheter with spacing of 2-2-2 mm was advanced into the coronary sinus (CS), with distal electrode at the anterior interventricular vein (AIV) and the proximal electrode at approximately 5 o'clock along the mitral annulus in the left anterior oblique view. Quadripolar catheters were placed in the His-bundle region, the right ventricular basal septum, and high right atrium. The patient underwent EPS demonstrating inducible

Section of Electrophysiology, Division of Cardiology, University of California San Francisco, San Francisco, CA, USA

* Corresponding author. Cardiac Electrophysiology, University of California San Francisco, 500 Parnassus Avenue, MUE 431, San Francisco, CA 94143-1354, USA.
E-mail address: badhwar@medicine.ucsf.edu

Card Electrophysiol Clin 4 (2012) 521–525
http://dx.doi.org/10.1016/j.ccep.2012.08.032
1877 9182/12/$ – see front matter

orthodromic AVRT. After the patient resumed sinus rhythm, ventricular pacing was performed at 2 remote sites (**Fig. 1**A), both resulting in earliest retrograde atrial activation near CS electrodes 10,9. Pacing from the posterior base of the right ventricle activated the lateral left ventricle (LV) in the direction from CS proximal to distal electrodes, with local ventriculoatrial (VA) timing of 70 milliseconds at CS electrodes 10,9. Pacing from the distal CS catheter in the AIV activated the lateral LV from CS distal electrodes to proximal, with local VA timing of 90 milliseconds at CS electrodes 10,9.

A single transseptal puncture was performed using an SL1 transseptal sheath (St Jude Medical, Sylmar, CA) and Baylis transseptal needle (Baylis Medical, Montreal, Canada) using 1 application of radiofrequency at 10 W. Mapping along the mitral annulus was performed using the Thermocool D/F curve externally irrigated catheter (Biosense Webster, Diamond Bar, CA). However, because of catheter instability, the SL1 sheath was exchanged over a wire for the SL3 sheath.

Based on the activation pattern of both the ventricular and atrial signals when pacing from the AIV, the ventricular insertion was determined to be near CS electrodes 16,15. Careful mapping along the lateral mitral annulus using a 3-dimensional electroanatomic mapping system (ESI; St Jude Medical, St Paul, MN) and the Thermocool ablation catheter was performed between ventricular insertion (CS 16,15) and atrial insertion (CS 10,9). A small, high-frequency signal on the bipolar ablation channel between the ventricular and atrial signals was observed near CS 16,15, corresponding to a small secondary negative deflection on the ablator tip unipolar channel. Ablation was performed in power-controlled setting at 25 W during ventricular pacing, just opposite to CS electrodes 15,16 (**Fig. 2**). Loss of retrograde conduction was seen in less than 2 seconds on initiation of ablation. A second lesion was placed in the same region for a total of 1 minute each. After 1 hour of observation, retrograde conduction was no longer observed. Burst pacing and extra-stimuli testing from the left atrium, right atrium, CS, and LV failed to induce any arrhythmias.

QUESTIONS

1. How is the presence of a "slant" in the AP determined from **Fig. 1**B?
2. How is the direction of the AP conduction determined from **Fig. 1**B?
3. Based on ventricular and atrial signals from the CS electrograms in **Fig. 1**B, how were both ventricular and atrial insertion sites identified?

DIAGNOSIS

Slanted, retrograde conducting left lateral AP, with anterior atrial insertion (CS 10,9), and posterior ventricular insertion (CS 16,15), which was successfully ablated at the ventricular insertion.

DISCUSSION

Previously failed ablation attempts for a left lateral AP may be suggestive of an AP with a slant. It has been shown that most APs are inserted obliquely along the annulus, and pacing techniques for successful mapping and ablation of AP potential have been described.[1,2] With a multipolar electrode catheter bracketing the atrial insertion of the pathway, ventricular pacing sites should be identified that will create a ventricular activation wavefront that travels in the opposite direction to pathway activation. Obliquely inserted AP is diagnosed by the prolongation of local VA interval by more than 15 milliseconds at the site of earliest atrial activation direction (measured by the first sharp ventricular deflection to the earliest atrial signal).[2] **Fig. 3** represents activation patterns seen with reversed ventricular pacing in a slanted AP. Simulating a left lateral pathway with a CS catheter bracketing the pathway, pacing in the posterior base of the right ventricle creates a ventricular wavefront from CS proximal to distal. The pathway activation is parallel to the ventricular activation wavefront. The atrial insertion is near CS 4,3, but yields a relatively narrow local VA interval owing to parallel activation. When the ventricular activation wavefront is reversed, with activation from CS distal to proximal, the atrial signal is again earliest at CS 4,3, but the local VA timing is longer than with parallel activation. As seen in **Fig. 3**B, the ventricular wavefront passes CS 4,3 first before reaching the ventricular insertion at CS 8,7, activating the AP until it reaches the atrial insertion at CS 4,3. When extrapolating the slope of atrial signals to the ventricular signals, the intersection of this extrapolated line to the first ventricular signal likely indicates the ventricular insertion of the AP that is the optimal site for ablation.

In this patient, the right panel of **Fig. 1**B shows longer local VA timing with CS distal to proximal ventricular activation, indicating that ventricular activation is the reverse of AP activation. Here, the red line in the figure extends the atrial activation past CS 10,9 until it intersects the ventricular signal at CS 16,15, highlighting the location of the ventricular insertion. Although the same information can be identified more accurately with mapping the earliest ventricular signal when antegrade conduction is present, lack of antegrade

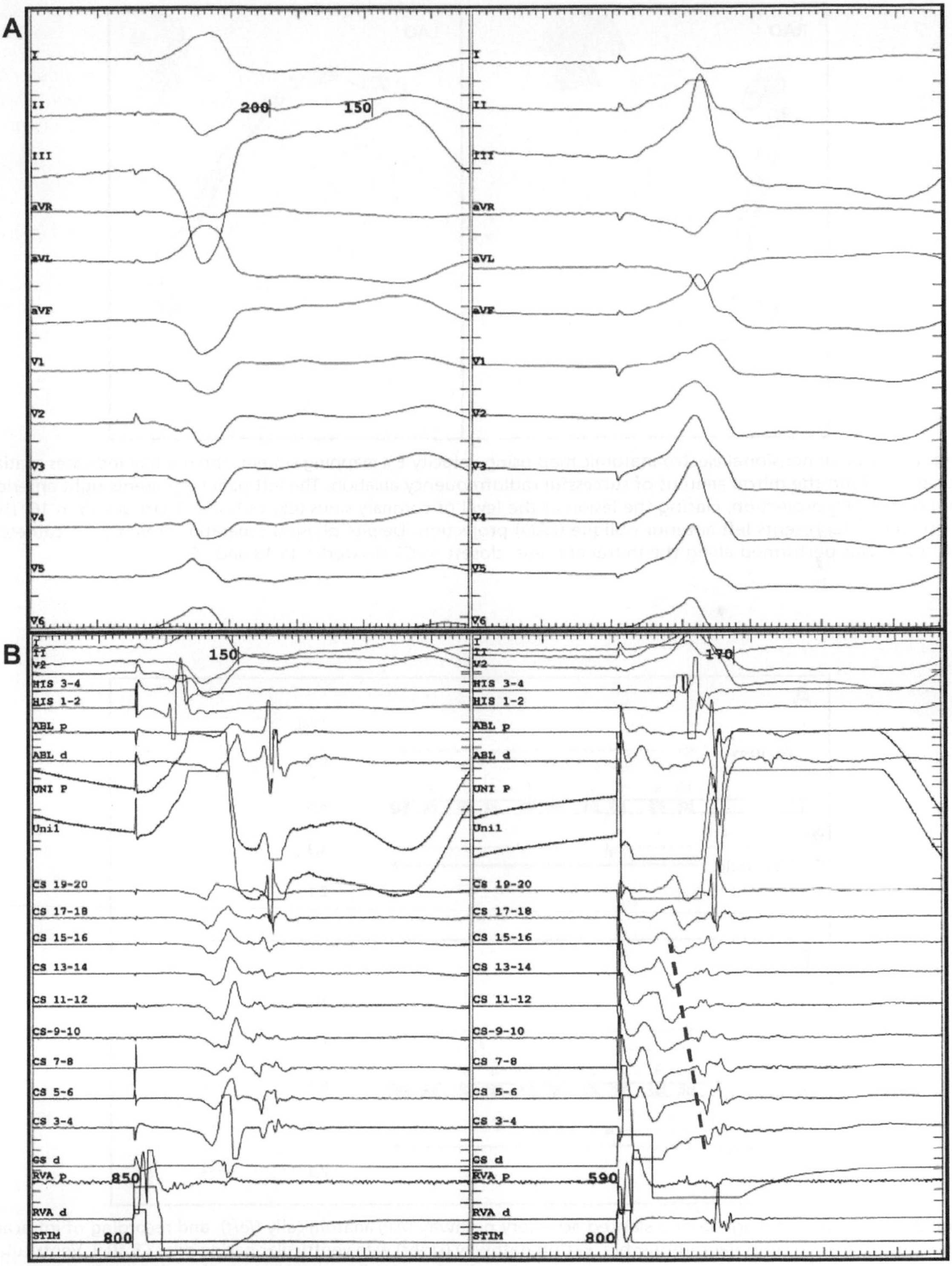

Fig. 1. (*A*) Twelve-lead electrocardiogram QRS morphologies pacing from 2 distinct right ventricular (RV) sites. The panel on the left represents QRS morphology pacing from the RV posterior base. The right panel represents QRS morphology pacing from the anterior interventricular vein. (*B*) Intracardiac electrogram recordings corresponding to the same 2 RV sites shown in *A*. The red dashed line shows the direction of activation of the accessory pathway. ABL, ablator signal recordings; CS, coronary sinus recordings; HIS, His-bundle recordings; RVA, right ventricular recordings; UNI, unipolar recordings from ablator proximal and distal electrodes.

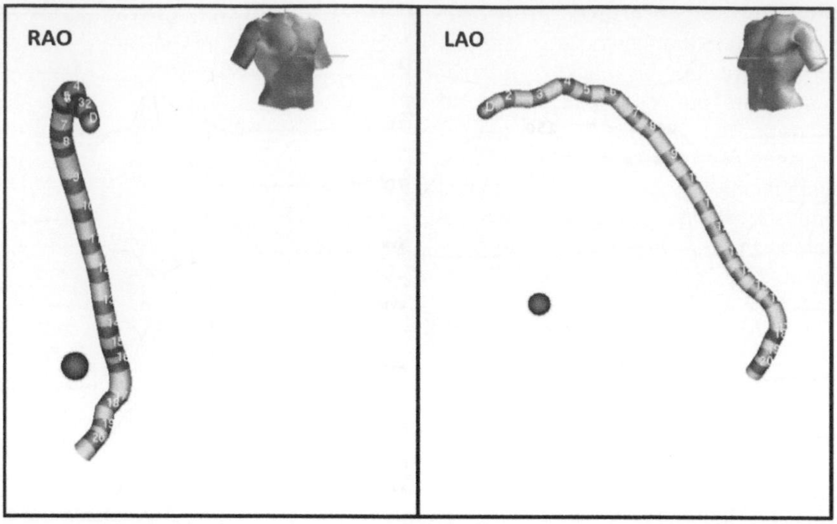

Fig. 2. Three-dimensional electroanatomic map using velocity ESI mapping system. The red ball indicates spatial location along the mitral annulus of successful radiofrequency ablation. The left panel represents right anterior oblique (RAO) projection, placing the lesion at the level of coronary sinus (CS) catheter electrodes 15 to 16. The right panel represents left anterior oblique (LAO) projection. Despite physical separation from the CS catheter, ablation was performed along the mitral annulus, closest to CS electrodes 14,13 and 15,16.

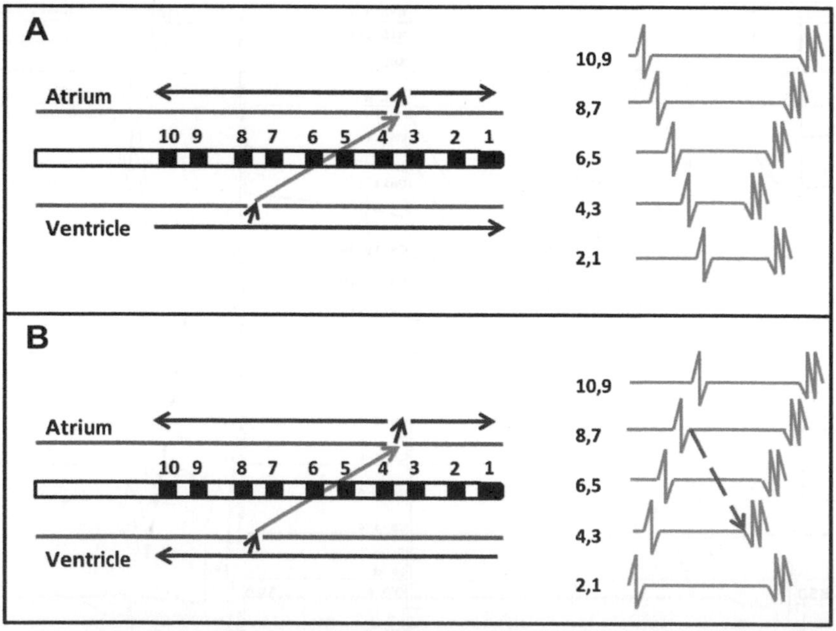

Fig. 3. (*A*) Anatomic diagram of a slanted accessory pathway (AP) anatomically (*left*), and recording of intracardiac signals from multipolar catheter bracketing pathway (*right*) with ventricular pacing near CS 10,9. Ventricular activation wavefront is activated in parallel to AP activation, resulting in relatively short local ventriculoatrial (VA) timing at atrial insertion site CS 4,3. (*B*) Anatomic diagram of the same slanted AP anatomically (*left*), and recording of intracardiac signals from multipolar catheter bracketing pathway (*right*) with ventricular pacing near CS 2,1. Ventricular activation wavefront is activated in reverse to AP activation, resulting in longer VA timing at atrial insertion site CS 4,3 compared with *A*. The dashed red line represents AP activation timing by following the slope of atrial activation. By extending this line backward until it intersects the ventricular signal, the ventricular insertion of the AP can be estimated to occur near CS electrodes 8,7.

conduction precludes this evaluation. Every attempt should be made to identify the AP potential, including pacing from the opposite ventricular wavefront to separate out local ventricular and atrial signals near the pathway, and pacing maneuvers to dissociate AP potential from ventricular and atrial signals. However, if the AP potential cannot be identified, empiric ablation near ventricular insertion along the pathway may also result in successful ablation.

SUMMARY

This case illustrates that oblique insertion of AP can lead to unsuccessful catheter ablation in a patient with retrograde conducting left lateral AP. Based on previous publications the authors demonstrate the technique of variable ventricular pacing to diagnose an oblique AP and identify both ventricular and atrial insertions. The ventricular pacing site that activates the ventricular signals opposite to the AP insertion leads to prolongation of VA interval at the site of earliest atrial activation. This prolongation allows identification of the AP potential that is extrapolated to the ventricular insertion site, which is the optimal site for successful ablation in such patients.

REFERENCES

1. Jackman WM, Friday KJ, Yeung-Lai-Wah JA, et al. New catheter technique for recording left free-wall accessory atrioventricular pathway activation. Identification of pathway fiber orientation. Circulation 1988;78:598–611.
2. Otomo K, Gonzalez MD, Beckman KJ, et al. Reversing the direction of paced ventricular and atrial wavefronts reveals an oblique course in accessory AV pathways and improves localization for catheter ablation. Circulation 2001;104: 550–6.

Failed Posteroseptal Accessory Pathway: Where to Ablate?

Marwan Refaat, MD[a], Nitish Badhwar, MBBS[b,*]

KEYWORDS

• Catheter ablation • Orthodromic reentrant tachycardia • Diverticulum

KEY POINTS

- Posteroseptal accessory pathways can be associated with coronary sinus (CS) venous abnormalities, including diverticulum and abnormal venous dilatations.
- Unsuccessful ablation of the accessory pathway in the right and left posteroseptal region should prompt a thorough coronary sinus occlusive venography with retrograde filling.
- Fusiform dilatation of the small cardiac vein can rarely be the site of the location of the posteroseptal pathway.
- Meticulous mapping in the coronary sinus venous anomalies for earliest atrial activation and accessory pathway potential can identify the target for successful epicardial ablation in the branches of the CS.

CLINICAL PRESENTATION

A 52-year-old man with a history of recurrent paroxysmal palpitations over several years remained symptomatic despite atrioventricular nodal blockade. The patient had previous electrophysiology studies and had been found to have an orthodromic reciprocating tachycardia (ORT) with retrograde conduction via a posteroseptal accessory pathway. The ORT was also noted to trigger atrial fibrillation. Three previous attempts at ablation of the posteroseptal accessory pathway in the right atrium and left atrium through transseptal and retrograde aortic approaches were unsuccessful. The patient was brought to the electrophysiology laboratory for another attempt at ablation because of his recurrent palpitations and limited exercise tolerance.

ELECTROPHYSIOLOGY STUDY

Multipolar electrode catheters were introduced percutaneously from the right femoral and internal jugular veins and positioned into the high right atrium, right ventricular apex, His bundle region, and coronary sinus (CS). Bipolar electrograms (30–500 Hz) and unipolar electrograms (0.5–500 Hz) were displayed and stored using a digital recording system (EP MedSystems, West Berlin, NJ). A quadripolar catheter was introduced from the left femoral vein and positioned in the inferior vena cava as a ground catheter for the unipolar signal, and a duodecapolar catheter was placed in the CS from the right internal jugular vein. The proximal electrodes of the duodecapolar catheter were in the main CS, and distal electrodes were in a posterolateral branch vein. Three-dimensional electroanatomic mapping was performed with CARTO (Biosense Webster, Diamond Bar, CA).

At baseline, the patient was in normal sinus rhythm. Baseline atrial-His and His-ventricular intervals were within normal limits, with no evidence of preexcitation. Sustained short R-P tachycardia was induced with catheter manipulation (**Fig. 1**). The diagnosis of ORT was confirmed, with the earliest atrial activation in the posteroseptal region of the coronary sinus (see **Fig. 1**).

[a] Section of Electrophysiology, Division of Cardiology, University of California, San Francisco, San Francisco, CA, USA; [b] Cardiac Electrophysiology, University of California San Francisco, 500 Parnassus Avenue, MUE 431, San Francisco, CA 94143-1354, USA
* Corresponding author.
E-mail address: badhwar@medicine.ucsf.edu

Card Electrophysiol Clin 4 (2012) 527–530
http://dx.doi.org/10.1016/j.ccep.2012.08.029
1877-9182/12/$ – see front matter

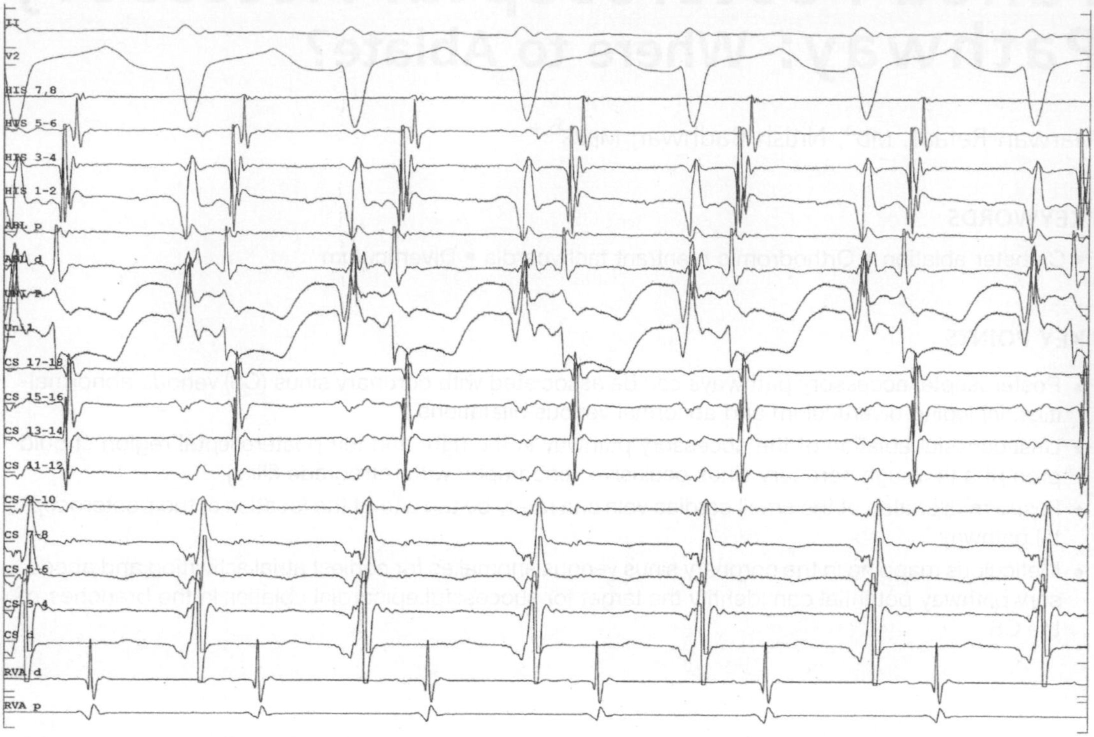

Fig. 1. Intracardiac electrogram recordings during orthodromic reciprocating tachycardia showing retrograde earliest atrial activation at the ablation catheter that is placed on the floor of the proximal coronary sinus near the small cardiac vein. ABL, ablator signal recordings near the small cardiac vein; CS, coronary sinus recordings with distal electrodes in the posterolateral vein and proximal electrodes in the coronary sinus; HIS, His bundle recordings; RVA, right ventricular recordings.

QUESTION

What is the most optimal mapping technique of this retrograde-only conducting posteroseptal accessory pathway?

DISCUSSION

A balloon occlusion technique was pursued by using a 6F balloon catheter over a 0.025-inch wire threading in the coronary sinus using an 8F SL3 sheath from the right femoral vein.

The LAO projection was adjusted to 50° to 55°, with the His catheter directed en face to adjust for cardiac rotation. A retrograde coronary sinus venography was done with manual injection of 15 mL without deflating the balloon. and with forceful pushing and retrograde filling documented on a 15-fps cine showing a fusiform bulbous dilatation of the small cardiac vein (SCV) close to the middle cardiac vein (MCV) (**Fig. 2**).

The SCV was targeted. A 7F D/F deflectable-tip Thermocool open-irrigated mapping/ablation catheter was maneuvered into position along the

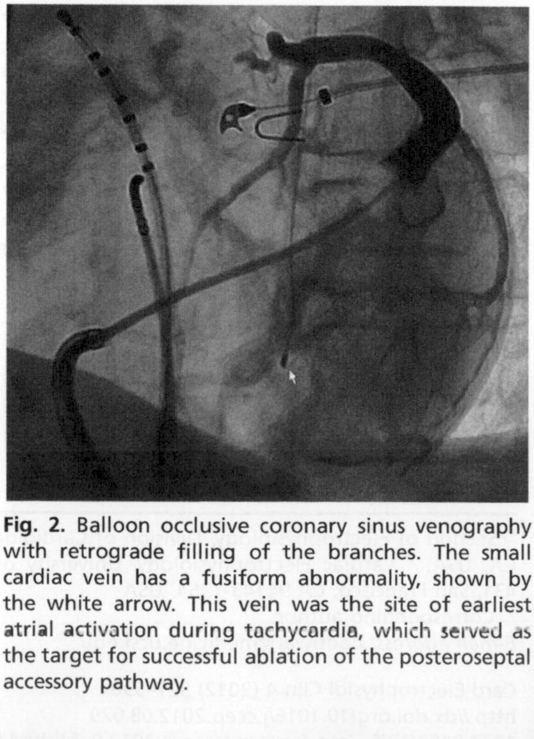

Fig. 2. Balloon occlusive coronary sinus venography with retrograde filling of the branches. The small cardiac vein has a fusiform abnormality, shown by the white arrow. This vein was the site of earliest atrial activation during tachycardia, which served as the target for successful ablation of the posteroseptal accessory pathway.

mouth of the SCV as well as the MCV within the CS. The SCV was chosen for radiofrequency energy application because of the presence of earliest retrograde atrial signal at this location during tachycardia that preceded all other atrial activations. Ventricular pacing during sinus rhythm with a duodecapolar catheter that had distal electrodes in a posterolateral branch vein of the CS also confirmed the presence of an accessory pathway potential and earliest retrograde atrial signal at this site. Retrograde conduction was lost over the posteroseptal pathway (change in retrograde atrial activation sequence) while mapping at the mouth of the SCV. The site was tagged on the mapping system and targeted for radiofrequency ablation with the open irrigated catheter. Power was dialed up to 45 W to achieve a 10 Ω impedance drop. ORT was not inducible after ablation at this site despite aggressive atrial pacing. Para-Hisian pacing confirmed a nodal response (**Fig. 3**). The patient has been symptom-free and off medications for 6 months.

This is a challenging ORT using a retrograde-only posteroseptal atrioventricular pathway, with several unsuccessful ablation attempts. The successful ablation of the pathway was achieved

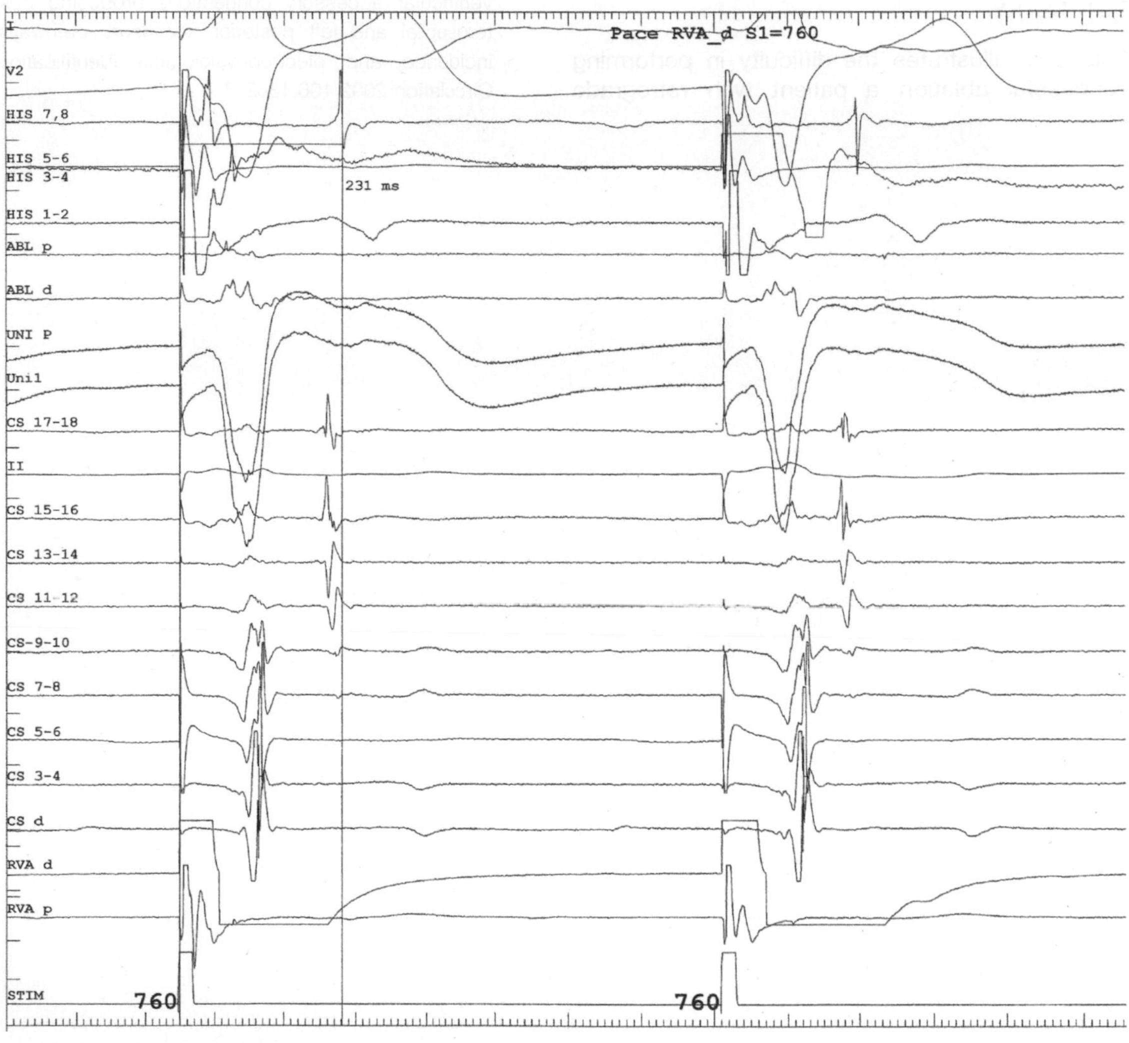

Fig. 3. Intracardiac electrogram recordings during para-Hisian pacing after successful catheter ablation of the posteroseptal accessory pathway showing AV nodal conduction. The first beat shows ventricle muscle capture with wide QRS, and the next beat shows ventricle and His capture with narrow QRS. The earliest retrograde atrial activation is at the His catheter that beats the ablation-catheter signal, and there is increase in VA timing with loss of His capture (first beat). ABL, ablator signal recordings near the small cardiac vein; CS, coronary sinus recordings with distal electrodes in the posterolateral vein and proximal electrodes in the coronary sinus; HIS, His bundle recordings; RVA, right ventricular recordings.

when CS venography was done with retrograde filling documenting the abnormal anatomy of a "sausage-shaped" SCV that was the target for ablation.

Venous anomalies were identified in 15 (9%) of 171 patients with coronary sinus accessory pathway.[1] CS venography showed fusiform enlargement of the terminal portion of the SCV in 3 patients and in both the SCV and MCV in 9 patients. This study reported that the accessory pathway was related to the enlarged region of the SCV or MCV in all 12 patients, and suggested a relationship between the fusiform enlargement and the CS accessory pathway as illustrated in the present case.

SUMMARY

This case illustrates the difficulty in performing successful ablation a patient with retrograde conducting posteroseptal accessory pathway. The presence of fusiform abnormality of the SCV that was the site of insertion of the posteroseptal accessory pathway was demonstrated. This site was identified by occlusive coronary sinus venography with retrograde filling. The site showed earliest activation during tachycardia and served as a target site for successful epicardial ablation of the posteroseptal accessory pathway.

REFERENCE

1. Sun Y, Arruda M, Otomo K, et al. Coronary sinus-ventricular accessory connections producing posteroseptal and left posterior accessory pathways: incidence and electrophysiological identification. Circulation 2002;106:1362–7.

Narrow QRS Tachycardia with Ventriculoatrial Block

Frederick T. Han, MD[a], Vasanth Vedantham, MD, PhD[b,*]

KEYWORDS

• Nodofascicular pathway • Nodoventricular pathway • Junctional tachycardia
• Narrow-complex tachycardia with atrioventricular dissociation

KEY POINTS

- Narrow-complex tachycardia with ventriculoatrial (VA) dissociation is rare.
- The differential diagnosis for narrow-complex tachycardia with VA dissociation includes junctional tachycardia, AV nodal reentrant tachycardia with upper common pathway block, and a circus-movement tachycardia using a concealed nodofascicular or nodoventricular pathway.
- Although baseline tachycardia characteristics can suggest one or another of these mechanisms, pacing maneuvers are required to make a definitive diagnosis in these difficult cases.

CLINICAL PRESENTATION

A 40-year-old athletic man presented for evaluation and management of exercise-induced palpitations. Initially the palpitations occurred only with strenuous exercise and resolved with rest. However, in the months before presentation, palpations occurred more frequently with less strenuous activity. Physical examination, laboratory studies, and an echocardiogram were all normal. Ambulatory monitoring revealed that palpitations correlated with a narrow-complex tachycardia that occurred during exercise (**Fig. 1**). The patient was referred for consideration of catheter ablation.

ELECTROPHYSIOLOGY STUDY AND ABLATION

Tachycardia Induction

Quadripolar electrode catheters were positioned in the high right atrium, right ventricular apex, and the His bundle region. A decapolar electrode catheter was placed in the coronary sinus. Normal intervals were recorded in sinus rhythm, and ventriculoatrial (VA) conduction was present with concentric retrograde activation and a long VA time. Tachycardia could not be induced with atrial overdrive pacing or programmed stimulation from the right atrium or coronary sinus with or without isoproterenol. Sustained narrow QRS complex tachycardia at a cycle length of 300 to 330 milliseconds was induced with ventricular overdrive pacing after isoproterenol infusion at 1 μg/min (**Fig. 2**). Strikingly and unexpectedly, narrow-complex tachycardia was induced and persisted with complete VA dissociation.

Question

What is the differential diagnosis for narrow-complex tachycardia with VA block and how can the tachycardia mechanism be established?

Tachycardia Characteristics

Two VA relationships were observed during tachycardia. Tachycardia showed either complete VA block or 2:1 VA conduction, occasionally transitioning from one to the other without interruption

[a] Division of Cardiology, University of Utah Health Sciences Center, 30 North 1900 East, Room 4A100, Salt Lake City, UT 84132, USA; [b] Cardiac Electrophysiology Section, Cardiology Division, University of California San Francisco, San Francisco, CA, USA
* Corresponding author. Cardiac Electrophysiology Section, Cardiology Division, University of California San Francisco, 505 Parnassus Avenue, M1179D, Box 0124, San Francisco, CA 94122-0124.
E-mail address: vedanthamv@medicine.ucsf.edu

Card Electrophysiol Clin 4 (2012) 531–536
http://dx.doi.org/10.1016/j.ccep.2012.08.030
1877-9182/12/$ – see front matter

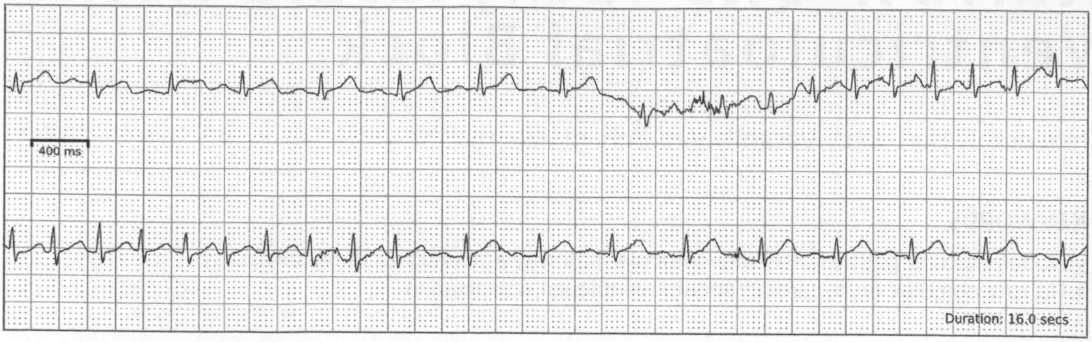

Fig. 1. Ambulatory monitor with narrow QRS tachycardia. Single-lead electrocardiogram shows initiation of narrow-complex tachycardia during mild exertion. P waves are not clearly visible during tachycardia, leaving a broad differential diagnosis.

of tachycardia (**Fig. 3**). When 2:1 AV conduction occurred, the atrial activation pattern was concentric and similar to what was observed during ventricular pacing. On beats with 2:1 VA conduction, the VA time was longer than half the tachycardia cycle length (long RP). During tachycardia, spontaneous cycle length variation occurred whereby changes in the His-His interval preceded changes in the R-R interval. The finding of AV dissociation and 2:1 VA conduction ruled out atrial tachycardia and atrioventricular nodal reentrant tachycardia (AVNRT) using an AV accessory pathway. The presence of

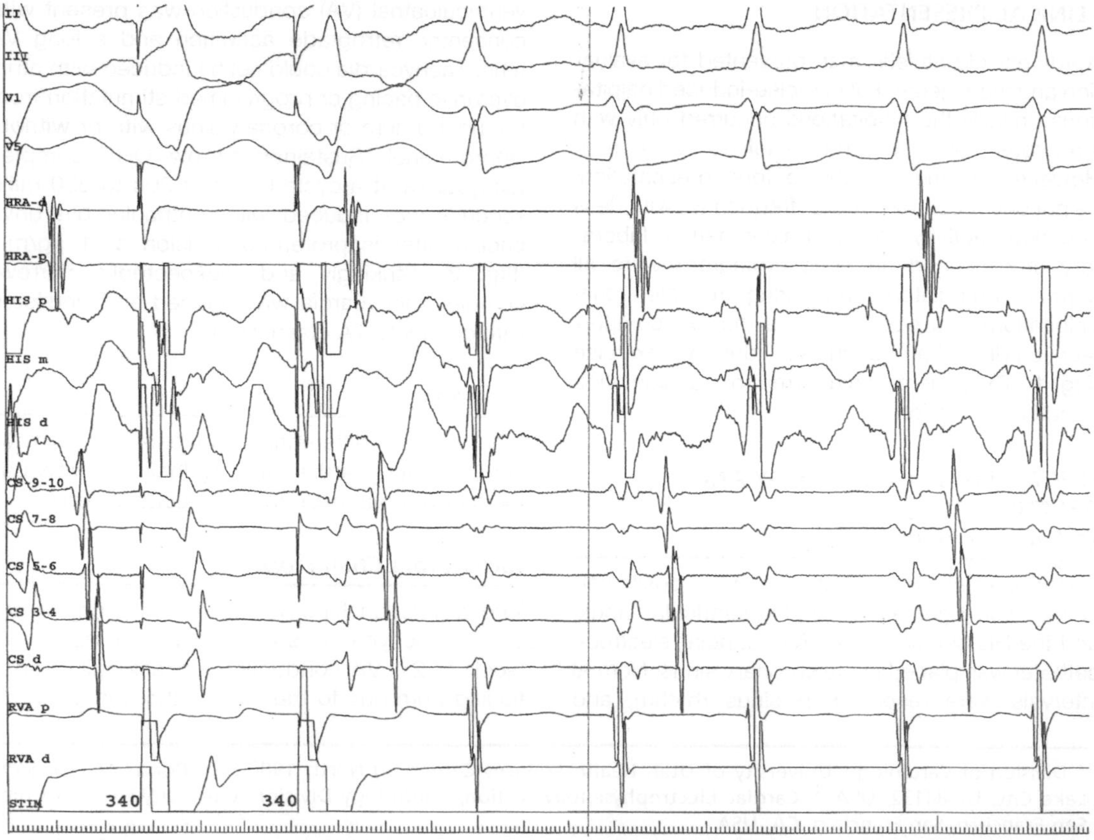

Fig. 2. Tachycardia initiation. Ventricular overdrive pacing at 340 milliseconds resulted in initiation of narrow-complex tachycardia at cycle length of 300 milliseconds whereby each QRS complex is preceded by a His deflection with a normal H-V interval. Ventriculoatrial (VA) conduction was absent during the pacing drive train, and atrial activation via the sinus node marches unperturbed through tachycardia initiation.

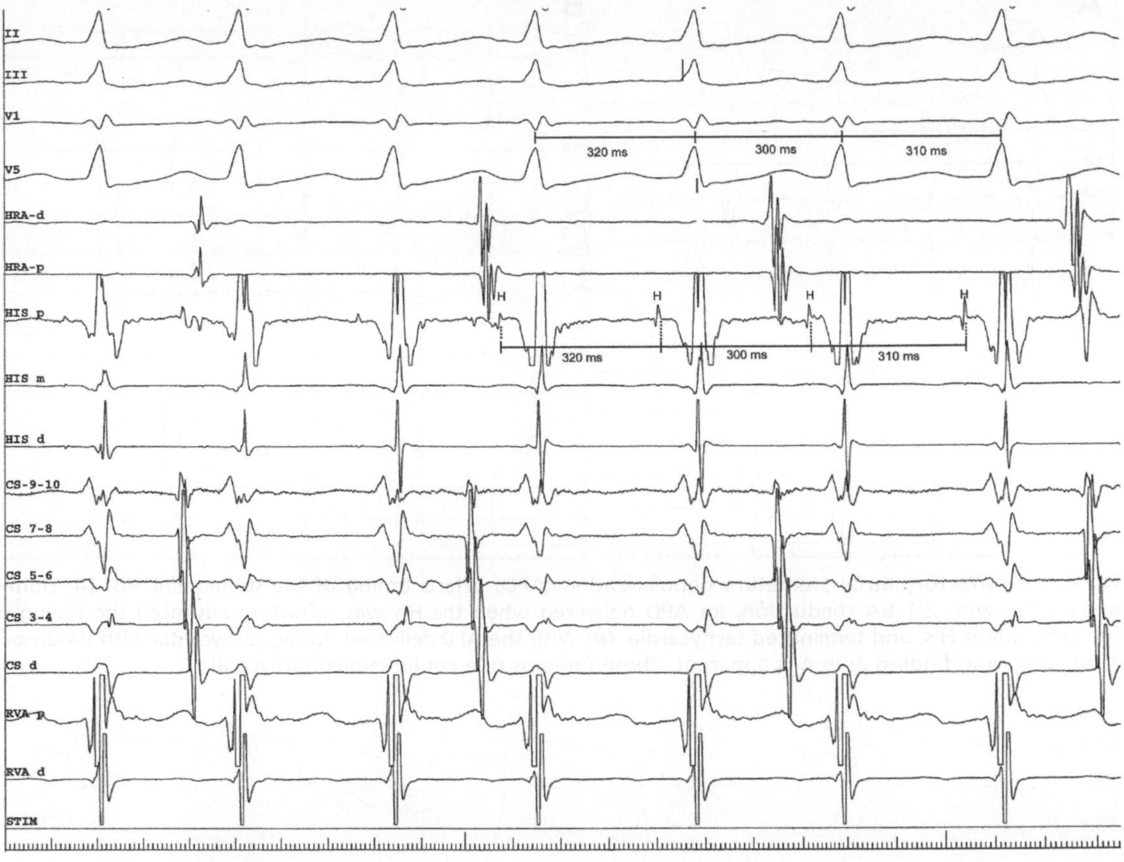

Fig. 3. Changing VA relationship during tachycardia. Tachycardia exhibited 2:1 VA conduction, with a retrograde activation pattern identical to that observed with ventricular pacing. In this trace, the first atrial activation is retrograde, with earliest activation in the proximal coronary sinus and high right atrial activation occurring proximal to distal. The 2 subsequent atrial activations are fusion beats, with earliest activation in coronary sinus but high right atrial activation proceeding distal to proximal. The fourth atrial activation is sinus in origin, completing the transition from 2:1 VA conduction to complete VA dissociation. Small changes in tachycardia cycle length are also evident on this tracing, with His-His interval changes predicting subsequent R-R interval changes, ruling out a ventricular origin for this tachycardia.

complete AV dissociation during some episodes of tachycardia ruled out an atrial tachycardia with double fire (1:2 AV conduction). Ventricular tachycardia was excluded by the narrow QRS complex and because variations in tachycardia cycle length were preceded by changes in the His-His interval.

Maneuvers During Tachycardia

The differential diagnosis of a narrow-complex tachycardia with VA dissociation includes AVNRT with upper common pathway block, junctional tachycardia (JT), and circus-movement tachycardia (CMT) using a concealed nodofascicular or nodoventricular (NF/NV) accessory pathway.[1] Ventricular overdrive pacing consistently terminated tachycardia, precluding the use of entrainment to identify the tachycardia mechanism.

JT can be distinguished from AVNRT by the response to atrial premature depolarizations.[2] A His-refractory atrial premature depolarization that affects the timing of the subsequent His confirms involvement of the AV node in the antegrade limb of a tachycardia circuit and rules out a focal JT. In the present case, late atrial premature depolarizations reproducibly advanced the subsequent His and terminated tachycardia, excluding JT as the tachycardia mechanism, and leaving AVNRT and CMT as the remaining possibilities (**Fig. 4**).

Administering His-refractory ventricular premature depolarizations (VPDs) can test for involvement of an accessory pathway in a tachycardia circuit. In the present case, His-refractory VPDs during periods of stable tachycardia cycle length delayed the inscription of the subsequent His (**Fig. 5**). On another occasion, spontaneous

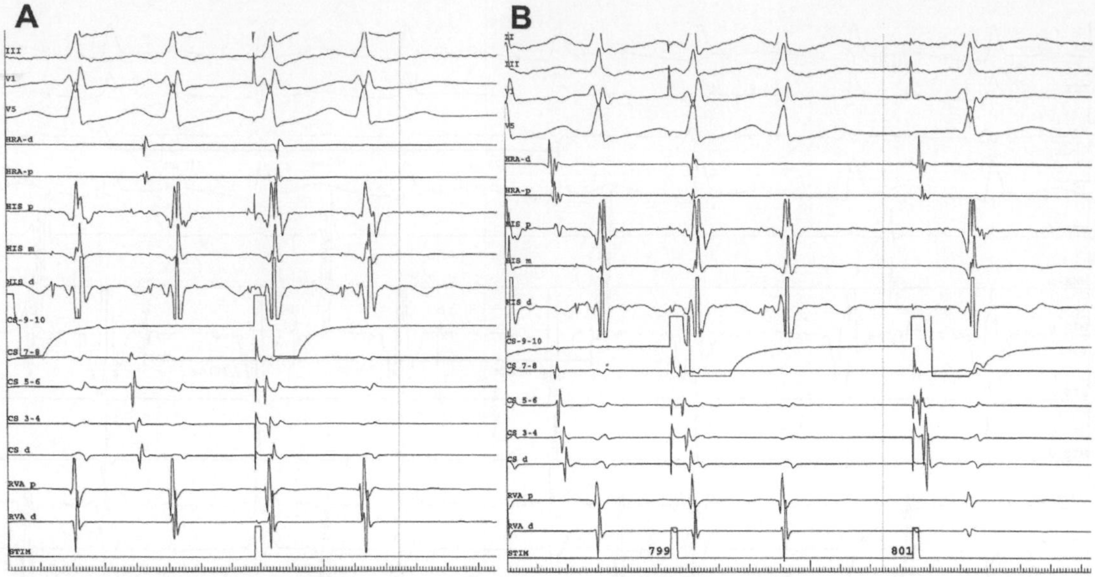

Fig. 4. His-refractory atrial premature depolarization (APD) affects timing of the subsequent His. (*A*) During tachycardia with 2:1 VA conduction, an APD delivered when the His was refractory advanced the timing of the subsequent His, and terminated tachycardia. (*B*) With the APD delivered during tachycardia with VA dissociation, the same finding as in *A* is apparent. These findings rule out junctional tachycardia.

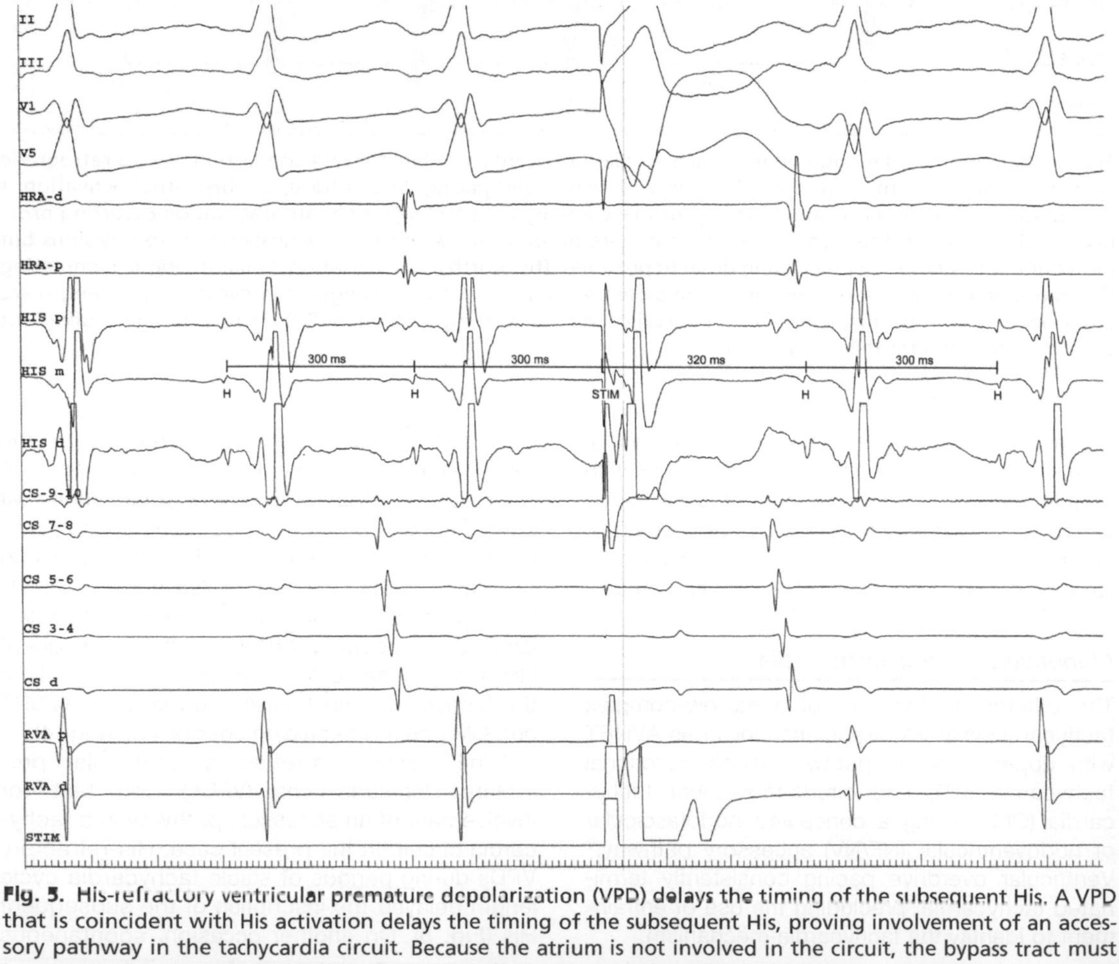

Fig. 5. His-refractory ventricular premature depolarization (VPD) delays the timing of the subsequent His. A VPD that is coincident with His activation delays the timing of the subsequent His, proving involvement of an accessory pathway in the tachycardia circuit. Because the atrium is not involved in the circuit, the bypass tract must insert into the AV node and is therefore a nodofascicular or nodoventricular pathway.

His-refractory VPDs terminated tachycardia. Either of these findings would be sufficient to prove involvement of a concealed accessory pathway in the tachycardia and exclude AVNRT. Because the atrium was not part of the tachycardia circuit, it was concluded that the accessory pathway inserted directly into the AV node, with retrograde conduction to the atrium most likely occurring via a slow retrograde AV nodal pathway, accounting for the long VA time on conducted beats. An alternative mechanism would be a slowly conducting NF/NV pathway inserting directly into the AV node.

Mapping and Ablation

A 4-mm quadripolar radiofrequency ablation catheter was used for mapping and ablation. Hypothesizing that that the NF/NV pathway inserted near the region of the slow AV nodal pathway, a strategy was pursued of identifying the site of earliest retrograde atrial activation, starting with the posteroseptal region of the tricuspid annulus and moving anterior and superior. Also, an attempt was made to identify a pathway potential that preceded retrograde atrial activation at candidate sites. The earliest atrial activation was localized to

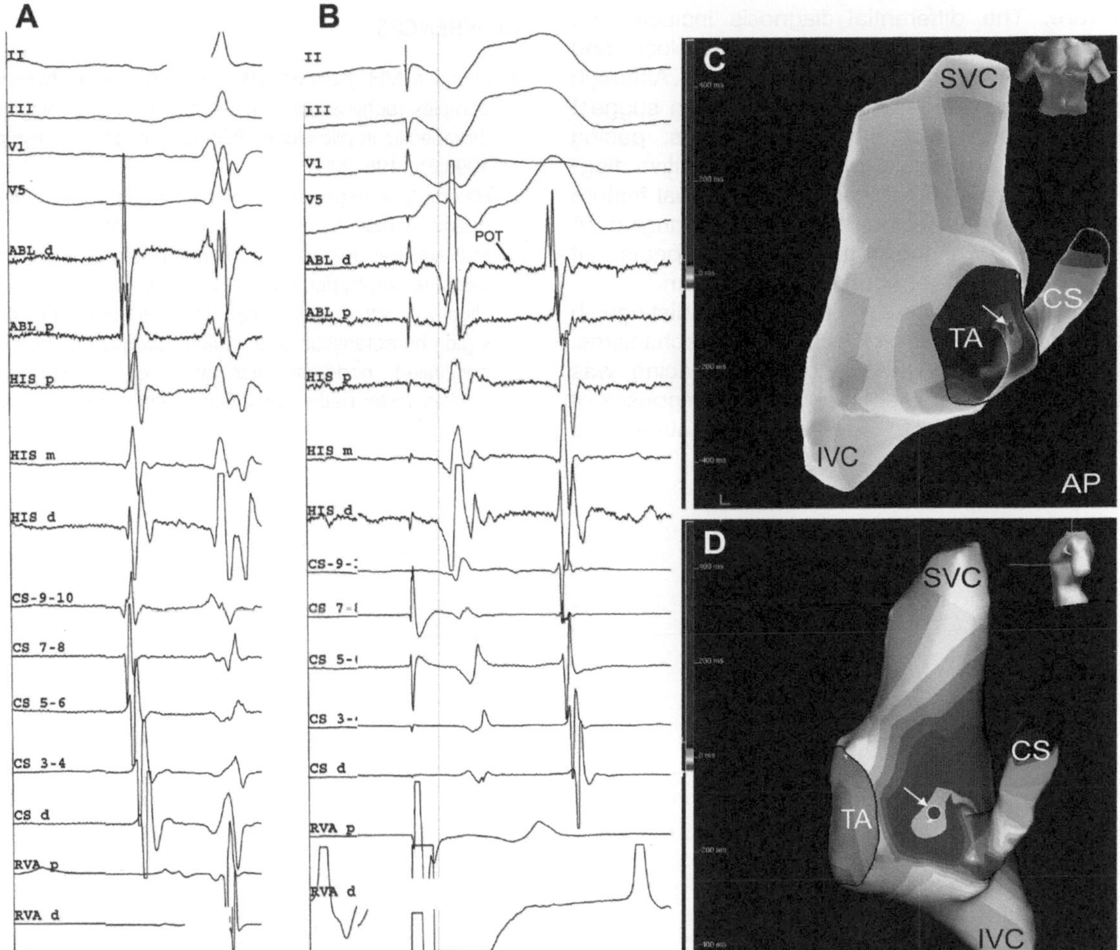

Fig. 6. Mapping and ablation. (*A*) With the ablation catheter at 3 o'clock on the tricuspid annulus positioned anterior and superior to the coronary sinus ostium, the electrogram in sinus rhythm shows an equal-amplitude atrial and ventricular signal without a His signal. (*B*) The same site during ventricular pacing shows earliest atrial activation and a low-amplitude signal that might reflect activation of a slow AV nodal pathway, or, less likely, a slowly conducting accessory pathway. (*C, D*) Ensite (St Jude Medical, St Paul, MN) activation maps in anteroposterior (*C*) and left lateral (*D*) orientation show the successful ablation lesion (*arrow*) at the site of earliest atrial activation during ventricular pacing. CS, coronary sinus; IVC, inferior vena cava; POT, pathway potential; SVC, superior vena cava; TA, tricuspid annulus.

a site anterior to the roof of the coronary sinus ostium, where electrograms revealed a 1:1 atrial to ventricular electrogram ratio in sinus rhythm and a low amplitude potential preceding atrial activation on ventricular paced beats (**Fig. 6**). Ablation was performed at this site, and subsequent ventricular overdrive pacing and programmed ventricular stimulation with and without isoproterenol infusion failed to induce the tachycardia. At 6 months after ablation, the patient has remained symptom-free and has resumed all of his usual activities without limitation.

DISCUSSION

Narrow-complex tachycardia with VA dissociation is rare. The differential diagnosis includes JT, AVNRT with upper common pathway block, and a CMT using a concealed NF/NV pathway. Although baseline tachycardia characteristics can suggest one or another of these mechanisms, pacing maneuvers are required to make a definitive diagnosis in these difficult cases.[1] An unusual feature in the present case, in addition to the changing VA relationship, was the long VA interval on beats that were conducted retrogradely to the atrium.

A standard maneuver performed to distinguish among narrow-complex tachycardia mechanisms, the response to ventricular overdrive pacing, was unhelpful in this case. However, the responses of the tachycardia to His-refractory atrial and ventricular depolarizations enabled the authors to make the diagnosis of CMT using a concealed NF/NV pathway and illustrate a diagnostic approach to this rare arrhythmia. Identification of an NF/NV pathway potential during tachycardia and ventricular pacing, the optimal mapping strategy for this arrhythmia, most commonly localizes the pathway insertion to the mid-septal region, very close to the successful ablation site.[2,3] When this approach is not possible, identification of the site of earliest atrial activation is an alternative strategy. In this case, the potential identified might have reflected activation of a slow AV nodal pathway or a slowly conducting NF/NV pathway.

REFERENCES

1. Hamdan MH, Kalman JM, Lesh MD, et al. Narrow complex tachycardia with VA block: diagnostic and therapeutic implications. Pacing Clin Electrophysiol 1998;21:1196–206.
2. Hluchy J, Schlegelmilch P, Schickel S, et al. Radiofrequency ablation of a concealed nodoventricular Mahaim fiber guided by a discrete potential. J Cardiovasc Electrophysiol 1999;10:603–10.
3. Hluchy J, Schickel S, Jorger U, et al. Electrophysiologic characteristics and radiofrequency ablation of concealed nodofascicular and left anterograde atriofascicular pathways. J Cardiovasc Electrophysiol 2000;11:211–7.

Ablation of Complex Atrial Flutters: Utilizing All of Our Tools

Gregory M. Marcus, MD, MAS

KEYWORDS

• Atrial flutter • Atypical flutter • Complex atrial flutter • Ablation

KEY POINTS

- Ablation of complex atrial flutters is likely to become increasingly more common, because most of these circuits are related to areas of slow conduction that result from discrete scars, such as from previous ablations or surgeries; essentially any patient who has undergone an invasive procedure in an atrium may be at risk.
- The exact prevalence and incidence of these atypical flutters remains unknown.
- Several tools are available to successfully ablate the majority of these complex flutters, including 3-dimensional electroanatomic mapping, intracardiac signals, and pacing maneuvers.
- It is important to use all of the information that can be obtained and not rely on a single technique or technology.

The mapping and ablation of a complex atrial flutter can involve many of the characteristics that attract us all to electrophysiology. The approach generally requires puzzle solving, an understanding of the underlying anatomy and physiology, correct interpretation of local signals, and appropriate use of the advanced technology available to us, while the successful ablation that results in abrupt termination of the tachyarrhythmia is often definitive and gratifying. However, these cases can sometimes represent some of the challenges we least enjoy about our field: pursuing these atrial flutters can be arduous and frustrating, particularly when more than one atypical flutter is observed or induced; at times, the results may be equivocal if it is difficult to be certain that the clinical flutter has been successfully addressed. This section provides a few cases that may offer some guidance regarding ways to approach and think about the mapping and ablation of these atypical circuits.

Ablation of complex atrial flutters is likely to become more and more common. As the majority of these circuits are related to areas of slow conduction that result from discrete scars, such as from previous ablations or surgeries, essentially any patient who has undergone some form of invasive procedure in an atrium may be at risk. Patients who have undergone an atriotomy for previous open heart surgery, those who have undergone correction of congenital heart disease, and those who have undergone left atrial ablation for atrial fibrillation are at particularly high risk. The epidemiology of these phenomena can be difficult to study because large datasets, such as Medicare or state-wide data as well as most National Institutes of Health–sponsored cohort studies, often group atypical and typical flutter together. Indeed, many simply lump these rhythms along with either atrial fibrillation or other supraventricular tachyarrhythmias. Experiences described by single centers are prone to both referral bias and inconsistent longitudinal follow-up. Therefore, the exact prevalence and incidence of these atypical flutters remains unknown. Without such data, it is difficult to determine particular risk factors and the general timing that these arrhythmias present after the original atrial intervention, and therefore to derive an understanding of the causal pathophysiology.

Electrophysiology Section, Division of Cardiology, University of California, San Francisco, 505 Parnassus Avenue, M-1180B, Box 0124, San Francisco, CA 94143-0124, USA
E-mail address: marcusg@medicine.ucsf.edu

Card Electrophysiol Clin 4 (2012) 537–538
http://dx.doi.org/10.1016/j.ccep.2012.08.001
1877-9182/12/$ – see front matter

Fortunately, there are several tools at our disposal to successfully ablate the majority of these complex flutters. It is important to use all of the information that can be obtained and not to rely on a single technique or technology. Three-dimensional electroanatomic mapping is critical in determining relative voltages (and therefore areas of scar, healthy tissue, and border-zone areas and/or channels in between scars) and can provide useful propagation maps. However, these maps are rarely, if ever, sufficient. Each point must first be interpreted correctly, using a meticulous and absolutely consistent approach. Certain information gleaned from the map must always be tempered by a healthy dose of skepticism: is that area of low voltage in fact due to poor contact (with awareness regarding far-field vs near-field signals)? When the entire cycle length is included in the map, might that represent a passive wavefront traversing slowly conducting tissue? Indeed, when we observe "early-meets-late," it can provide evidence that a macro-reentrant circuit is present, but this somewhat arbitrary area may not represent the best place to deliver ablation lesions.

The electroanatomic map must be complemented by a careful evaluation of the intracardiac signals. While a mid-diastolic fractionated signal can represent the critical isthmus and the ideal ablation target, a blind loop or even a distant, unrelated scar can also by chance coincide in time with the diastole of the flutter circuit. Similarly, if the electroanatomic map points to an area of scar with slow conduction, large signals indicating healthy tissue in that area should be interpreted with caution.

Finally, pacing maneuvers can be helpful and confirm the findings from the electroanatomic map and local signals. While entrainment mapping can help the operator to hone in on the area of interest relatively quickly, this is often at the risk of terminating or changing the tachycardia. Before any pacing, operators should familiarize themselves with both the intracardiac pattern and surface electrocardiogram flutter wave to be able to detect a change in the circuit. Moreover, when interpreting entrainment operators must not only confirm consistent atrial capture but also recognize exactly what component of the atrial signal has been captured when measuring the postpacing interval.

The authors are pleased to present the following cases in hopes of demonstrating these teaching points in an interesting and educational manner.

Intraisthmus Reentry

Kurt S. Hoffmayer, PharmD, MD[a,*],
Melvin M. Scheinman, MD[b]

KEYWORDS

• Catheter ablation • Atrial flutter • Intraisthmus reentry

KEY POINTS

- Intraisthmus reentry is a microreentrant atrial flutter circuit localized to the septal portion of the cavotricuspid isthmus (CTI), and is a common cause of recurrent flutter after CTI ablation.
- Diagnosis is confirmed when entrainment mapping of the lateral and mid CTI is out of the circuit (postpacing interval [PPI] − tachycardia cycle length [TCL] >30 milliseconds) and the septal CTI and coronary sinus ostium are in the circuit (PPI − TCL <30 milliseconds).
- Radiofrequency ablation in the region of the septal CTI successfully terminates tachycardia in the majority of cases.

CLINICAL PRESENTATION

A 70-year-old man presented with palpitations 2 years after an apparently successful cavotricuspid isthmus (CTI) ablation for typical atrial flutter. The surface electrocardiogram is shown in **Fig. 1**. He was referred for repeat electrophysiology study and catheter ablation.

ELECTROPHYSIOLOGY STUDY AND ABLATION

The patient presented to the electrophysiology laboratory in atrial flutter. An electrophysiology study was performed using a decapolar catheter positioned in the coronary sinus, a quadripolar catheter in the His bundle region, a duodecapolar placed in the right atrium along the tricuspid annulus, and a 3.5-mm open irrigated catheter for mapping and ablation. The tachycardia had a cycle length of 240 milliseconds. Electroanatomic mapping was performed with the CARTO system (Biosense Webster, Inc, Diamond Bar, CA, USA). An electroanatomic map was created during the tachycardia (**Fig. 2**). Entrainment mapping from the midisthmus at 6 o'clock on the tricuspid valve in the left anterior oblique view is shown in **Fig. 3**.

Question:

What is the most likely mechanism of the tachycardia? What is your primary approach to ablation?

DISCUSSION

The most likely diagnosis is intraisthmus reentry.[1] Intraisthmus reentry is a microreentrant atrial flutter circuit localized to the septal portion of the CTI, and involves the septal isthmus as well as the ostium of coronary sinus.[1] It is a common cause of recurrent flutter after CTI ablation and is estimated to be the culprit arrhythmia in 20% of these patients.[2]

The diagnosis is confirmed when entrainment mapping from the lateral and mid CTI demonstrates that those areas are outside of the circuit (postpacing interval [PPI]−tachycardia cycle length [TCL] >30 milliseconds), and when entrainment of the coronary sinus ostium and septal CTI is "in" (PPI−TCL <30 milliseconds).

[a] Section of Electrophysiology, Division of Cardiology, University of California, San Francisco, 500 Parnassus Avenue, MUE-434, Box 1354, San Francisco, CA 94143, USA; [b] Section of Electrophysiology, Division of Cardiology, University of California, San Francisco, 500 Parnassus Avenue, San Francisco, CA 94143, USA
* Corresponding author.
E-mail address: kurt.hoffmayer@ucsf.edu

Card Electrophysiol Clin 4 (2012) 539–543
http://dx.doi.org/10.1016/j.ccep.2012.08.002

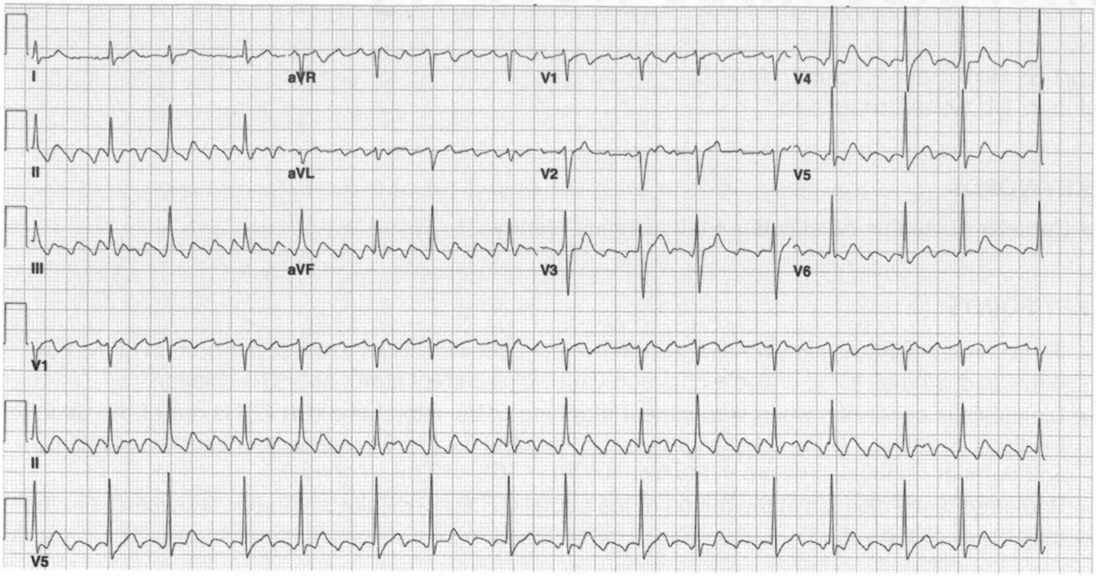

Fig. 1. Twelve-lead electrocardiogram of the clinical tachycardia. (A color version of this figure is available online.)

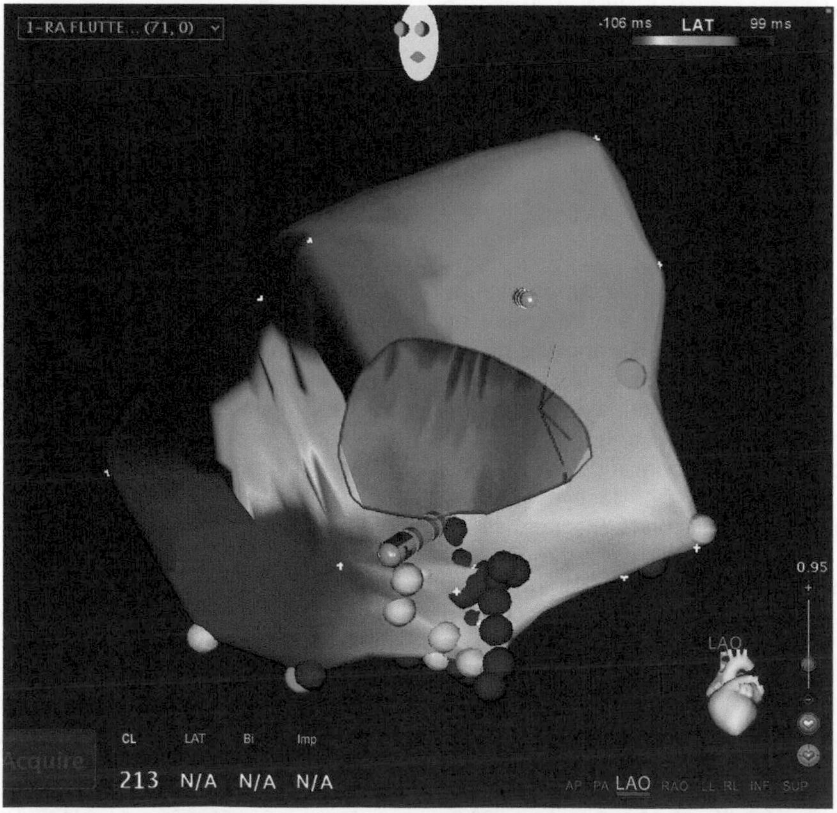

Fig. 2. CARTO electroanatomic map during the clinical tachycardia revealing counterclockwise activation around the tricuspid annulus in the left anterior oblique (LAO) projection. Ablation lesions are seen near 6 o'clock in the cavotricuspid isthmus (CTI). This map is consistent with counterclockwise flutter, with "early meets late" configuration around the tricuspid annulus and greater than 90% of the cycle length recorded.

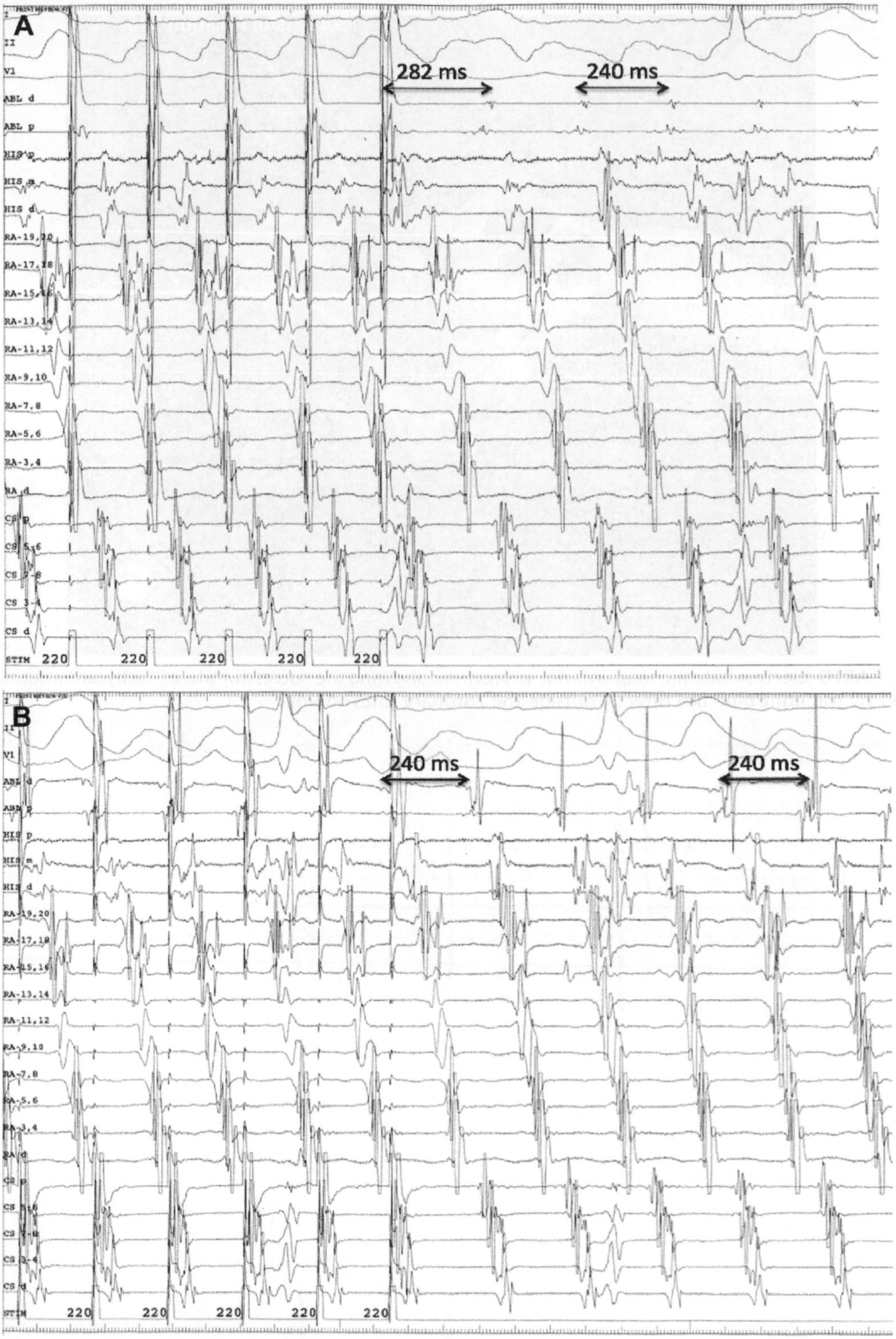

Fig. 3. (*A*) Entrainment pacing from the distal ablation catheter (ABL d) positioned at the mid CTI at 6 o'clock in the LAO projection 20 milliseconds faster than the tachycardia cycle length. The postpacing interval (PPI) is 282 milliseconds and the tachycardia cycle length (TCL) is 240 milliseconds, with resultant PP–TCL of 42 milliseconds, demonstrating that the mid CTI is out of the circuit. (*B*) Entrainment pacing from the distal ablation catheter (ABL d) positioned at the septal CTI is 20 milliseconds faster than the tachycardia cycle. The PPI is 240 milliseconds and the TCL is 240 milliseconds, with resultant PP–TCL of 0 milliseconds, demonstrating that the septal CTI is in the circuit.

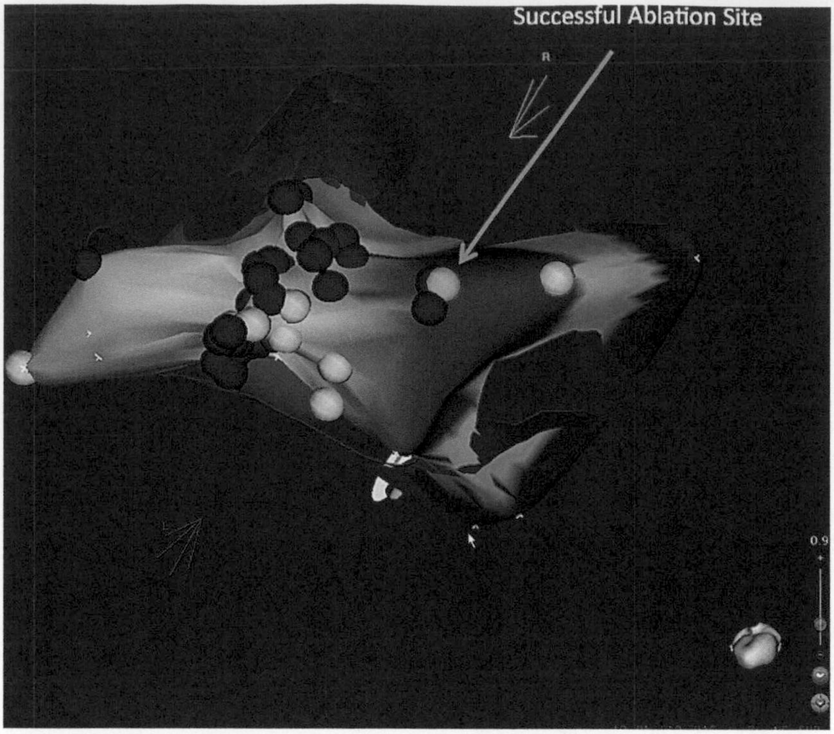

Fig. 4. CARTO electroanatomic map inferior projection, showing the successful site of tachycardia termination marked by the light blue ball directly outside the coronary sinus ostium.

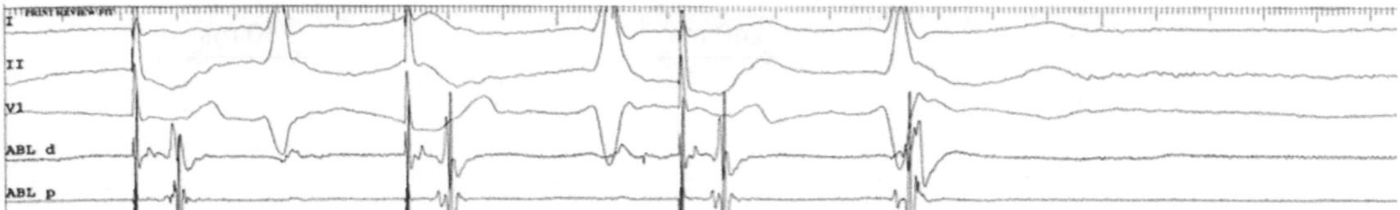

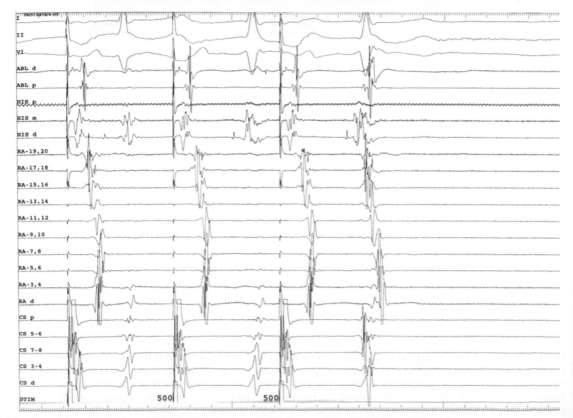

Fig. 5. Pacing from the coronary sinus (CS) ostium reveals a leak in the original CTI line.

Radiofrequency ablation in the region of the septal CTI successfully terminates tachycardia in more than 85% of cases, as was seen in our case (**Fig. 4**). Others have been shown to terminate in the mid or anteroinferior CTI regions.[2] The successful sites of ablation show the longest duration of fractionated potentials in areas of concealed entrainment.[1,2]

This case beautifully demonstrates these findings. The original CARTO electroanatomic map is consistent with typical counterclockwise flutter, with an "early meets late" configuration around the tricuspid annulus and greater than 90% of the cycle length recorded. Entrainment mapping reveals that most of the CTI is out of the circuit. Intraisthmus reentry is a microreentrant circuit and, because of unilateral block (or delay in the isthmus), may produce a 3-dimensional map that is "diagnostic" of macroreentry around the annulus. All patients who undergo repeat atrial flutter ablation should have the presence of isthmus bidirectional block confirmed, and in this case there was a leak from the original ablation that required further ablation lesions to produce bidirectional block.[3] Entrainment mapping in this case demonstrated that only the septal CTI was in the circuit, whereas the rest of the tricuspid annulus sites were out of the circuit, signifying that it was not the slow conduction or "leak" of the previous CTI line that was responsible for the tachycardia. After termination of the tachycardia, pacing from the coronary sinus showed evidence of a leak in the original CTI line (**Fig. 5**).

SUMMARY

Intraisthmus reentry is a microreentrant atrial flutter circuit localized to the septal portion of the CTI, and is a common cause of recurrent flutter after CTI ablation. Diagnosis is confirmed when entrainment mapping demonstrates that the lateral and mid CTI are out of the circuit (PPI−TCL >30 milliseconds) and that the septal CTI and coronary sinus ostium are in the circuit (PPI−TCL <30 milliseconds). Radiofrequency ablation in the region of the septal CTI successfully terminates tachycardia in the majority of cases.

REFERENCES

1. Yang Y, Varma N, Keung EC, et al. Reentry within the cavotricuspid isthmus: an isthmus dependent circuit. Pacing Clin Electrophysiol 2005;28(8):808–18.
2. Yang Y, Varma N, Badhwar N, et al. Prospective observations in the clinical and electrophysiological characteristics of intra-isthmus reentry. J Cardiovasc Electrophysiol 2010;21(10):1099–106.
3. Mangat I, Tschopp DR Jr, Yang Y, et al. Optimizing the detection of bidirectional block across the flutter isthmus for patients with typical isthmus-dependent atrial flutter. Am J Cardiol 2003;91(5):559–64.

Postsurgical Atrial Arrhythmia in a Patient with Partial Anomalous Pulmonary Venous Return

Emily Ruckdeschel, MD, Russell R. Heath, MD, William H. Sauer, MD, Duy Thai Nguyen, MD*

KEYWORDS

• Catheter ablation • Congenital heart disease • Atrial flutter • Anomalous pulmonary veins

KEY POINTS

• Knowledge of the patient's congenital anatomy and surgical correction, as well as a combination of entrainment and electroanatomic mapping, can help to efficiently define the tachycardia mechanism and identify the culprit area sustaining the tachycardia.

CLINICAL HISTORY

A 19-year-old man with a history of partial anomalous pulmonary venous return who was status post a Warden procedure presented with a supraventricular tachycardia (SVT). The Warden procedure is a surgical technique whereby the superior vena cava (SVC) is divided, and the cephalic portion is directly anastomosed to the right atrial appendage. Furthermore, the caudal SVC serves as a conduit for the pulmonary veins to drain into the left atrium after a baffle is created from the caudal SVC through an atrial septal defect (either preexisting or surgically created) into the left atrium.

Several months after his surgery, the patient presented with an SVT with variable block and hypotension (**Fig. 1**). The patient had no presurgical history of arrhythmias. He underwent a cardioversion and was placed on sotalol. However, after the arrhythmia recurred with significant symptoms, he was referred for electrophysiologic (EP) study and ablation.

IMAGING FINDINGS

EP Study and Treatment

Multipolar catheters were placed in the right atrium (RA), His-bundle region, right ventricle, and coronary sinus (CS). At baseline, the patient was in SVT with a tachycardia cycle length (TCL) of 292 milliseconds. Variable atrioventricular (AV) block was present, thus ruling out AV reentrant tachycardia. AV nodal reentrant tachycardia with lower common pathway block is rare and was essentially excluded by a high to low atrial activation. Hence, atypical atrial flutter was the most likely diagnosis. Entrainment from the distal CS and from the cavotricuspid isthmus showed that these areas were out of the tachycardia circuit. Activation mapping (CARTO electroanatomic navigation system; Biosense Webster, Diamond Bar, CA) confirmed a macro-reentrant circuit, with the entire TCL within the right atrium with an "early meets late" transition in the posterior RA (**Fig. 2**A). The boundaries of the patient's baffle, bordering the superior and septal RA, were out of the tachycardia circuit. Mapping

Disclosures: None.
Cardiac Electrophysiology, Cardiology Division, Anschutz Medical Campus, University of Colorado, Denver, 12401 East 17th Avenue, B-132, Aurora, CO 80045, USA
* Corresponding author.
E-mail address: duy.t.nguyen@ucdenver.edu

Card Electrophysiol Clin 4 (2012) 545–548
http://dx.doi.org/10.1016/j.ccep.2012.08.003
1877-9182/12/$ – see front matter

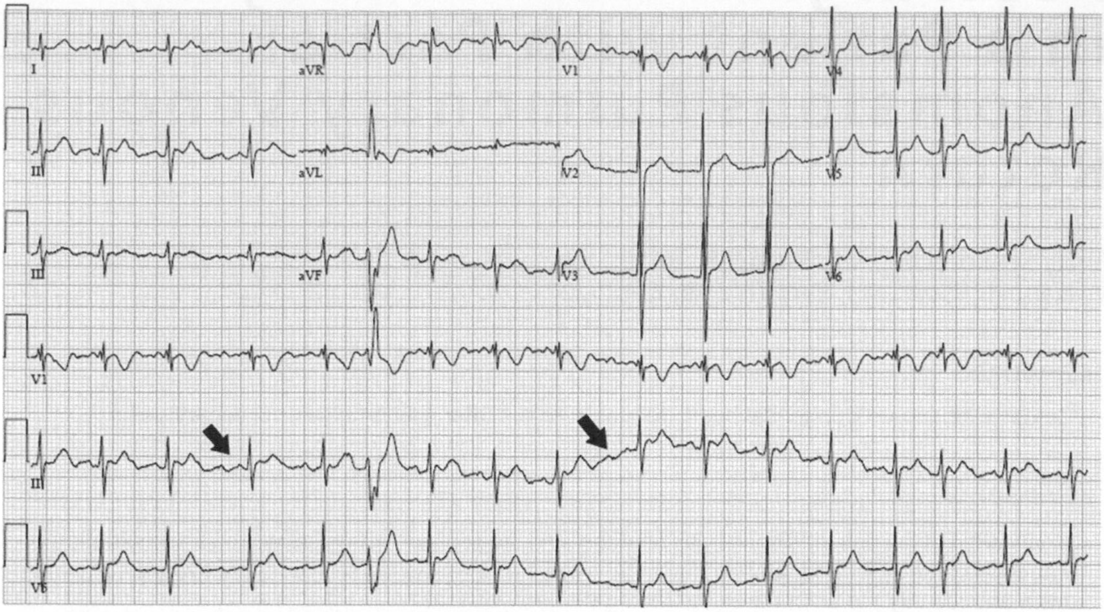

Fig. 1. Twelve-lead electrocardiogram of a narrow-complex tachycardia with variable block. Atrial activity (*arrows*) was more visible with the variable block.

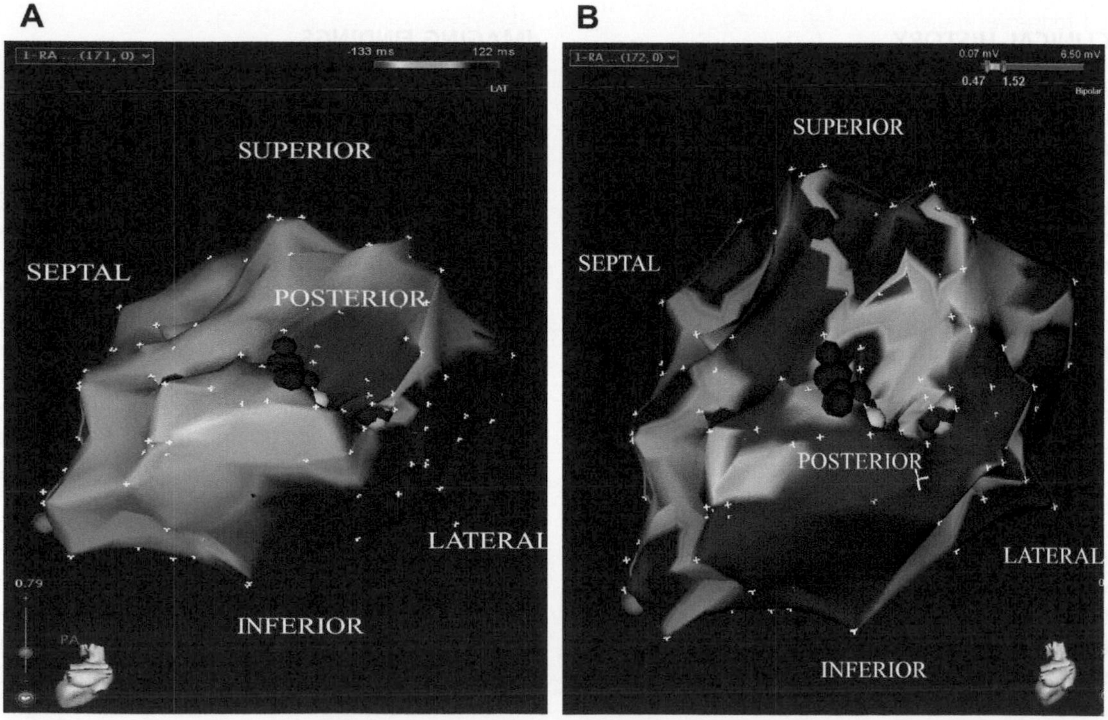

Fig. 2. (*A*) Posteroanterior view of CARTO electroanatomic map of patient's right atrium (RA). Atrial activation timing was obtained, with red as earliest activation and purple as latest activation. The tachycardia circuit revolved around areas of scar in the posterior right atrium, with the site of latest activation meeting site of earliest activation in an area of isthmus between 2 large areas of scar in the posterior RA. Sites of ablation are shown as red circles. The patient's baffle was superior and septally directed. (*B*) Posteroanterior view of CARTO electroanatomic map of RA. Voltage was obtained, with red as areas of scar (<0.47 mV) and purple as healthy myocardium (>1.52 mV). The tachycardia circuit revolved around 2 large areas of scar in the posterior RA. Ablations (*red circles*) within the isthmus between these 2 areas of scar in the posterior RA rendered the tachycardia noninducible.

of the posterior RA showed a mid-diastolic potential in an isthmus between 2 areas of scar. Entrainment from this isthmus resulted in a postpacing interval (PPI) that equaled the TCL (**Fig. 3**). Ablation at this site terminated the tachycardia (**Fig. 4**), and the tachycardia could not be reinduced with atrial burst pacing or multiple extra-stimuli, on and off isuprel. An ablation line was drawn across the isthmus between these 2 areas of scar (**Fig. 2**B). The patient has remained arrhythmia-free for more than 1 year.

DISCUSSION

Atrial arrhythmias occur commonly after cardiac surgery in patients with congenital heart disease (CHD). The most common tachycardias in postsurgical CHD patients include scar-based intra-atrial reentrant tachycardia (IART) or atriotomy incision-related tachycardias, as well as typical isthmus-dependent atrial flutter.[1] IARTs can develop weeks to years after surgery and are more often seen with greater degrees of scar, atrial dilation, and atrial thickening. Atrial rates of IARTs tend to be slower than typical atrial flutter and can frequently conduct 1:1 to the ventricles. Atrial arrhythmias in CHD can cause variable symptoms but, even when they are asymptomatic, can compromise ventricular function over time, especially in patients with systemic right ventricles and single ventricles. Rapid atrial arrhythmias can cause syncope as well as precipitate ventricular arrhythmias and sudden cardiac death.

Partial anomalous pulmonary venous return is a relatively uncommon congenital heart defect whereby the venous drainage from 1 or more lung lobes returns to an area other than the left atrium. Most commonly, it is the right upper or middle lobe that drains into the SVC. Anomalous veins may also drain into a vertical vein (such was the case with this patient), the inferior vena cava, or the CS. Patients may remain asymptomatic for many years or present with exertional symptoms, pulmonary hypertension, or right heart enlargement. The Warden procedure was developed in the 1980s to treat partial anomalous venous connection. In particular, it was designed to avoid excessive atrial manipulation during surgery, which can lead to high rates of supraventricular arrhythmias as well as pulmonary vein and SVC stenosis.[2] Rates of IART following repair of partial anomalous pulmonary venous connection are not well defined. It has been shown that a right atriotomy incision approach has a lower rate of dysrhythmias,

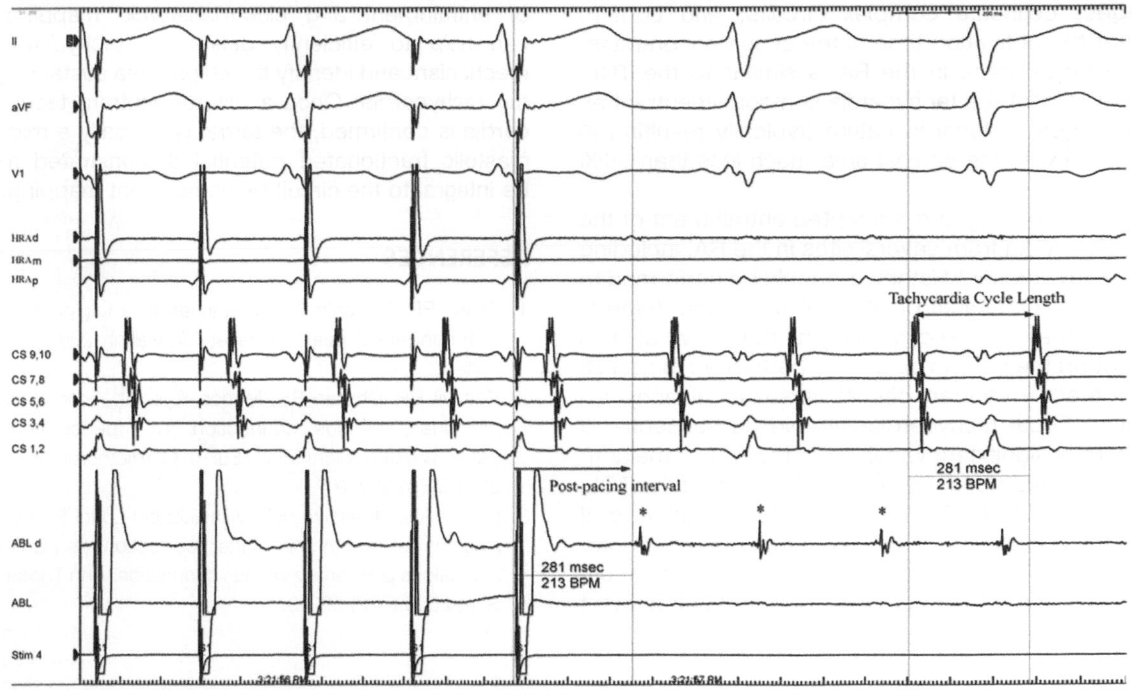

Fig. 3. Atypical atrial flutter with variable AV block and a high to low atrial activation pattern. Mid-diastolic signals (*asterisk*) were found in an isthmus between 2 areas of scar in the posterior right atrium. Entrainment was performed, and the postpacing interval minus tachycardia cycle length (PPI−TCL) was essentially zero, with concealed fusion of the atrial activation pattern. ABL, ablator; CS, coronary sinus with 1, 2 as most distal and 9, 10 as most proximal; d, distal; HRA, high right atrium; m, mid; p, proximal.

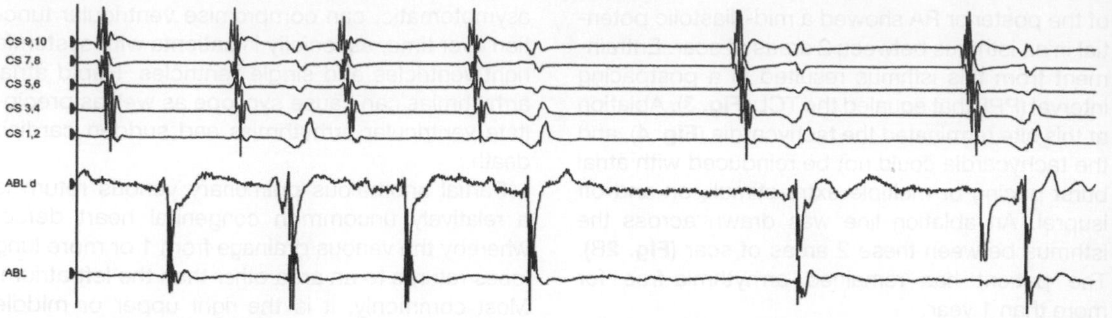

Fig. 4. Ablation at the site of entrainment in **Fig. 3** terminated the tachycardia within seconds (ablation signals maximally gained).

compared with an extended incision from the RA through the cavoatrial junction.[3] In the present patient there was an extended incision made during surgery to better define his left atrium, which likely led to an increased burden of scar. His tachycardia did not involve the atrial baffle; this is not unusual, given that presumably there was little scar and less heterogeneity of the baffle tissue only a few months after its creation.

The approach to suspected atrial arrhythmias in postsurgical CHD patients should use a combination of entrainment, electroanatomic activation, and voltage mapping. Initially electroanatomic mapping can be used to define areas of low voltages, delineate complex circuits, and confirm that the activation time of the circuit encompassing large areas in the RA is similar to the TCL, that is, that the tachycardia is macro-reentrant as opposed to focal in nature (typically resulting in a map with the earliest area much less than 50% of TCL).

Next, pacing and attempted entrainment of the tachycardia from several sites in the RA, including the cavotricuspid isthmus, should be performed to assess for typical or atypical right atrial flutters. Pacing at several cycle lengths from several sites around the RA can be quickly performed to assess for macro-reentrant circuits versus focal tachycardias. Focal tachycardias should be suspected if there is significant variability in the TCL, if the activation map does not account for most of the TCL, if there is lack of early meets late activation, or if there is an inability to show that 2 sites greater than 2 cm apart are part of the tachycardia circuit. Finally, if the response to pacing and entrainment suggests a macro-reentrant tachycardia and no site in the RA is found to be in the circuit, entrainment from the atrial septum and from the distal CS should be done to assess for left atrial tachycardias, although left atrial tachycardias are less common in CHD patients with right-sided atrial abnormality.

SUMMARY

The key features of this case are relevant to the majority of atypical flutters in CHD patients. Knowledge of the patient's congenital anatomy and surgical correction, as well as a combination of entrainment and electroanatomic mapping, can help to efficiently define the tachycardia mechanism and identify the culprit area sustaining the tachycardia. Once a macro-reentrant tachycardia is confirmed, the target is typically a mid-diastolic fractionated potential demonstrated to be integral to the circuit by entrainment mapping.

REFERENCES

1. Walsh EP, Cecchin F. Arrhythmias in adult patients with congenital heart disease. Circulation 2007;115: 534–45.
2. Kottayil BP, Dharan BS, Menon S, et al. Anomalous pulmonary venous connection to superior vena cava: Warden technique. Eur J Cardiothorac Surg 2011;39(3):388–91.
3. Buz S, Alexi-Meskishvili V, Villavicencio-Lorini F, et al. Analysis of arrhythmias after correction of partial anomalous pulmonary venous connection. Ann Thorac Surg 2009;87(2):580–3.

Incisional Atrial Flutter in a Patient with Repaired Tetralogy of Fallot

Frederick T. Han, MD*, Walter Li, MD, Melvin M. Scheinman, MD, Ronn E. Tanel, MD

KEYWORDS

• Incisional reentry atrial flutter • Congenital heart disease • Tetralogy of Fallot

KEY POINTS

- Patients who have undergone surgical repair of congenital heart disease often have multiple substrates for atrial arrhythmia.
- An electroanatomic mapping system can be useful for mapping areas of low voltage consistent with a previous atriotomy or scar that may serve as the substrate for the atrial tachyarrhythmia.
- In patients with multiple tachyarrhythmias, successful ablation of the primary atrial flutter may allow secondary flutter circuits to become manifest.

CLINICAL HISTORY

A 40-year-old man born with tetralogy of Fallot presented for an electrophysiology study and ablation of an atrial tachyarrhythmia refractory to sotalol. As an infant, he underwent a Waterston shunt to augment his pulmonary arterial circulation. This shunt was followed by a tetralogy of Fallot repair: ventricular septal defect repair, Waterston shunt takedown, and right ventricular outflow tract reconstruction. In a separate surgery, the ascending aorta stenosis (at the previous Waterston shunt site) was revised. As an adult, the patient developed bacterial endocarditis. After medical therapy for the endocarditis, the patient had an ascending and transverse aortic arch reconstruction, a bioprosthetic pulmonic valve replacement, right pulmonary artery patch augmentation, a right atrial maze procedure, and a transvenous dual-chamber pacemaker implanted for high-grade atrioventricular (AV) block. At the time of presentation, the Maze operative report was not available for review. Despite sotalol, the patient complained of persistent daily palpitations with exercise intolerance correlating with atrial high-rate episodes on his pacemaker. Given the patient's age, history of restrictive lung disease, and hypothyroidism, the patient deferred further antiarrhythmic medical therapy and elected to pursue electrophysiology study and ablation for his atrial tachyarrhythmia.

IMAGING FINDINGS

Echocardiogram revealed a bioprosthetic valve in the right ventricular outflow tract with trivial stenosis and insufficiency. There was mild tricuspid insufficiency with a pacemaker lead visualized in the right ventricle. The right ventricle was mildly dilated with mild hypertrophy and mild systolic dysfunction. There was mild right atrial dilatation. The left ventricle was of normal size. There was mild aortic insufficiency.

LABORATORY FINDINGS

Complete blood count, electrolytes, and renal and hepatic function were within normal limits. Thyroid

Section of Electrophysiology, Division of Cardiology, University of California San Francisco Medical Center, 500 Parnassus Avenue, MUE – 434, Box 1354, San Francisco, CA 94122, USA
* Corresponding author.
E-mail address: Frederick.Han@ucsf.edu

Card Electrophysiol Clin 4 (2012) 549–555
http://dx.doi.org/10.1016/j.ccep.2012.08.005
1877-9182/12/$ – see front matter © 2012 Published by Elsevier Inc.

function studies were within normal limits on thyroid hormone replacement therapy.

PHYSICAL EXAMINATION FINDINGS

Blood pressure 103/62 mm Hg, pulse 88, respiratory rate 18 breaths per minute, pulse oximetry 92%.

The patient was a well-appearing, acyanotic man. There was no jugular venous distention with a normal carotid upstroke. The patient's breathing was unlabored with normal breath sounds bilaterally. The patient had a regular rate and rhythm with a normal S1, split S2, and a 2/6 systolic ejection murmur at the left upper sternal border. The abdomen was soft, nontender, and nondistended. There was no clubbing, cyanosis, or edema.

CLINICAL COURSE

Electrophysiology Study

A duodecapolar electrode catheter was placed around the tricuspid valve annulus with the distal pole in the midcoronary sinus. Quadripolar electrode catheters were positioned at the His bundle region and at the right ventricular apex. An 8-mm tip radiofrequency ablation catheter was used for mapping and ablation. The baseline presenting rhythm was an ectopic atrial rhythm from the low lateral tricuspid annulus conducted with a right bundle branch block QRS complex at a cycle length of 1270 milliseconds. Atrial flutter was induced with double atrial extrastimuli from the midcoronary sinus at an S1/S2/S3 coupling interval of 400/320/330 milliseconds. The flutter cycle length was 390 milliseconds (**Fig. 1**). The atrial flutter was conducted with 2:1 AV block, which excluded the possibility of AV reentrant tachycardia. AV nodal reentrant tachycardia with lower common pathway block was ruled out by the atrial activation sequence during tachycardia, which was earliest at the midlateral right atrium (RA) adjacent to electrode pair M10 during tachycardia (**Fig. 1**). Activation mapping of the RA characterized more than 90% of the flutter cycle length, consistent with a macroreentrant atypical atrial flutter (**Fig. 2**A). Attempted entrainment of the atrial flutter from the proximal coronary sinus and the low septal RA dissociated atrial activation at these sites from the tachycardia in the lateral RA, confirming that these sites were not part of the tachycardia circuit. Pacing from the midcavotricuspid isthmus (CTI) during the baseline ectopic atrial rhythm and during the atrial tachyarrhythmia failed to capture the atrial myocardium at this site. Entrainment from the midlateral RA and the low lateral RA indicated that these sites were part of a macroreentrant atrial flutter circuit with a postpacing interval (PPI) within 10 milliseconds of the tachycardia cycle length (TCL). In addition, entrainment from the midlateral RA (**Fig. 3**) showed concealed entrainment. Split atrial electrograms, suggesting a prior surgical incision, were also noted along the lateral RA, especially at electrode pair M9 (**Fig. 1**). At the low lateral RA, there was a triphasic signal observed on the ablation catheter from the low lateral RA (**Fig. 3**).

The activation pattern in **Fig. 2** suggests the presence of a dual-loop incisional macroreentrant atrial flutter with each loop sharing a common protected isthmus. Data to support this diagnosis include the following findings: (1) the coronary sinus ostium and posteroseptal RA were dissociated from the atrial tachycardia during atrial overdrive pacing from these sites (ruling out CTI-dependent atrial flutter), (2) the CTI could not be captured with atrial pacing at baseline and during the atrial tachycardia, and (3) the atrial flutter was entrained at both the midlateral and inferolateral RA. The case was challenging because of areas of low bipolar voltage in the posterolateral RA and the CTI that impaired activation mapping with the duodecapolar catheter. As a result, dense fine mapping of the lateral RA with the ablation catheter was required to define the circuit. Activation mapping allowed us to define an activation sequence proceeding from the inferior RA through a central isthmus that exited in the midlateral RA. The posterolateral RA demonstrated a faster conduction velocity and served to maintain the dominant atrial macroreentrant circuit at a cycle length of 390 milliseconds. The atrial activation for this circuit proceeded posteriorly from the exit site and inferiorly along the posterolateral RA to the entrance site (**Fig. 2**B, arrow A). The superior, posterior, and medial RA were activated passively as the wavefront of atrial activation proceeded posteriorly around a line of block, presumably created either by the right atrial maze or a surgical atriotomy. As seen in **Fig. 2**, there was also a secondary circuit with a slower conduction velocity that propagated anteriorly toward the tricuspid valve, then inferiorly toward the entrance site into the critical isthmus (**Fig. 2**B, arrow B). The secondary slower circuit did not become manifest until the dominant flutter circuit was interrupted. The set of linear ablation lesions was started posterior to the position of the duodecapolar catheter where entrainment was shown. The ablation lesions were extended posteriorly to a region of low voltage, designated as scar. During ablation adjacent to the site of concealed entrainment, a change in the atrial flutter cycle length to 417 milliseconds was

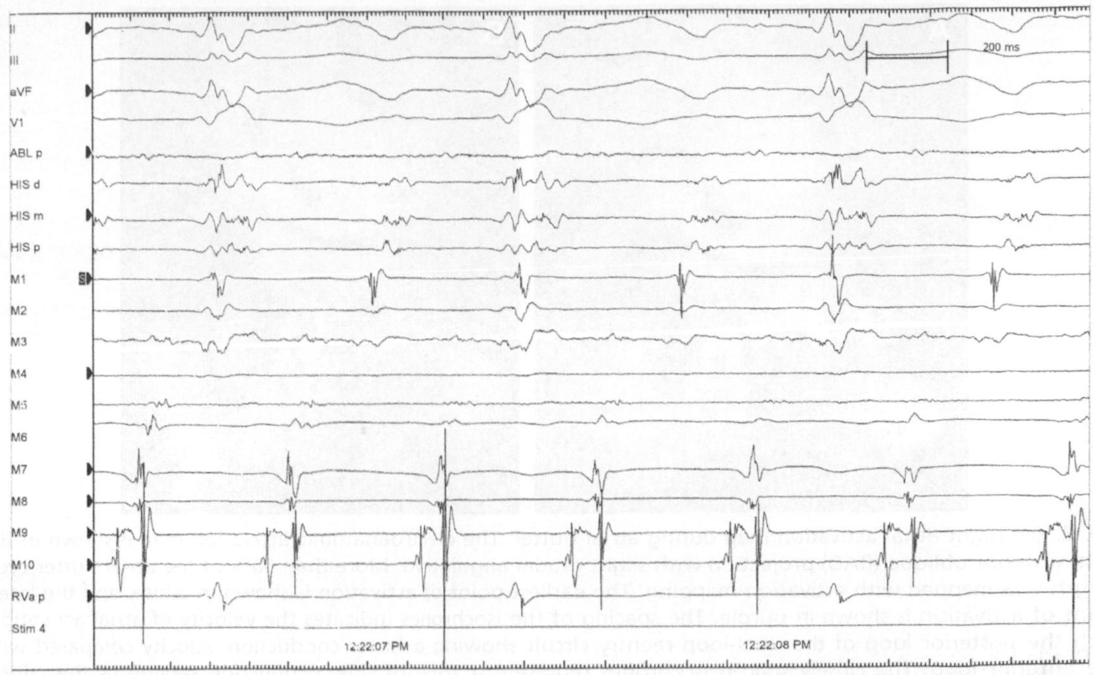

Fig. 1. Surface electrocardiogram (ECG) and intracardiac electrograms during atrial flutter. Surface ECG leads are arranged in descending order of leads II, III, avF, and V1. The duodecapolar catheter was arranged with the distal tip (M1) in the midcoronary sinus and M4 in the cavotricuspid isthmus. The surface atrial flutter cycle length was 390 milliseconds. The earliest atrial activation was in the midlateral right atrium at M10. ABLp, proximal ablation catheter bipole; HISd, His distal bipole; HISm, His midbipole; HISp, His proximal bipole; M1, duodecapolar 1 to 2 bipole; M2, duodecapolar 3 to 4 bipole; M3, duodecapolar 5 to 6 bipole; M4, duodecapolar 7 to 8 bipole; M5, duodecapolar 9 to 10 bipole; M6, duodecapolar 11 to 12 bipole; M7, duodecapolar 13 to 14 bipole; M8, duodecapolar 15 to 16 bipole; M9, duodecapolar 17 to 18 bipole; M10, duodecapolar 19 to 20 bipole; RVAp, proximal right ventricular apex bipole.

observed. There was no change in the activation sequence recorded by the duodecapolar catheter. To address the second atrial flutter, the line of lesions was extended anteriorly to the tricuspid valve annulus. Although the tachycardia terminated several times during delivery of these anterior lesions, atrial flutter remained inducible with a longer cycle length (up to 438 milliseconds) while maintaining the same intracardiac electrogram activation sequence. The increase of the flutter cycle length correlated with a delay in activation of electrode pairs M7 to M5 on the duodecapolar catheter, consistent with a delay in the circuit without complete block across the critical isthmus. We then returned to mapping of the flutter circuit in the midlateral RA at the site of concealed entrainment. With further mapping in a site that had been previously identified as scar and low voltage, we discovered a site with a mid-diastolic atrial electrogram on the ablation catheter (**Fig. 4**). Based on the previous entrainment results along with the atrial flutter circuit activation map, we assumed that this was the critical site within the protected isthmus responsible for maintenance of this circuit. Ablation at this site subsequently terminated the atrial flutter and rendered it noninducible.

Post ablation atrial burst pacing and atrial extrastimuli testing failed to induce any additional atrial tachyarrhythmias.

DISCUSSION

The mechanism of postoperative incisional atrial tachyarrhythmias (and therefore the approach to mapping and ablation) depends on the patient's previous surgical history and potential barriers to conduction that may have been created by atriotomies, baffles, and surgical ablation lesions. Regardless of the previous surgery, cavotricuspid isthmus-dependent atrial flutter is the most common atrial flutter observed in patients with the more common types of congenital heart disease.[1–3] Regardless of the mechanism, patients with a history of prior cardiac surgery are at higher risk of recurrent atrial tachyarrhythmias despite

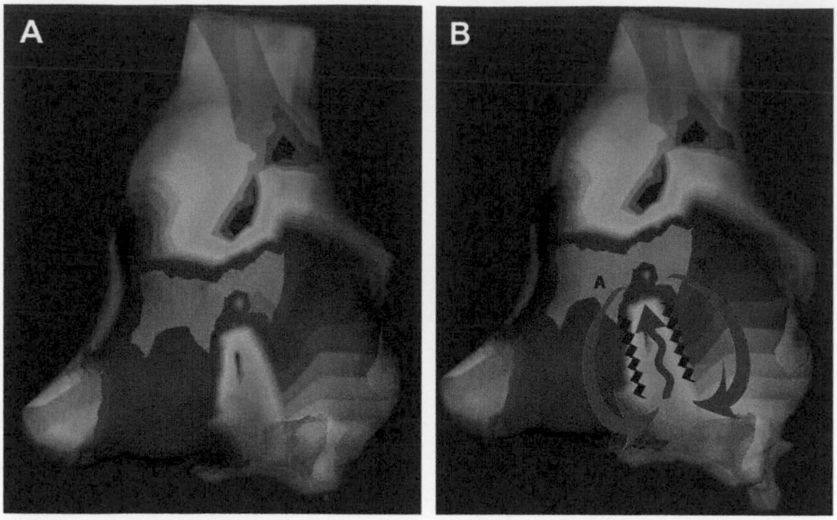

Fig. 2. (*A*) Right atrial activation map during atrial flutter. The electroanatomic activation map is shown in the right anterior oblique (RAO) projection with slight caudal angulation. More than 90% of the atrial flutter cycle length was mapped with activation mapping. The earliest point of activation is shown in white, and the latest point of activation is shown in purple. The spacing of the isochrones indicates the velocity of atrial activation, with the posterior loop of the dual-loop reentry circuit showing a faster conduction velocity compared with the anterior loop. The closely spaced isochrones represent a zone of slow conduction serving as the critical isthmus maintaining the atrial flutter. (*B*) Right atrial activation map with atrial flutter circuit diagram. The electroanatomic activation map is shown in the RAO projection with slight caudal angulation. The earliest point of activation is shown in white, and the latest point of activation is shown in purple. The anterior and posterior barriers of the protected isthmus are identified by the black wavy lines, which presumably represent suture lines from the patient's previous atriotomies. The blue arrow (A) is the dominant loop of the flutter circuit responsible for the atrial flutter cycle length of 390 milliseconds. After ablation of the posterior loop, the second loop with the blue arrow (B) became the manifest circuit with an initial flutter cycle length of 417 milliseconds. Ablation of the anterior loop increased the flutter cycle length to 438 milliseconds. Ablation in the central isthmus identified by the pink wavy arrow terminated the flutter and rendered it noninducible.

successful ablation of the clinical arrhythmia.[3–5] Details of any previous cardiac surgeries, regarding atriotomy locations, shunt/anastomosis sites, baffle construction, valve repair or replacements, and Maze lesion sets can help to guide vascular access as well as the intraprocedural mapping and ablation strategy. In addition, electroanatomic mapping with activation and voltage mapping are especially important for defining the circuit and the substrate of the arrhythmias,[6] because the surface electrocardiogram (ECG) flutter wave may be misleading.[7]

Because the substrate for atrial tachyarrhythmias in patients with congenital and acquired heart disease can facilitate multiple atrial tachyarrhythmias, performing an activation map first can allow (1) determination of whether the atrial activation pattern shows an early-meets-late pattern (suggesting a macroreentrant mechanism) or a focal origination with a centrifugal spread (suggesting a microreentrant, automatic, or triggered mechanism), (2) definition of the percentage of the cycle length within the chamber(s) of interest, (3) avoid premature termination of the arrhythmia with pacing or entrainment. In addition, a simultaneous bipolar voltage map can be created and used to define areas of scar that serve as the anatomic substrate for macroreentrant atrial flutter circuits.

Comparison of the voltage map with the activation map can also be helpful. With activation mapping, more than 85% of the automatic markings of endocardial activation timing can be inaccurate at sites of low-amplitude fractionated potentials.[6] These sites require manual adjustment of the activation timing. In addition, far-field electrical events, especially with a larger tip distal electrode, are prone to imprecise measurements of activation timing.[6] Superimposition of a bipolar voltage map on the activation map can help to define the significance of low-amplitude fractionated potentials, because these areas may correlate with local myocardial activation within myocardial scar and thus suggest a macroreentrant atrial tachyarrhythmia.[6] After creation of an electroanatomic map, entrainment mapping from the various sites in the right and left atria is

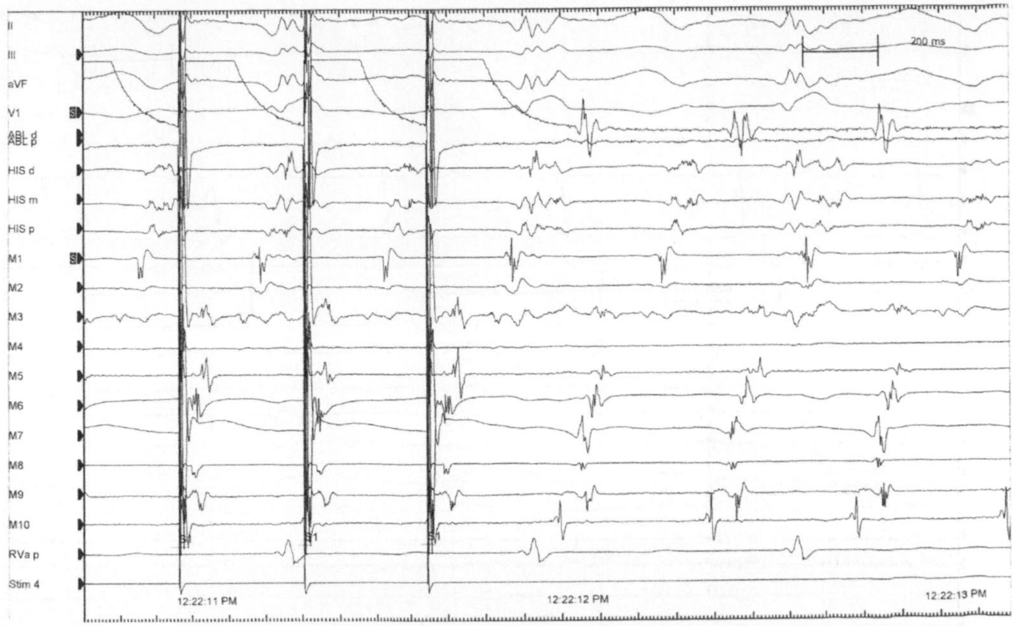

Fig. 3. Surface ECG and intracardiac electrograms during atrial flutter. Surface ECG leads are arranged in descending order of leads II, III, avF, and V1. The duodecapolar catheter was arranged with the distal tip (M1) in the midcoronary sinus and M4 in the cavotricuspid isthmus. Atrial flutter cycle length was 390 milliseconds, and the postpacing interval at the distal ablation catheter was 391 milliseconds. Entrainment from the ablation catheter positioned at M7 replicated the intracardiac electrogram activation sequence during atrial flutter on M8 to M1. ABLd, distal ablation catheter bipole; ABLp, proximal ablation catheter bipole; HISd, His distal bipole; HISm, His midbipole; HISp, His proximal bipole; M1, duodecapolar 1 to 2 bipole; M2, duodecapolar 3 to 4 bipole; M3, duodecapolar 5 to 6 bipole; M4, duodecapolar 7 to 8 bipole; M5, duodecapolar 9 to 10 bipole; M6, duodecapolar 11 to 12 bipole; M7, duodecapolar 13 to 14 bipole; M8, duodecapolar 15 to 16 bipole; M9, duodecapolar 17 to 18 bipole; M10, duodecapolar 19 to 20 bipole; RVAp, proximal right ventricular apex bipole.

performed to define the mechanism and to localize the circuit of the atrial tachyarrhythmia.

After CTI-dependent flutter, incisional reentry flutters are the second most common type of atrial tachyarrhythmia in patients with previous cardiac surgery.[3,5] With a right lateral atriotomy, the most common circuit of an incisional reentry atrial flutter is around the atriotomy scar. With activation mapping, the site of the atriotomy can be identified by the presence of split potentials that fuse to a single potential at the cranial and caudal ends of the atriotomy. In this case, the history of multiple cardiac surgeries, the history of a surgical right atrial maze procedure, and the presence of low voltage in the posterolateral RA impaired precise mapping of the atriotomy dimensions. In addition, the history of multiple previous surgeries in conjunction with the atrial flutter activation map suggests that 2 adjacent atriotomies created a protected central isthmus facilitating a dual-loop reentry atrial flutter circuit (**Fig. 4**). The electroanatomic activation map of the atrial flutter and the result of the flutter ablation suggest that the posterior limb of the dual-loop circuit likely represented the dominant limb. This conclusion is based on the evidence that (1) the activation map of the posterior limb shows larger isochrones along the posterior limb of the circuit (indicating a faster conduction velocity); (2) the initial ablation lesions from the posterolateral RA to the site of entrainment produced a spontaneous lengthening of the atrial flutter cycle length (indicating successful ablation of the posterior limb and transition to the anterior limb for maintenance of the second atrial flutter); and (3) despite spontaneous termination of the slower cycle length flutter during ablation of the anterior limb, the flutter remained inducible, suggesting a protected isthmus that had not been ablated. The ablation lesion that terminated the atrial flutter and rendered the flutter noninducible was a lesion in the midposterolateral RA adjacent to the original site of concealed entrainment with a favorable PPI versus TCL. Previous mapping at this site was notable for the presence of low-amplitude electrograms and likely represented poor myocardial contact with the trabeculated RA. This case shows the importance of ensuring adequate myocardial contact during voltage and activation mapping of low-voltage myocardium. Intracardiac echocardiography can be useful to

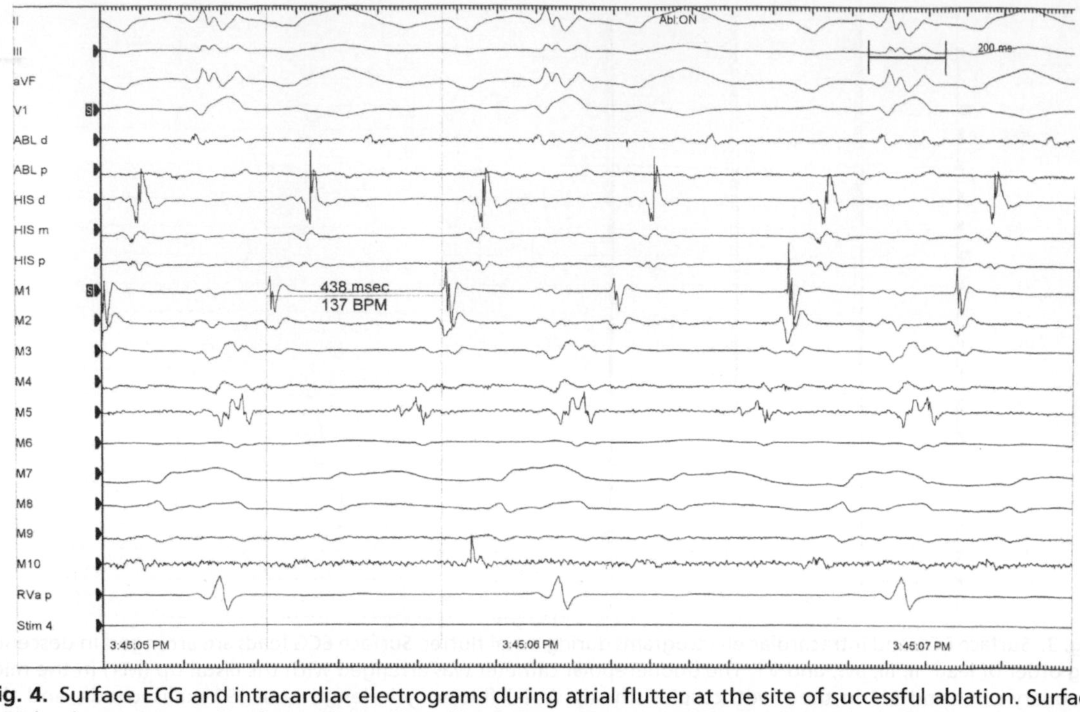

Fig. 4. Surface ECG and intracardiac electrograms during atrial flutter at the site of successful ablation. Surface ECG leads are arranged in descending order of leads II, III, avF, and V1. The duodecapolar catheter was arranged with the distal tip (M1) in the midcoronary sinus and M4 in the cavotricuspid isthmus. The atrial flutter cycle length was 438 milliseconds. Note the mid-diastolic electrogram on ABLd that was mapped to a site adjacent to the site of concealed entrainment in **Fig. 3**. Ablation at this site terminated the atrial flutter within 7 seconds and rendered it noninducible. ABLd, distal ablation catheter bipole: ABLp, proximal ablation catheter bipole; HISd, His distal bipole; HISm, His midbipole; HISp, His proximal bipole; M1, duodecapolar 1 to 2 bipole; M2, duodecapolar 3 to 4 bipole; M3, duodecapolar 5 to 6 bipole; M4, duodecapolar 7 to 8 bipole; M5, duodecapolar 9 to 10 bipole; M6, duodecapolar 11 to 12 bipole; M7, duodecapolar 13 to 14 bipole; M8, duodecapolar 15 to 16 bipole; M9, duodecapolar 17 to 18 bipole; M10, duodecapolar 19 to 20 bipole; RVAp, proximal right ventricular apex bipole.

verify catheter contact in areas of interest and reduce errors in mapping secondary to poor contact.[8]

SUMMARY

Multiple atrial tachyarrhythmias are common in patients with previous cardiac surgery. These arrhythmias are usually macroreentrant circuits that require a combination of activation and entrainment mapping to define the circuit and the site for successful ablation. Electroanatomic mapping is useful for defining the circuit and the substrate of these tachyarrhythmias. High-density mapping of myocardial scar can identify the protected isthmus of macroreentrant circuits critical to the tachycardia.

REFERENCES

1. Chan DP, Van Hare GF, Mackall JA, et al. Importance of atrial flutter isthmus in postoperative intra-atrial reentrant tachycardia. Circulation 2000; 102:1283–9.
2. Kalman JM, VanHare GF, Olgin JE, et al. Ablation of 'incisional' reentrant atrial tachycardia complicating surgery for congenital heart disease. Use of entrainment to define a critical isthmus of conduction. Circulation 1996;93:502–12.
3. Lukac P, Pedersen AK, Mortensen PT, et al. Ablation of atrial tachycardia after surgery for congenital and acquired heart disease using an electroanatomic mapping system: which circuits to expect in which substrate? Heart Rhythm 2005;2:64–72.
4. Seiler J, Schmid DK, Irtel TA, et al. Dual-loop circuits in postoperative atrial macro re-entrant tachycardias. Heart 2007;93:325–30.
5. Verma A, Marrouche NF, Seshadri N, et al. Importance of ablating all potential right atrial flutter circuits in postcardiac surgery patients. J Am Coll Cardiol 2004;44:409–14.
6. de Groot NM, Schalij MJ, Zeppenfeld K, et al. Voltage and activation mapping: how the recording technique

affects the outcome of catheter ablation procedures in patients with congenital heart disease. Circulation 2003;108:2099–106.
7. Akar JG, Al-Chekakie MO, Hai A, et al. Surface electrocardiographic patterns and electrophysiologic characteristics of atrial flutter following modified radiofrequency MAZE procedures. J Cardiovasc Electrophysiol 2007;18:349–55.
8. Kean AC, Gelehrter SK, Shetty I, et al. Experience with CartoSound for arrhythmia ablation in pediatric and congenital heart disease patients. J Interv Card Electrophysiol 2010;29:139–45.

Atypical Atrial Flutter with Typical-Appearing Pattern on ECG

Raphael K. Sung, MD, Gregory M. Marcus, MD, MAS*

KEYWORDS

• Catheter ablation • Atrial flutter • Atypical flutter • Pulmonary vein isolation

KEY POINTS

- Atypical left atrial flutter, particularly near the septum, may mimic typical cavotricuspid isthmus–dependent flutter on 12-lead electrocardiogram.
- Careful examination of lead V_1 may help identify atypical flutter, particularly when V_1 is broad based or has a double hump.
- Entrainment criteria only indicate the location of the circuit and not the critical limb of the tachycardia. Further evaluation is needed to identify the critical area to terminate the arrhythmia.
- When using 3-dimensional electroanatomic mapping, high-density mapping in the regions of interest is needed to help identify potential channels, identifying the critical limb of the tachycardia.

CLINICAL HISTORY

A 67-year-old man was referred to the electrophysiology (EP) service for evaluation of atrial flutter. He noted an episode of chest discomfort associated with palpitations for 15 to 20 minutes. Exercise stress testing was performed and revealed that the patient had atrial flutter that reproduced most of his symptoms. The patient was subsequently referred for EP study and ablation.

IMAGING FINDINGS

A 12-lead electrocardiogram (ECG) demonstrated broad, positive flutter wave deflections in V_1 as well as negative flutter waves in the inferior leads, consistent with typical flutter (**Fig. 1**).

LABORATORY FINDINGS

All are within normal limits.

PHYSICAL EXAMINATION FINDINGS

All are within normal limits.

CLINICAL COURSE

A duodecapolar catheter was placed around the tricuspid annulus, quadripolar catheters placed in the His-bundle region and the right ventricular apex, and a decapolar catheter into the coronary sinus. The initial activation sequence within the right atrium was not consistent with typical cavotricuspid isthmus (CTI)–dependent atrial flutter (**Fig. 2**). Entrainment from within the CTI as well as both lateral and septal to the CTI showed that this area was outside of the circuit, with a postpacing interval (PPI) greater than 30 ms of the tachycardia cycle length (TCL).

Several additional sites within the right atrium were selected for entrainment mapping and showed that the midseptum was the only location with a PPI within 30 ms of TCL. An area in the

Section of Electrophysiology, Division of Cardiology, University of California, San Francisco, San Francisco, CA, USA

* Corresponding author. UCSF Cardiac Electrophysiology, 500 Parnassus, MUE 434, San Francisco, CA, 94143.
E-mail address: marcusg@medicine.ucsf.edu

Card Electrophysiol Clin 4 (2012) 557–562
http://dx.doi.org/10.1016/j.ccep.2012.08.004
1877-9182/12/$ – see front matter

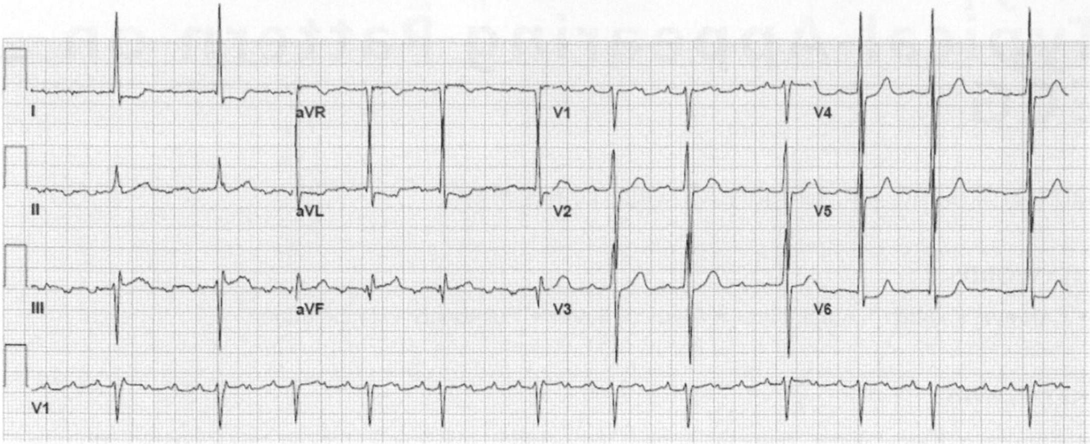

Fig. 1. Twelve-lead ECG performed during clinical atrial flutter. The overall pattern of flutter waves are consistent with typical counterclockwise atrial flutter, with positive deflections in V_1 and negative deflections in II, III and aVF. However, on closer analysis of V_1, the positive deflection is broad with a double hump, consistent with atypical atrial flutter near the left atrial septum.

midright septum with a PPI equal to the TCL and low-amplitude complex fractionation (see **Fig. 2**) was identified, but delivery of radiofrequency energy using an internally irrigated 4-mm catheter (Chili, Boston Scientific, Natick, Massachusetts) had no effect. A single transseptal puncture was then performed to pursue activation and substrate mapping of the left atrium. Entrainment mapping was again performed at several sites within the left atrium, including the left superior and inferior pulmonary veins; right common pulmonary vein (RCPV); lateral, posterior, and septal walls; and left atrial roof. The PPI was within 30 ms around the RCPV antrum, with the PPI closely matching the TCL near the inferior border of the RCPV (at the 3-o'clock position).

Mapping with a 3-dimensional (3D) electroanatomic mapping system (ESI, St Jude Medical, St Paul, Minnesota) confirmed a macroreentrant circuit around the area of the RCPV that encompassed the tachycardia cycle length (**Fig. 3**). A linear ablation line was performed connecting the inferior border of the RCPV to the mitral annulus without affecting the tachycardia. A higher-density 3D mapping was performed evaluating the potential tachycardia circuit around the right common pulmonary vein. An area in the anterosuperior aspect of the RCPV was shown to have low-amplitude, complex diastolic fractionation (**Fig. 4**). On careful evaluation of the resulting map, a figure-of-8 circuit was hypothesized as depicted in **Fig. 3**. The decision was made to perform a full pulmonary vein isolation rather than segmental ablation of the RCPV to prevent any future atrial arrhythmias that may result from the RCPV. During the pulmonary vein isolation ablation, the tachycardia cycle length slowed down from 240 ms to 280 ms, with ablation in the posterosuperior aspect of the RCPV. The tachycardia terminated with ablation in the anterosuperior aspect. However, pulmonary vein potentials demonstrating a connection to the left atrium persisted, and a complete circumferential ablation was performed until entrance and exit block was demonstrated.

Following electrical isolation of the RCPV, burst pacing and extrastimuli testing from the left atrium, right atrium, and coronary sinus failed to induce any arrhythmias.

QUESTIONS

1. Are there any ECG findings that help distinguish typical right atrial cavotricuspid isthmus–dependent flutter from atypical left-sided atrial flutter?
2. What findings from the intracardiac electrograms in **Fig. 2** indicate that this is likely a poor site for flutter termination?

DIAGNOSIS

The diagnosis was atypical left-sided atrial flutter, likely with a figure-of-8 double loop around the right common pulmonary vein (see **Fig. 3**).

DISCUSSION

The initial 12-lead ECG analysis is helpful to determine whether the atrial flutter is suggestive of typical atrial flutter. As is well recognized, typical counterclockwise (CCW) flutter is characterized

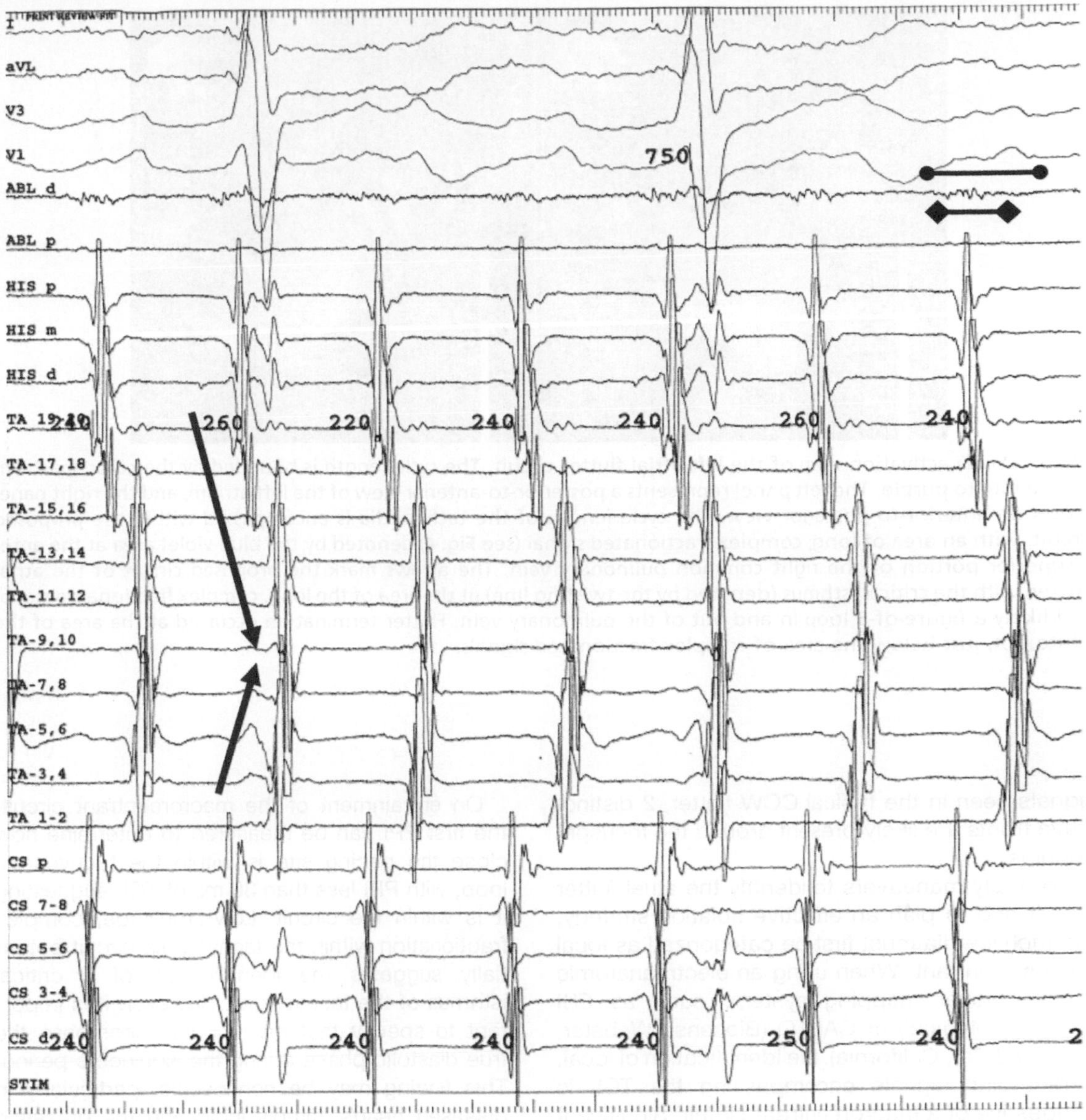

Fig. 2. Intracardiac electrograms demonstrating an activation sequence that is not consistent with typical counterclockwise atrial flutter. The 2 single arrows indicate that there are 2 wave fronts of atrial activation around the tricuspid annulus. On the top right, the line bounded by 2 circles indicates the duration of the flutter waves on the surface leads. The line bounded by 2 diamonds denotes duration of the complex, low-amplitude atrial signal at the midright atrial septum on the ablator distal electrodes. Surface leads I, aVL, V3, and V_1 are shown. ABL, ablator; CS, coronary sinus (with 1–2 as most distal and 9–10 as most proximal); d, distal; HIS, His bundle; m, mid; p, proximal; TA, duodecapolar around the tricuspid annulus (with 1–2 as most distal [lateral to the cavotricuspid isthmus] and 19–20 as most proximal).

by a negative flutter wave in the inferior leads and positive or biphasic (positive-negative) flutter waves in V_1 and the reverse for typical clockwise flutter. However, atypical left atrial flutter may mimic the typical CCW flutter pattern as seen in this patient, with positive deflection in V_1 and negative deflection in the inferior leads.[1,2] It has been suggested that this type of atypical flutter can be identified by the presence of a broad-based positive flutter deflection in V_1, sometimes with a double hump.[1,2] On closer inspection of the patient's 12-lead ECG, this finding is, in fact, observed. The intracardiac activation pattern of the duodecapolar catheter in the tricuspid annulus position demonstrates a non–CTI-dependent tachycardia (see **Fig. 2**). Rather than a linear activation pattern of

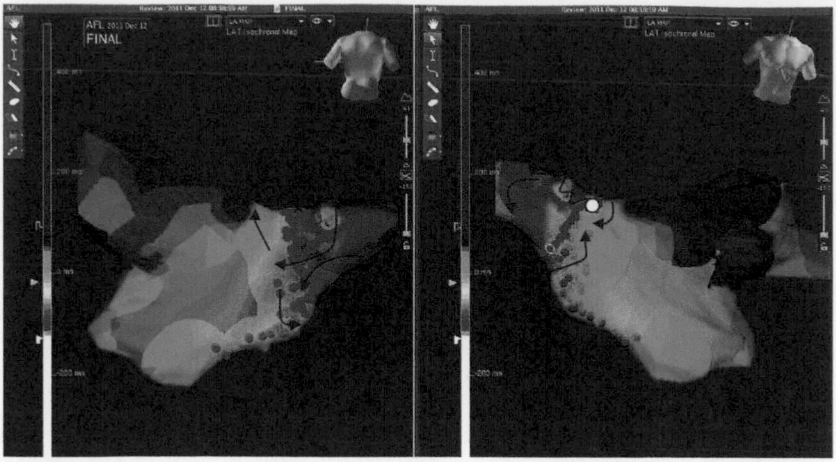

Fig. 3. ESI 3D activation map of the left atrial flutter circuit. The cycle length is bounded by the color spectrum from white to purple. The left panel represents a posterior-to-anterior view of the left atrium, and the right panel shows an anterior-to-posterior view. The cycle length of the tachycardia is encompassed within the proposed circuit, with an area of long, complex fractionated signal (see **Fig. 4**) denoted by the blue-violet area at the anterosuperior portion of the right common pulmonary vein. The arrows mark the proposed circuit of the atrial flutter, with the critical isthmus (denoted by the twisting line) at the area of the long, complex fractionated signal and likely a figure-of-8 loop in and out of the pulmonary vein. Flutter termination occurred at the area of the white dot, just below the area of complex fractionated signals.

signals seen in the typical CCW flutter, 2 distinct wave fronts are likely present around the tricuspid annulus.

To apply maneuvers to identify the atrial flutter circuit and to plan an effective ablation strategy, the tachycardia must first be categorized as focal versus reentrant. When using an electroanatomic 3-dimensional mapping system, such as ESI (St Jude Medical) or CARTO (Biosense Webster, Diamond Bar, California), the identification of local, intracardiac signals encompassing the TCL is suggestive of a macroreentrant circuit. Significant myocardial disease with slowed atrial conduction can mimic this phenomenon despite a focal origin. A more specific criterion of reentrant rhythms is fulfilled when entrainment criteria are met.[3] During overdrive pacing the tachycardia at a slightly faster cycle length than TCL, 3 characteristics must be present: (1) constant fusion during pacing assessed from either intracardiac electrograms (ICE) or ECG; (2) progressive fusion as the pacing rate is increased (either ICE or ECG); and (3) orthodromic wave front block terminates tachycardia and changes the activation sequence. It is important to apply these criteria because focal atrial tachycardia may exhibit consistent PPI-TCL intervals. In addition, a microreentrant circuit may appear focal on an electroanatomic map but will still fulfill these entrainment criteria.

On entrainment of the macroreentrant circuit, the first PPI can be measured to determine how close the pacing site is within the tachycardia loop, with PPI less than 30 ms of TCL suggesting it is within the circuit. Low-amplitude, complex fractionation within the tachycardia circuit potentially suggests the identification of a critical isthmus of the tachycardia. However, it is important to specify that this should encompass the true diastolic phase during the isoelectric period. This finding may be nonspecific, particularly in diseased hearts, simply indicating the presence of scar. **Fig. 2** shows that the complex fractionation starts at the beginning and ends at the middle of the flutter wave; although unlikely to terminate tachycardia, ablation was still attempted before performing a transseptal puncture.

In this case, at first glance, the ESI activation map (see **Fig. 3**) suggests a focal atrial tachycardia originating from within the RCPV and exiting the vein at the posteroinferior aspect. However, rigorous entrainment criteria demonstrated a macroreentrant circuit as described earlier. On closer inspection of the activation map in **Fig. 3**, just inside the site of termination marked by a white dot, there was an area of low-amplitude, complex fractionation spanning throughout the atrial flutter diastolic period (see **Fig. 4**), implicating its functional role as the zone of slow conduction

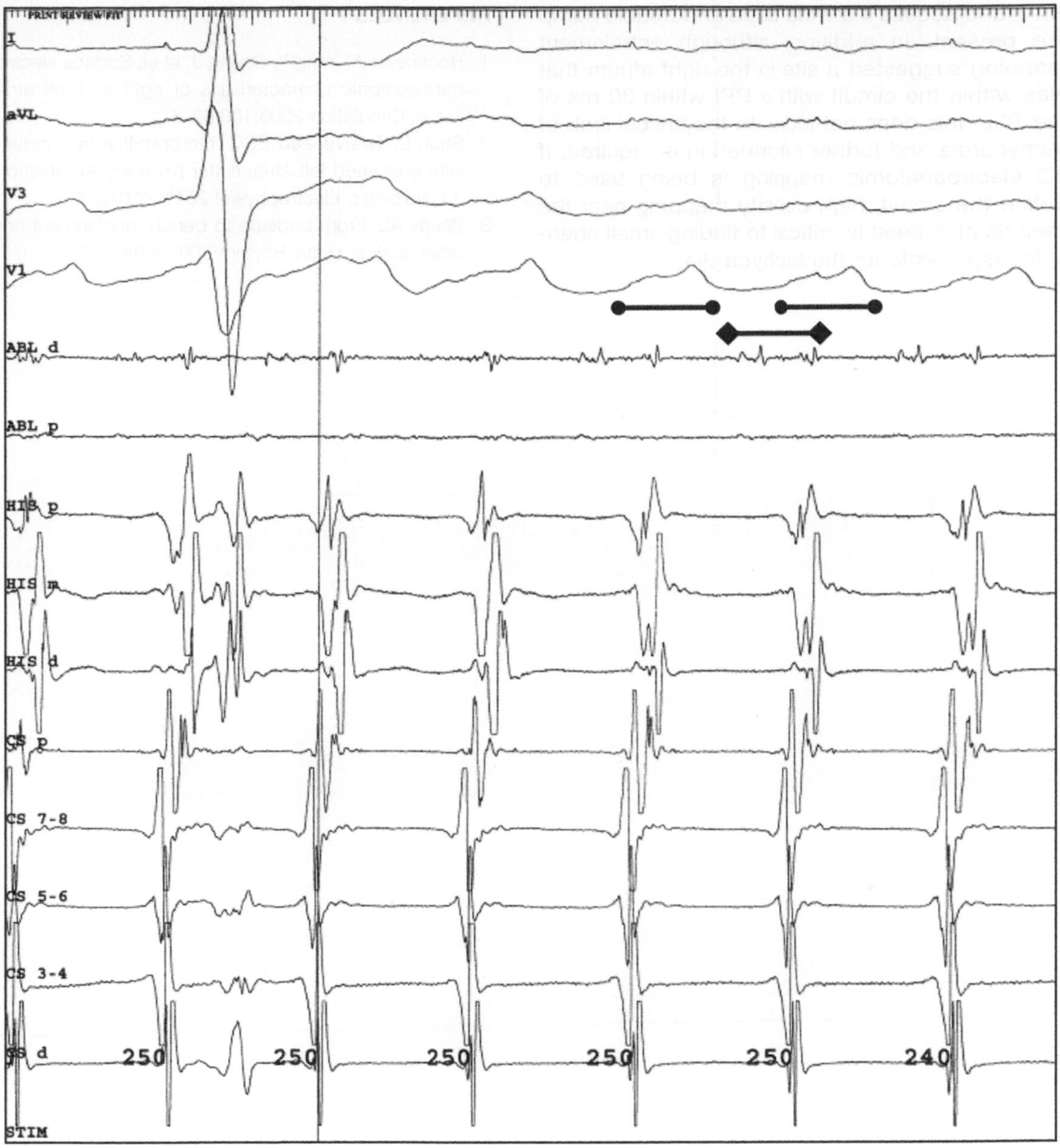

Fig. 4. Intracardiac electrograms demonstrating long, small-amplitude, complex fractionated signal at the anterosuperior region of the right common pulmonary vein. This corresponds to the area of the twisting line just above the white dot in **Fig. 3**. The line bounded by 2 circles indicates the duration of the flutter waves on the surface leads. The line bounded by 2 diamonds denotes the duration of the complex, low-amplitude atrial signal at the anterosuperior region of the RCPV on the ablator distal electrodes, just above where ablation terminated tachycardia during pulmonary vein isolation. Surface leads I, aVL, V3, and V_1 are shown. ABL, ablator; CS, coronary sinus (with 1–2 as most distal and 9–10 as most proximal); d, distal; HIS, His bundle; m, mid; p, proximal.

(isthmus). Consequently, the flutter was not terminated by a mitral annular line connecting the RCPV to the mitral annulus and only terminated when that area was transected during the pulmonary vein isolation.

SUMMARY

This case clearly describes an atypical atrial flutter that at first glance seems to have a typical flutter appearance on ECG. However, careful inspection of lead V_1 is necessary, with the preparation of left-sided access if a wide base and double hump are present. In addition, although entrainment mapping suggested a site in the right atrium that was within the circuit with a PPI within 30 ms of the TCL, this does not indicate the critical limb of tachycardia and further information is required. If 3D electroanatomic mapping is being used to define the circuit, high-density mapping near the regions of interest is critical to finding small channels responsible for the tachycardia.

REFERENCES

1. Bochoeyer A, Yang Y, Cheng J, et al. Surface electrocardiographic characteristics of right and left atrial flutter. Circulation 2003;108:60–6.
2. Shah D. Twelve-lead ECG interpretation in a patient with presumed left atrial flutter following AF ablation. J Cardiovasc Electrophysiol 2011;22:613–7.
3. Waldo AL. From bedside to bench: entrainment and other stories. Heart Rhythm 2004;1:94–106.

Cycle Length Alternans During Ablation of Cavotricuspid Isthmus–Dependent Atrial Flutter

Bharat K. Kantharia, MD, FRCP, FESC

KEYWORDS

• Atrial flutter • Cavotricuspid isthmus • Radiofrequency ablation

KEY POINTS

- A beat-by-beat cycle length alternans of cavotricuspid atrial flutter is a rare phenomenon.
- Cycle length alternans seen in atrial flutter may occur due to an exaggerated mechanoelectric feedback (ie, variation in atrial pressure and volume on a beat-to-beat basis).
- Cycle length alternans observed during ablation of cavotricuspid isthmus (CTI) for atrial flutter may occur as a result of dissociation of conduction within the isthmus resulting from changes in the electrophysiologic properties that may occur from the ablation lesions.

CASE PRESENTATION

A 55-year-old man with a history of hypertensive heart disease and symptomatic atrial flutter (AFL) was referred for radiofrequency (RF) ablation therapy. The patient was taking ramipril for hypertension and only digoxin for AFL. Physical examination was unremarkable. Transthoracic echocardiogram revealed mild left atrial enlargement with left ventricular hypertrophy and normal ejection fraction.

Invasive electrophysiology study performed with a duodecapolar catheter, a decapolar catheter, and a quadripolar catheter placed at the lateral right atrium (RA) along the tricuspid valve annulus, coronary sinus (CS), and septally at the His bundle region, respectively, showed typical counterclockwise AFL at a steady and stable cycle length of 210 milliseconds with 2:1 and 3:1 ventricular conduction. The intracardiac electrogram recordings, a 3-D electroanatomic CARTO (Biosense-Webster, Diamond Bar, California) activation mapping performed during tachycardia, and concealed entrainment at CTI confirmed the tachycardia to be a typical counterclockwise CTI-dependent AFL. To make a linear line of conduction block through CTI, RF ablation was commenced along the CTI using an open-irrigated 3.5-mm–tip ThermoCool catheter (Biosense-Webster, Diamond Bar, California) at a power setting of 30 W. RF lesions were applied for 60 seconds and were guided by local electrograms, fluoroscopy, and CARTO imaging. The initial lesion was applied at the ventricular aspect, and the catheter was dragged toward the atrial aspect on marked diminution and/or elimination of atrial electrograms. Potential mechanisms for the observed change/s that occurred after initial

Disclosure for conflict of interest: None.
Division of Clinical Cardiac Electrophysiology, The University of Texas Health Science Center at Houston, 6431 Fannin Street, Suite MSB 1.246, Houston, TX 77030, USA
E-mail address: bkantharia@yahoo.com

Card Electrophysiol Clin 4 (2012) 563–566
http://dx.doi.org/10.1016/j.ccep.2012.08.006
1877-9182/12/$ – see front matter

RF lesions, as shown in **Fig. 1**, and further course during the procedure are discussed.

DISCUSSION

Fig. 1 shows recordings from the surface ECG leads and intracardiac electrograms that were obtained after initial RF lesions. A regular irregularity in the AFL cycle length (ie, cycle length alternans [250 milliseconds and 210 milliseconds]) in the duodecapolar catheter, with similar atrial activation sequence as recorded by the His, duodecapolar, ablation, and CS catheters with 2:1 ventricular conduction is seen. The cycle length, however, as recorded in the septal (His) and the left atrium (CS poles), remains virtually fixed at 250 milliseconds.

The observed cycle length alternans seen in this case may be due to an exaggerated mechanoelectric feedback that occurred after creation of RF lesions. It is possible that with 2:1 ventricular conduction, a greater beat-by-beat volume change occurs in the normal-sized RA than a dilated left atrium. The cycle length in the left atrium, therefore, remains fixed. Typical AFL is considered a highly regular rhythm, barring some reports on small variations in cycle length.[1–3] During spontaneous oscillations, the variability of AFL cycle length has been demonstrated as small (ie, approximately 5 milliseconds).[2,3] The mechanoelectric feedback influenced by (1) ventricular contraction, (2) the phases of respiration, and (3) the autonomic nervous system can potentially cause variation in atrial pressure, volume, and, thus, cycle length of AFL on a beat-to-beat basis. Studies conducted before the era of RF ablation that used power spectral analysis techniques have shown that there is an inherent periodic pattern to spontaneous AFL cycle length, with beat-to-beat cycle length variability composed of 2 oscillations: 1 prevalent at the frequency of ventricular contraction and 1 at the

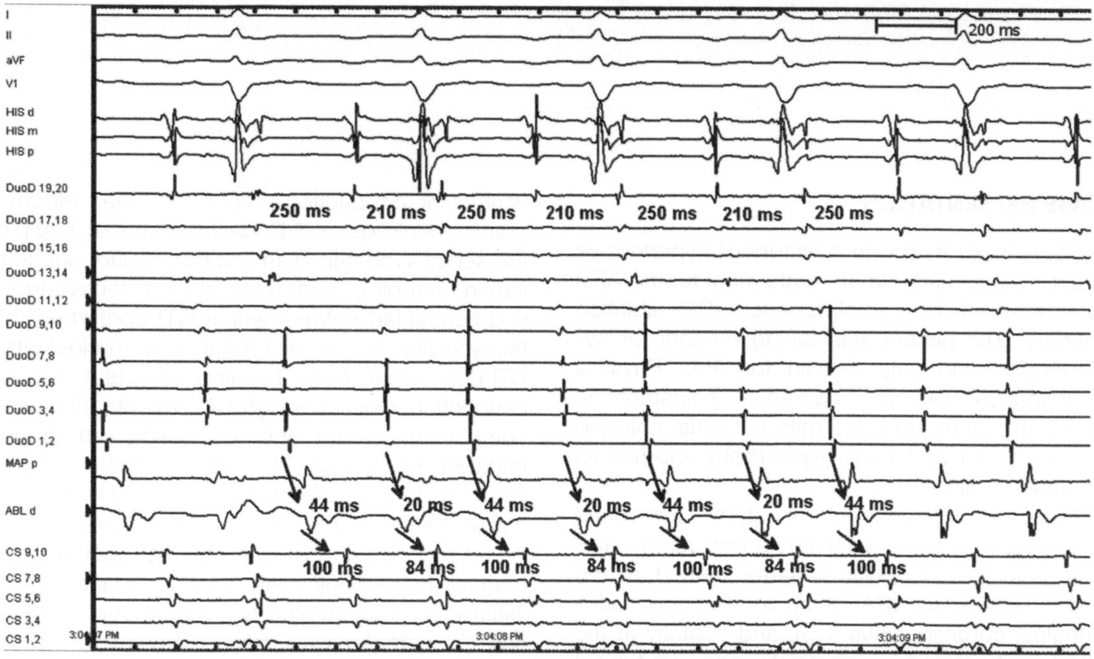

Fig. 1. Intracardiac recordings of the arrhythmia during ablation are shown (paper speed, 100 mm/s). The channels show recordings from surface leads I and II, aVF, and V1; the His bundle: His d (distal), His m (mid), and His p (proximal); duodecapolar catheter placed along the tricuspid annulus: DuoD (1–2 = distal, 9–10 = mid, and 19–20 = proximal); the proximal and distal ablation poles: MAP (mapping) p and ABL (ablation) d; and the CS (1–2 = distal, 5–6 = mid, and 9–10 = proximal). Cycle length alternans (250 milliseconds and 210 milliseconds), but with the same counterclockwise atrial activation sequence of atrial flutter, is seen in the duodecapolar catheter. In the CS and His channels, tachycardia at fixed cycle length of 250 milliseconds is seen. Total activation time from the lower lateral RA through the isthmus to the CS os is longer at 144 milliseconds (the lower lateral RA pole of the duodecapolar catheter to the ablation catheter at the mid-isthmus (*vertically slanted arrows*) = 44 milliseconds and the ablation catheter to the CS os (*horizontally slanted arrows*) = 100 milliseconds) and is longer for the wavefront after shorter cycle length compared with 104 milliseconds (the lower lateral RA pole of the duodecapolar catheter to the ablation catheter at the midisthmus = 20 milliseconds and the ablation catheter to the CS os = 84 milliseconds) for the wavefront after longer cycle length.

frequency of respiration.[2,3] Both ventricular and respiratory oscillations are independent of autonomic tone because they persist after autonomic blockade and can be observed in patients after heart transplantation.[2,3]

Independent of mechanical function, several "electrophysiological" mechanisms can be postulated and considered, such as the lower loop and upper loop reentries and the intraisthmus reentry.[4,5]

Fig. 2 shows a schematic representation of different wavefronts to explain changes observed in **Fig. 1**. Early breakthroughs at duodecapolar 5–6 poles indicate the possibility of short-circuiting of the orthodromic wavefront through the low terminal crest and reentry to the RA from the posterior aspect of the inferior vena cava (IVC). Such short-circuiting of the wavefront, coupled with dissociation of electric conduction of activation wavefront through 2 zones within the CTI due to different conduction properties after RF ablation, remains a likely explanation of the observation. The 2 zones were composed of (1) a gap between the lesions in the anterior CTI and (2) the remaining atrial aspect of the posterior CTI posterior to RF lesion #2. Possibly due to acute effects of RF energy, significant slowing in conduction of the wavefront occurred in the anterior CTI zone near the gap compared with the posterior CTI. The total activation time from the lower lateral RA to the CS os was longer at 144 milliseconds (44 milliseconds from the lower lateral RA pole of the duodecapolar catheter to the ablation catheter at the midisthmus

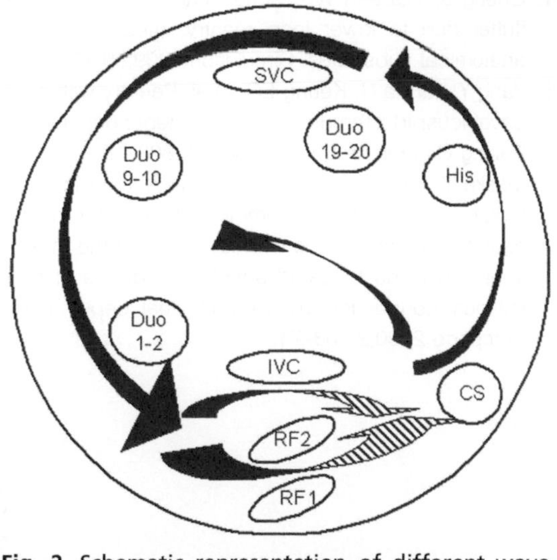

Fig. 2. Schematic representation of different wavefronts to explain changes observed in **Fig. 1**. RA and CTI represented in the left anterior oblique view. Duo, duodecapolar; His, His bundle region; RF, RF ablation lesion; SVC, superior vena cava.

and 100 milliseconds from the ablation catheter to the CS os) and was longer for the wavefront after short cycle length traveling though the gap compared with 104 milliseconds (20 milliseconds from the lower lateral RA pole of the duodecapolar catheter to the ablation catheter at the midisthmus and 84 milliseconds from the ablation catheter to the CS os) after longer cycle length when traveling through the nonablated posterior CTI (see **Fig. 1**). Thus, the cycle length of AFL in the left atrium remains fixed.

Entrainment mapping individually at these 2 sites would have strengthened the contended explanation of intraisthmus dissociation of conduction. Alternatively, it could be argued that given the small area involving conduction dissociation and smaller difference of 40 milliseconds between the cycle lengths, it would have been difficult to flawlessly delineate 2 circuits if pacing had captured adjacent circuit and/or the difference between the postpacing interval and the tachycardia cycle length measured 30 milliseconds (rather than zero), a number that is acceptable to define concealed entrainment. Likewise, creating 2 new separate activation CARTO maps taking individual cycle length would have helped. Again, the shortcomings were the situations of performing high-density maps involving a small area and capturing correct electrograms for individual tachycardia of different cycle length within the similar window of interest settings. For these reasons, repeat entrainment or activation CARTO mapping was not performed.

In some patients with dual conduction physiology of the CTI, a sudden jump in cycle length of AFL during segmental RF ablation of CTI may be observed. Such a jump in cycle length, however, is also associated with change in the activation sequence of the AFL wavefront. Such a phenomenon has been thought to result from dual septal exits both anterior and posterior to the CS os from dual circumferential muscle bundles in the CTI.[6]

With application of contiguous RF lesions in the zone of faster conduction property in the posterior CTI, the arrhythmia terminated (**Fig. 3**). Bidirectional conduction block through CTI was accomplished subsequently on further application of RF lesion at the gap between RF lesions #1 and #2.

Many times, changes in activation and cycle length of AFL during ablation are unnoticed or, when recognized, may lead to dilemmas in ablation strategies. Proper understanding of the exact mechanism, however complex, of any phenomenon is highly desirable but may not always be possible. In the case presented in this article, the explanations of the mechanisms of altered pattern

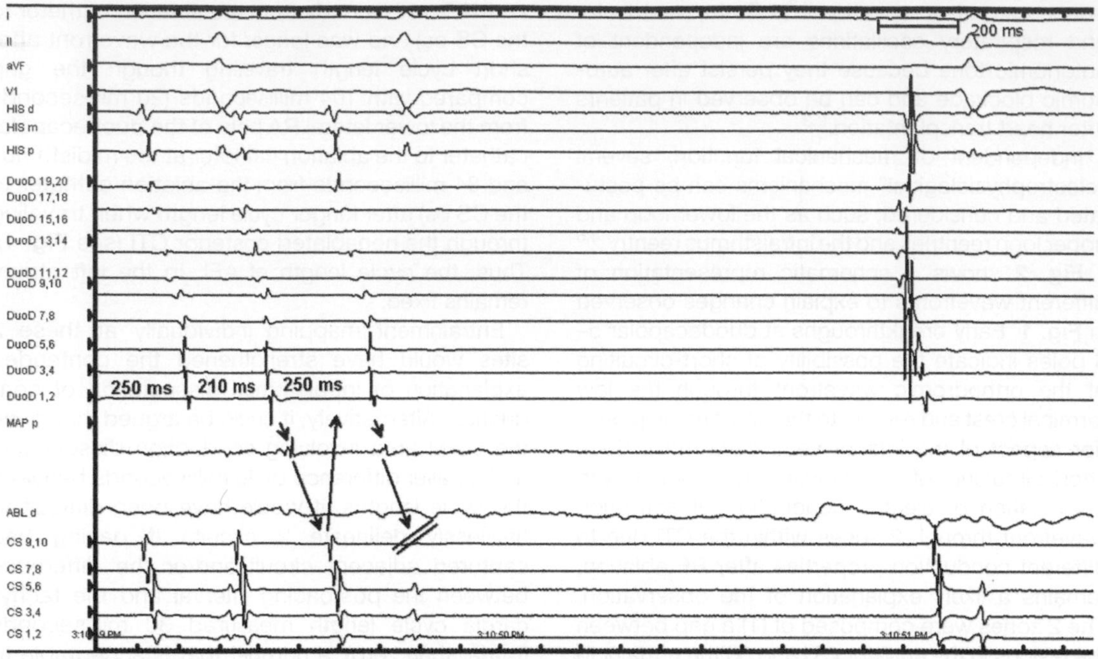

Fig. 3. Recording format (as in **Fig. 1**). The arrows (*two contiguous downward pointing small arrows and one larger upward pointing arrow*) indicate conduction and activation pattern through cavotricuspid isthmus (CTI). With application of contiguous RF lesions in the zone of faster conduction property in the posterior CTI, conduction through CTI is interrupted (*symbolically represented with two horizontally slanted bars after two contiguous small arrows*) resulting in termination of the arrhythmia.

and cycle length change discussed remain potentially circumstantial rather than absolutely conclusive. Nonetheless, such an exercise in considering and exploring different potential mechanisms to explain uncommon findings often yields valuable results and should be the standard of practice for electrophysiologists performing complex ablations.

REFERENCES

1. Wells JL, MacLean WA, James TN, et al. Characterization of atrial flutter: studies in man after open heart surgery using fixed atrial electrodes. Circulation 1979;60:665–73.
2. Stambler BS, Ellenbogen KA. Elucidating the mechanisms of atrial flutter cycle length variability using power spectral analysis techniques. Circulation 1996;94:2515–25.
3. Ravelli F, Mase M, Disertori M. Mechanical modulation of atrial flutter cycle length. Prog Biophys Mol Biol 2008;97:417–34.
4. Cheng J, Cabeen WR, Scheinman MM. Right atrial flutter due to lower loop reentry; mechanism and anatomical substrates. Circulation 1999;99:1700–5.
5. Yang Y, Varma N, Keung EC, et al. Reentry within the cavotricuspid isthmus: an isthmus dependent circuit. Pacing Clin Electrophysiol 2005;28:808–18.
6. Iesaka Y, Yamane T, Goya M, et al. A jump in cycle length of orthodromic common atrial flutter during catheter ablation at the isthmus between the inferior vena cava and tricuspid annulus; evidence of dual isthmus conduction directed to dual septal exits. Europace 2000;2:163–71.

Atrial Fibrillation

Fred Morady, MD

KEYWORDS

- Ablation • Atrial fibrillation • Pulmonary vein potentials

KEY POINTS

- A basic component of virtually all ablation strategies for atrial fibrillation is electrical isolation of the pulmonary venous muscle sleeves.
- The end point of pulmonary vein isolation is elimination of all pulmonary vein potentials, which indicates complete entrance block and exit block.
- It is important to distinguish pulmonary vein potentials from electrograms that can mimic them.

Catheter ablation of atrial fibrillation has become an increasingly used therapeutic option for patients who have been troubled with this arrhythmia. A basic component of virtually all ablation strategies for atrial fibrillation is electrical isolation of the pulmonary venous muscle sleeves. Pulmonary vein isolation typically is sufficient to eliminate paroxysmal atrial fibrillation and usually is a necessary component of the ablation strategy for persistent or longstanding persistent atrial fibrillation.[1]

During catheter ablation procedures, a multipolar ring catheter is positioned within the antrum or proximal portion of a pulmonary vein, where both atrial and pulmonary vein potentials are recorded. The end point of pulmonary vein isolation is elimination of all pulmonary vein potentials, which indicates complete entrance block and exit block. Although entrance block usually is accompanied by exit block, it is possible for the former to occur in the absence of the latter. Exit block is verified by the absence of atrial capture when pacing within a pulmonary vein or by the failure of spontaneous depolarizations within a pulmonary vein to conduct to the atrium.[2]

Pulmonary vein potentials must be distinguished from the atrial electrograms that can be recorded by the ring catheter. In the left pulmonary veins, an atrial electrogram recorded along the anterior aspect of the pulmonary veins can represent a far-field electrogram originating in the left atrial appendage. These electrograms can mimic pulmonary vein potentials but can be recognized as left atrial appendage electrograms by pacing within the left atrial appendage.[3] If an electrogram recorded within a pulmonary vein is drawn into the pacing stimulus, this confirms that it is a left atrial appendage electrogram. In the right superior pulmonary vein, small high-frequency electrograms recorded along the anterior aspect of the vein may originate in the superior vena cava or high right atrium, which lie immediately anterior to the right superior pulmonary vein. If the interval between the onset of the sinus P wave and the electrogram in question is less than 40 milliseconds, this indicates that the electrogram is most likely originating in the superior vena cava or right atrium, not in the right superior pulmonary vein.[4]

REFERENCES

1. Calkins H, Kuck KH, Cappato R, et al. 2012 HRS/EHRA/ECAS expert consensus statement on catheter and surgical ablation of atrial fibrillation: recommendations for patient selection, procedural techniques, patient management and follow-up, definitions,

University of Michigan Health System, 1500 East Medical Center Drive, Ann Arbor, MI 48109, USA
E-mail address: fmorady@med.umich.edu

Card Electrophysiol Clin 4 (2012) 567–568
http://dx.doi.org/10.1016/j.ccep.2012.08.008
1877-9182/12/$ – see front matter

endpoints, and research trial design. J Interv Card Electrophysiol 2012;33:171–257.

2. Gerstenfeld E, Dixit S, Callans D, et al. Utility of exit block for identifying electrical isolation of the pulmonary veins. J Cardiovasc Electrophysiol 2002;13:971–9.
3. Shah D, Haissaguerre M, Jais P, et al. Left atrial appendage activity masquerading as pulmonary vein potentials. Circulation 2002;105:2821–5.
4. Shah D, Burri H, Sunthorn H, et al. Identifying far-field superior vena cava potentials within the right superior pulmonary vein. Heart Rhythm 2006;3:898–902.

Is the Right Superior Pulmonary Vein Isolated?

Aman Chugh, MD[a,*], Fred Morady, MD[b]

KEYWORDS

• Atrial fibrillation • Catheter ablation • Pulmonary vein isolation • Far-field electrograms

KEY POINTS

- After pulmonary vein isolation, one may encounter potentials on the ring catheter recording of unclear origin and significance.
- The origin of these potentials can be determined with activation mapping or pacing maneuvers.
- These observations/maneuvers may help prevent unnecessary ablation of the pulmonary veins.

CASE HISTORY

A 58-year-old man underwent pulmonary vein (PV) isolation for paroxysmal atrial fibrillation. At the end of the procedure, the PVs were examined for reconnection. **Fig. 1**A shows the recording from the right superior PV, which shows sharp potential

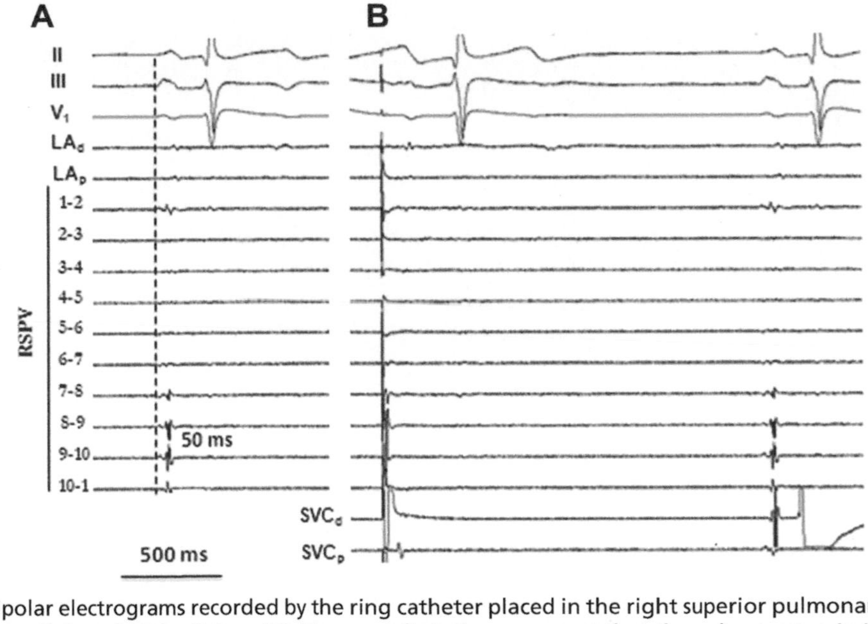

Fig. 1. (*A*) Bipolar electrograms recorded by the ring catheter placed in the right superior pulmonary vein (RSPV). The sharp potentials on bipoles 8–9 and 9–10 may at first glance suggest that the pulmonary vein is not isolated. The dashed line corresponds to the onset of the p-wave. LA, left atrial. Also displayed are electrocardiographic leads II, III, and V1. (*B*) Pacing from the superior vena cava (SVC) advances the potentials in question to the stimulus artifact, confirming an SVC origin. Hence, the pulmonary vein is isolated and no further ablation is required.

[a] Department of Internal Medicine, Cardiovascular Center, 1500 East Medical Center Drive, Floor 3, Ann Arbor, MI 48109, USA; [b] University of Michigan Health System, 1500 East Medical Center Drive, Cardiovascular Center, SPC 5853, Ann Arbor, MI 48109, USA
* Corresponding author.
E-mail address: achugh@med.umich.edu

Card Electrophysiol Clin 4 (2012) 569–570
http://dx.doi.org/10.1016/j.ccep.2012.08.014

on bipoles 8–9 and 9–10. Is the right superior PV isolated?

COMMENTARY

The possible origins of the potentials in question include the right atrium, superior vena cava (SVC), left atrium, and a PV connection. Pacing from the coronary sinus or the left atrial appendage is helpful in determining whether left-sided PVs are isolated, but pacing from these sites is not as helpful for right-sided PVs. A study by Shah and colleagues[1] showed that potentials recorded from right superior PVs that are within 30 milliseconds from the onset of the p-wave are likely (sensitivity 92%, specificity 100%) to be due to activation of the SVC. In this case, activation of the potentials in question is 50 milliseconds after the p-wave onset (see **Fig. 1**A), which may suggest a left atrial or PV origin. However, pacing (at an output just above the capture threshold) from the SVC advances these potentials to the pacing stimulus, confirming an SVC origin (**Fig. 1**B). In this case, delayed conduction into the SVC was responsible for the potentials being recorded >30 milliseconds after the onset of the p-wave. This maneuver confirmed complete isolation of the right superior PV and obviated the need for further radiofrequency ablation.

REFERENCE

1. Shah D, Burri H, Sunthorn H, et al. Identifying far-field superior vena cava potentials within the right superior pulmonary vein. Heart Rhythm 2006;3:898–902.

Is This Pulmonary Vein Isolated?

Fred Morady, MD

KEYWORDS

• Pulmonary vein • Atrium • Left superior pulmonary vein • Atrial fibrillation • Catheter ablation

KEY POINTS

- Unidirectional block is infrequent in pulmonary veins but is important to recognize because it may be responsible for recurrent atrial fibrillation after catheter ablation.
- If there is no automatic activity arising in a pulmonary vein after isolation, the only way to recognize unidirectional block is to pace inside the pulmonary vein through the electrodes of a ring catheter to look for conduction to the atrium.

CASE HISTORY

Circumferential antral ablation was performed in a 56-year-old man with paroxysmal atrial fibrillation. The electrograms shown in **Fig. 1** were recorded after circumferential ablation around the left superior pulmonary vein (LSPV). Is this pulmonary vein electrically isolated from the left atrium?

COMMENTARY

There is slow automatic activity arising in the LSPV, and this activity is dissociated from the sinus beats, indicating that there is complete entrance block. However, depending on the coupling interval between the last sinus beat and the pulmonary vein potentials, there is conduction

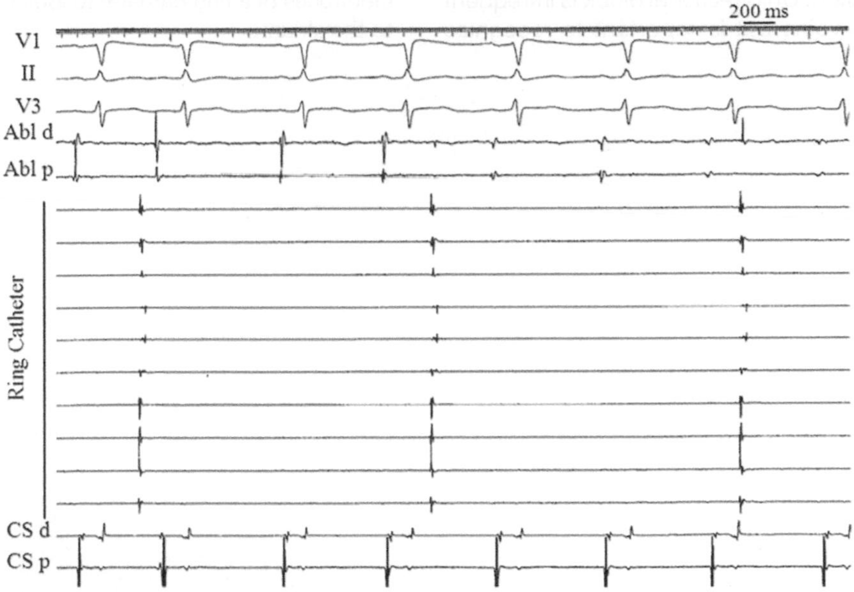

Fig. 1. Electrograms recorded with a ring catheter within the left superior pulmonary vein after circumferential antral ablation. The ablation catheter was positioned in the body of the left atrium. Abl, ablation catheter; cs, coronary sinus; d, distal; p, proximal.

University of Michigan Health System, 1500 East Medical Center Drive, Ann Arbor, MI 48109, USA
E-mail address: fmorady@med.umich.edu

Card Electrophysiol Clin 4 (2012) 571–572
http://dx.doi.org/10.1016/j.ccep.2012.08.015

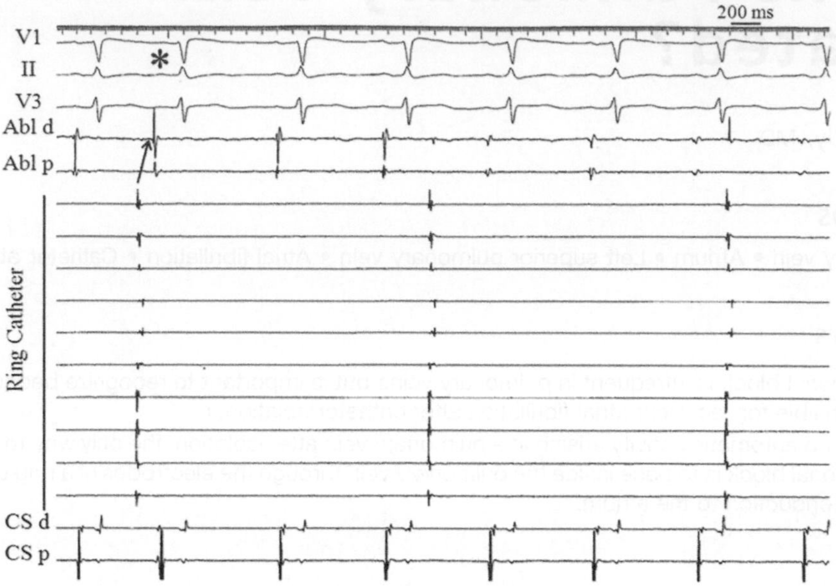

Fig. 2. The arrow marks the pulmonary vein potentials that are conducted from the left superior pulmonary vein to the left atrium, resulting in a premature atrial depolarization (*asterisk*).

from the LSPV to the left atrium, resulting in a premature atrial depolarization (**Fig. 2**). Therefore, this pulmonary vein is not completely isolated.

This case is an example of unidirectional block in a pulmonary vein. Unidirectional block is infrequent in pulmonary veins but is important to recognize because it may be responsible for recurrent atrial fibrillation after catheter ablation. If there is no automatic activity arising in a pulmonary vein after isolation, the only way to recognize unidirectional block is to pace inside the pulmonary vein through the electrodes of a ring catheter to look for conduction to the atrium.

Risks Associated with Extensive Left Atrial Ablation

Rakesh Latchamsetty, MD*, Aman Chugh, MD,
Fred Morady, MD

KEYWORDS

- Left atrial ablation • Atrial fibrillation • Pulmonary veins

KEY POINTS

- With extensive left atrial ablation, isolation or delayed activation of structures in addition to the pulmonary veins is possible.
- Caution should be used with further ablation.

CASE HISTORY

A 56-year-old man with 3 prior left atrial ablations for atrial fibrillation (AF) was referred for ablation for recurrent paroxysmal AF. **Fig. 1** shows a spontaneous premature atrial depolarization when the ring catheter was positioned in the left inferior pulmonary vein and a decapolar catheter was in the coronary sinus. Is this vein isolated?

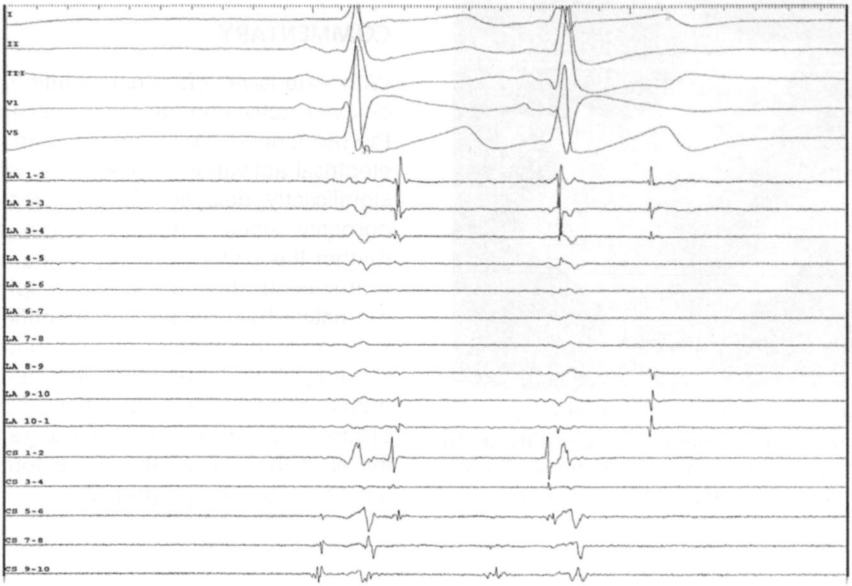

Fig. 1. A sinus beat followed by a premature atrial depolarization. The ring catheter is within the left inferior pulmonary vein. A decapolar catheter is positioned in the coronary sinus. CS, coronary sinus; La, lasso.

Department of Internal Medicine, University of Michigan Health System, 1500 East Medical Center Drive, Ann Arbor, MI 48109, USA
* Corresponding author.
E-mail address: rakeshl@umich.edu

Card Electrophysiol Clin 4 (2012) 573–574
http://dx.doi.org/10.1016/j.ccep.2012.08.016
1877-9182/12/$ – see front matter

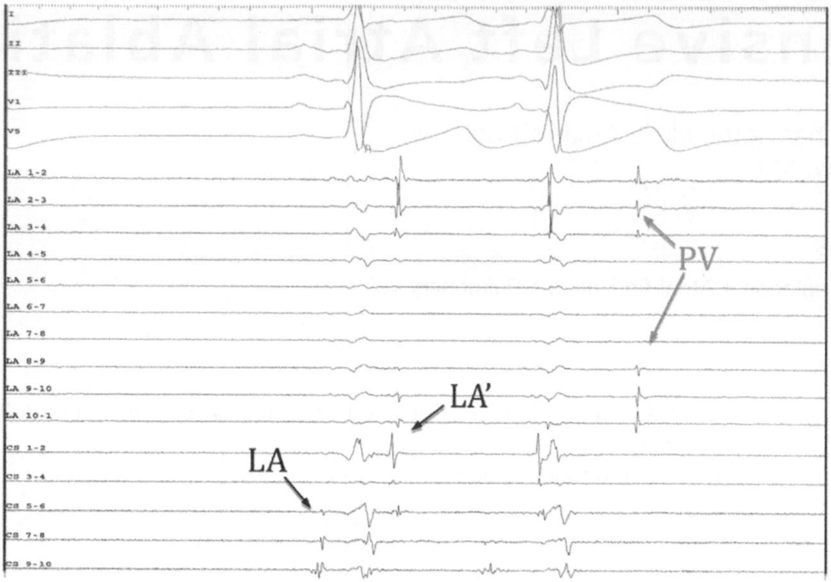

Fig. 2. Early (LA) and late (LA') left atrial activation is seen on the coronary sinus catheter. Pulmonary vein (PV) potentials are delayed following a premature atrial contraction.

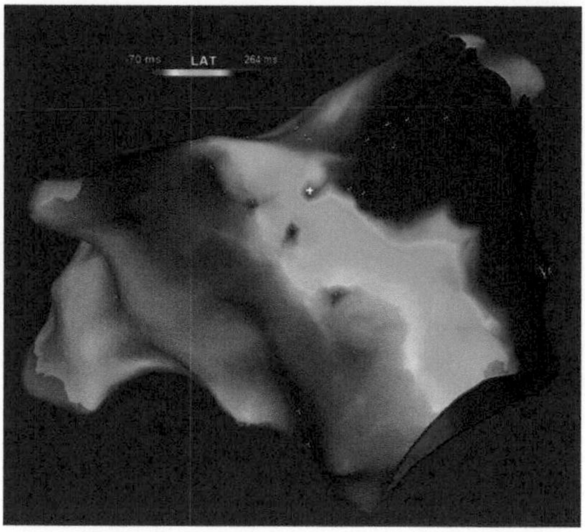

Fig. 3. Activation map using the Carto (Biosense Webster) electroanatomical mapping system illustrating the delayed activation of the lateral left atrium. The left atrium is shown in the anteroposterior projection.

What particular caution should be taken with further ablation in this patient?

COMMENTARY

With extensive left atrial ablation, isolation or delayed activation of structures in addition to the pulmonary veins is possible. In this example, electrical activation of the lateral left atrium was significantly delayed. This is depicted on the coronary sinus catheter, where during sinus rhythm the distal coronary sinus atrial electrograms occur after the QRS complex (**Fig. 2**). A premature beat delays and identifies the pulmonary vein potentials on the lasso catheter. Caution should be used with further ablation because of the risk of isolation of the lateral left atrium and left atrial appendage, which may increase the risk of thrombus formation in the left atrial appendage (**Fig. 3**).

Is This a Good Target Site for Ablation of an Atrial Tachycardia?

Aman Chugh, MD[a,*], Fred Morady, MD[b]

KEYWORDS

• Atrial fibrillation • Atrial tachycardia • Global capture • Mapping

KEY POINTS

- Tachycardia termination during pacing that does not result in global atrial capture is a very specific finding for identification of the critical site of the reentrant circuit.
- Radiofrequency energy delivery at such a site is highly effective in eliminating the tachycardia.

CASE HISTORY

A 68-year-old woman who had previously undergone pulmonary vein (PV) isolation for paroxysmal atrial fibrillation (AF) at another institution was referred for recurrent AF and tachycardia. After elimination of AF, which required reisolation of the PVs and radiofrequency (RF) ablation at the right atrial (RA) appendage, she developed a sustained atrial tachycardia (AT). A potential ablation site was found at the high posterior RA. Before RF energy delivery, phrenic nerve capture was ruled out by high-output pacing (**Fig. 1**). Should RF energy be delivered at this site?

COMMENTARY

Fig. 1 shows an AT at a cycle length of 400 milliseconds. There is also a very low-amplitude electrogram recorded by the distal bipole of the ablation catheter, which precedes the p wave. Despite pacing at a longer cycle length (600 milliseconds) than that of the AT, the tachycardia terminated. The key observation is that the tachycardia terminated despite the fact that the pacing stimulus did not result in atrial capture. This finding is very specific for identifying a critical site in a reentry circuit. Although the stimulus did not result in global atrial

[a] Department of Internal Medicine, Cardiovascular Center, University of Michigan Health System, 1500 East Medical Center Drive Floor 3, Ann Arbor, MI 48109, USA; [b] University of Michigan Health System, 1500 East Medical Center Drive, Cardiovascular Center, SPC 5853, Ann Arbor, MI 48109, USA
* Corresponding author.
E-mail address: achugh@med.umich.edu

Card Electrophysiol Clin 4 (2012) 575–576
http://dx.doi.org/10.1016/j.ccep.2012.08.034
1877-9182/12/$ – see front matter

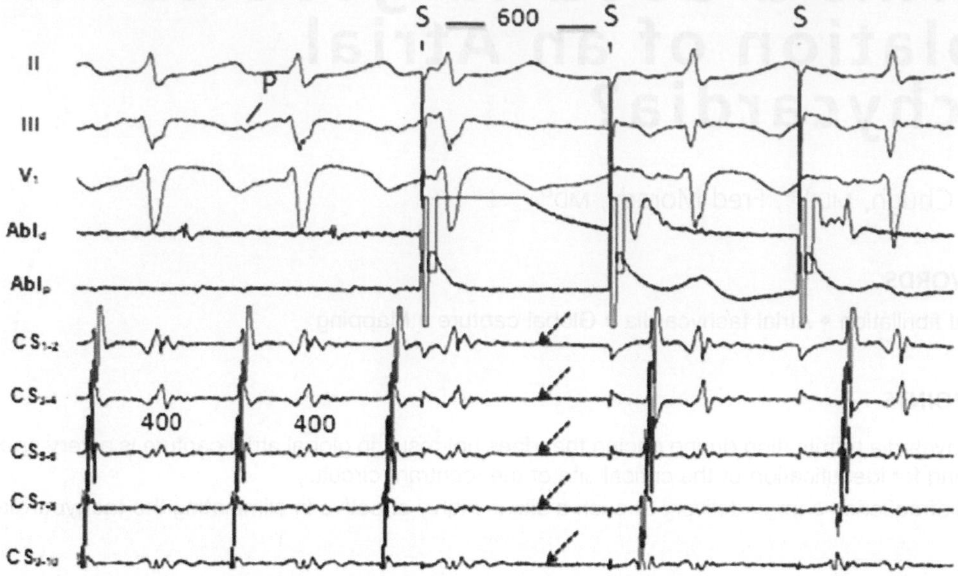

Fig. 1. Bipolar electrograms recorded by the distal and proximal bipoles of the ablation catheter (Abl) and coronary sinus (CS). Also displayed are electrocardiographic leads II, III, and V1. P, p wave; S, stimulus. Arrows indicate termination of the tachycardia.

capture, it resulted in local capture of the critical site, which rendered the site refractory to the subsequent reentrant wavefront, terminating the tachycardia. A single RF lesion was delivered at this site and rendered the tachycardia noninducible.

Pulmonary Vein Isolation in a 63-year-old Man with Paroxysmal Atrial Fibrillation

Rakesh Latchamsetty, MD*, Fred Morady, MD

KEYWORDS

• Pulmonary vein isolation • Atrial fibrillation • Catheter ablation

KEY POINTS

- Using a ring catheter in the pulmonary vein facilitates targeted antral pulmonary vein isolation by identifying the site of earliest pulmonary vein activation.
- However, signals from the ring catheter in the RSPV can represent pulmonary vein potentials, far-field left atrial potentials, or far-field superior vena cava/right atrial potentials.
- It is important to recognize that sometimes enough decremental conduction occurs into the pulmonary vein to cause conduction block.

CASE HISTORY

Pulmonary vein (PV) isolation was performed in a 63-year-old man with paroxysmal atrial fibrillation. The electrograms shown in **Fig. 1** were recorded during antral ablation around the right superior pulmonary vein (RSPV). **Fig. 2** shows the response

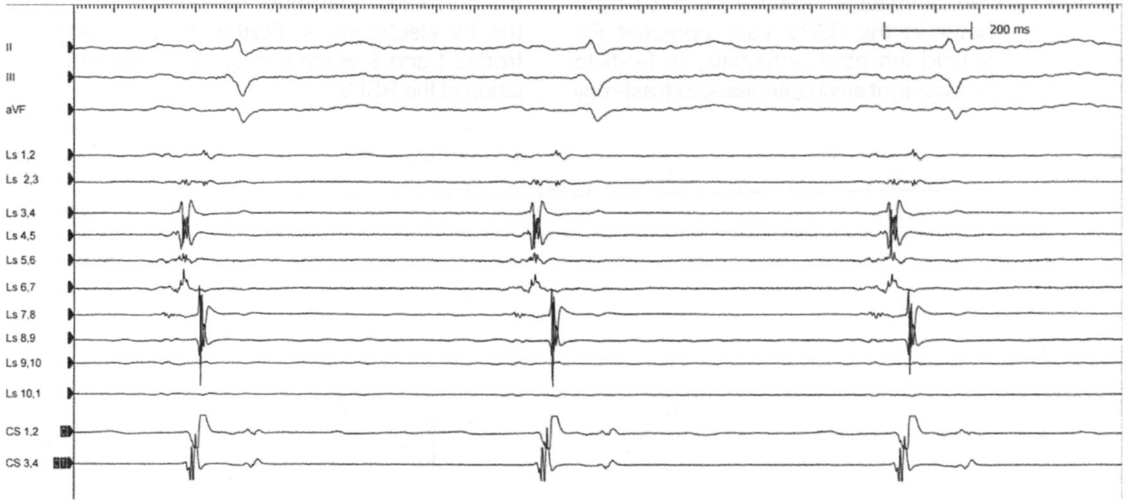

Fig. 1. Electrograms recorded with a ring catheter within the right superior pulmonary vein during antral ablation. A quadripolar catheter is positioned in the coronary sinus. CS, coronary sinus; Ls, lasso.

Department of Internal Medicine, University of Michigan Health System, 1500 East Medical Center Drive, Ann Arbor, MI 48109, USA
* Corresponding author.
E-mail address: rakeshl@umich.edu

Card Electrophysiol Clin 4 (2012) 577–578
http://dx.doi.org/10.1016/j.ccep.2012.08.017
1877-9182/12/$ – see front matter

cardiacEP.theclinics.com

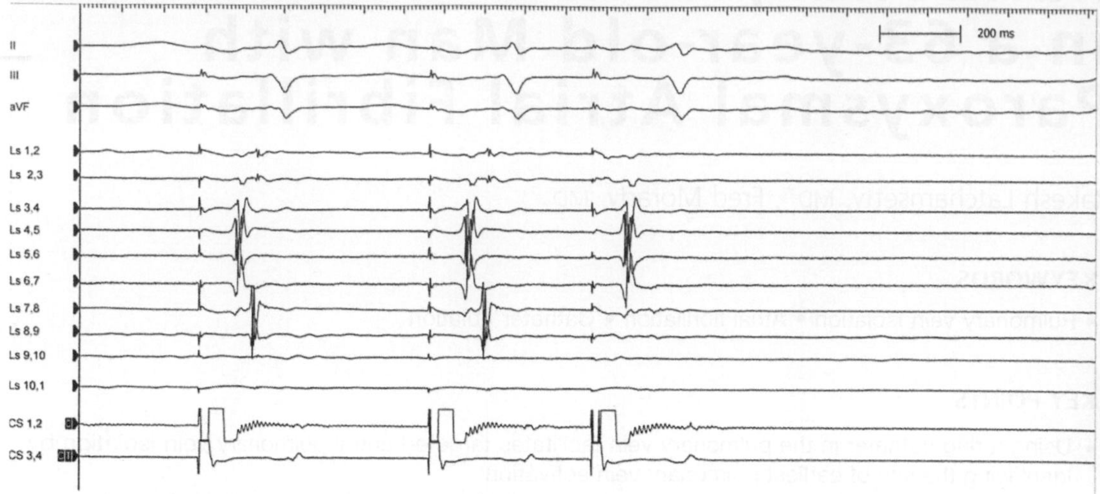

Fig. 2. Pacing with a premature atrial stimulus is performed from the coronary sinus catheter with the ring catheter positioned in the right superior pulmonary vein. CS, coronary sinus; Ls, lasso.

to an atrial extrastimulus from the coronary sinus. Is this vein already isolated? If not, which electrodes of the ring catheter should be targeted next?

COMMENTARY

Using a ring catheter in the PV facilitates targeted antral PV isolation by identifying the site of earliest pulmonary vein activation. However, signals from the ring catheter in the RSPV can represent PV potentials, far-field left atrial potentials, or far-field superior vena cava/right atrial potentials. Extrastimuli from the left atrium often leads to decremental conduction into the PV and can be used to distinguish PV potentials from far field potentials.

In this case, it is important to recognize that sometimes enough decremental conduction occurs into the PV to cause conduction block. With the premature stimulus, block is induced into the RSPV, but the far field atrial signals remain (**Fig. 3**). Therefore the preceding beat must be looked at to identify the PV electrograms. Further ablation near electrodes 1 and 8 of the ring catheter resulted in isolation of the RSPV.

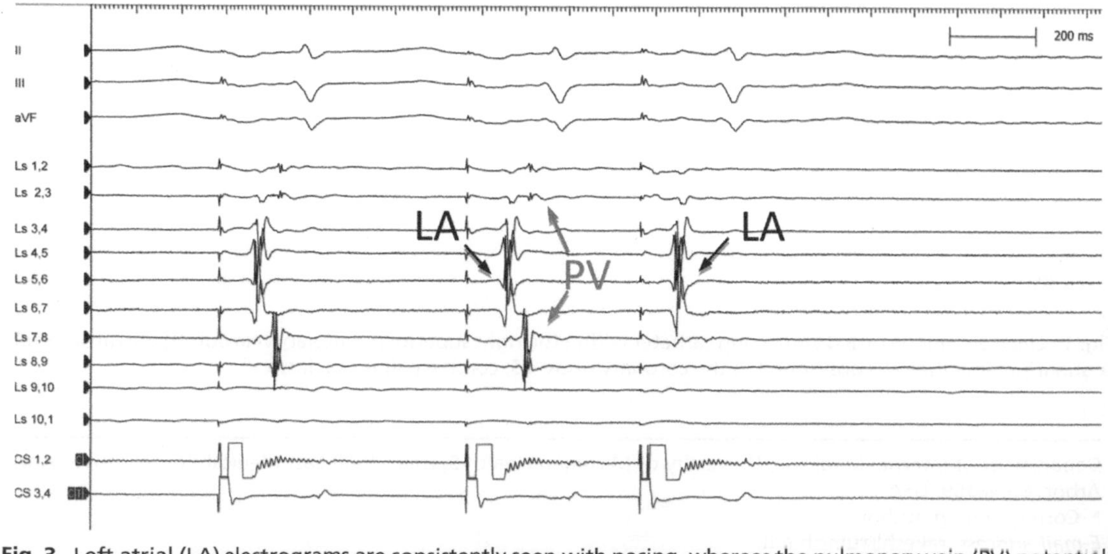

Fig. 3. Left atrial (LA) electrograms are consistently seen with pacing, whereas the pulmonary vein (PV) potentials drop out with the premature stimulus. CS, coronary sinus; Ls, lasso.

Introduction to Pediatric Arrhythmias

Ronn E. Tanel, MD

KEYWORDS

• Pediatric arrhythmias • Catheter ablation • Reentrant tachycardia • Congenital heart disease

KEY POINTS

- Because intra-atrial reentrant tachycardia is especially common in patients who have had a Fontan operation for single-ventricle physiology or a Mustard or Senning operation for transposition of the great arteries, anatomic considerations and surgical techniques are particularly important to understand when planning an invasive electrophysiology procedure in such a patient.
- Although success rates for ablation of complex intra-atrial reentrant tachycardia circuits in patients with congenital heart disease are lower than in those with more routine arrhythmias, close attention to unusual electrophysiologic and anatomic details can result in significant modification of the arrhythmia substrate.

Adults with congenital heart disease often develop atrial arrhythmias during long-term follow-up, with some specific anatomic lesions having a higher incidence. There are currently more than 1 million patients who have survived to adulthood after being treated for congenital heart disease as a child (Hoffman JI, Kaplan S, Liberthson RR. Prevalence of congenital heart disease. Am Heart J 2004; 147:425–39). Atrial flutter, also termed intra-atrial reentrant tachycardia or incisional atrial tachycardia in this cohort, is the most common arrhythmia mechanism in these patients. This macro-reentrant circuit within abnormal atrial muscle has some electrophysiologic characteristics that are similar to atrial flutter in patients with structurally normal hearts, but the cycle length, P-wave morphology, number of reentrant circuits, and anatomic course of the circuit may have very different properties. As opposed to a circuit that propagates around the tricuspid annulus in typical atrial flutter, intra-atrial reentrant tachycardia may use surgical patches, atriotomy incisions, cannulation sites, and other natural anatomic structures to define the reentry circuit.

Because intra-atrial reentrant tachycardia is especially common in patients who have had a Fontan operation for single-ventricle physiology or a Mustard or Senning operation for transposition of the great arteries, anatomic considerations and surgical techniques are particularly important to understand when planning the invasive electrophysiology procedure. Echocardiography and angiography can help provide an understanding of distorted anatomy, unusual surgical interventions, and the location of the true atrioventricular annulus. In addition, it is important to identify atypical locations of the atrioventricular node and His bundle to avoid inadvertent damage to normal conduction tissue. Three-dimensional mapping equipment can be particularly helpful during ablation procedures in these complex patients, and high-resolution magnetic resonance or computed tomography imaging merged with 3-dimensional maps may provide enhanced anatomic definition. Ablation often requires large-tip catheters, high-output generators, and irrigated catheters to create sufficient lesions in scarred and hypertrophied atrial tissue. Although success rates for ablation of complex intra-atrial reentrant tachycardia circuits in patients with congenital heart disease are lower than in those with more routine arrhythmias, close attention to unusual electrophysiologic and anatomic details can result in significant modification of the arrhythmia substrate.

Division of Pediatric Cardiology, Pediatric Arrhythmia Center, UCSF School of Medicine, UCSF Children's Hospital, 521 Parnassus Ave, Box 0632, San Francisco, CA 94143, USA
E-mail address: Ronn.Tanel@ucsf.edu

Card Electrophysiol Clin 4 (2012) 579
http://dx.doi.org/10.1016/j.ccep.2012.08.019

Intra-Atrial Reentrant Tachycardia in an Adult with Ebstein Anomaly

Walter Li, MD*, Ronn E. Tanel, MD

KEYWORDS

- Implantable cardioverter-defibrillator • Supraventricular tachycardia • Catheter ablation

KEY POINTS

- Adults with congenital heart disease, especially those who have had prior surgical procedures, often have multiple arrhythmia substrates.
- Electroanatomic mapping and entrainment maneuvers are helpful in defining the arrhythmia substrate.
- Successful ablation of the primary arrhythmia substrate may subsequently reveal other secondary arrhythmia substrates.

CLINICAL PRESENTATION

A 42-year-old woman with Ebstein anomaly of the tricuspid valve previously underwent bioprosthetic tricuspid valve replacement, a surgical biatrial Maze procedure, and placement of an epicardial dual-chamber pacemaker. That procedure was complicated by a right coronary artery occlusion requiring a saphenous vein graft. She later developed atrial arrhythmias that recurred following cardioversion. Medical therapy was not tolerated because of side effects. Although the patient was in full-time employment, she had severe exercise intolerance. She was referred for electrophysiology study and catheter ablation therapy.

PHYSICAL EXAMINATION FINDINGS

Vital signs revealed a heart rate of 73 beats/min, blood pressure of 108/70 mm Hg, and pulse oximetry on room air of 97%. She was a well-appearing, acyanotic, overweight woman with no baseline respiratory distress. Jugular venous distension was present to 10 to 12 cm with prominent v-waves. The cardiac examination had a regular rhythm. There was a split first heart sound and a soft, physiologically split second heart sound. There was a 1/6 holosystolic murmur at the left lower sternal border. The distal pulses were full and equal without radiofemoral delay. The abdomen was soft and nondistended without hepatomegaly. Extremities were warm and well perfused without clubbing or edema.

IMAGING FINDINGS

Echocardiography showed moderate dilation of the right atrium and right ventricle. Moderate tricuspid regurgitation and stenosis were present at the bioprosthetic tricuspid valve. The predicted right ventricular systolic pressure was normal. Both right and left ventricles had moderate systolic dysfunction. The ventricular septum was dyskinetic, and the left ventricular volume was decreased because of compression from the dilated right ventricle. No atrial or ventricular level shunts were present.

LABORATORY STUDIES

The electrocardiogram showed atrial flutter at a cycle length of 260 milliseconds. The flutter waves were negative in the inferior leads and

Disclosure: Dr Li receives fellowship funding support from Medtronic and St Jude Medical.
Division of Pediatric Cardiology, Department of Pediatrics, UCSF School of Medicine, UCSF Benioff Children's Hospital, San Francisco, CA, USA
* Corresponding author. University of California, San Francisco, 505 Parnassus Avenue, RM 1235, San Francisco, CA 94143.
E-mail address: walter.li@ucsf.edu

Card Electrophysiol Clin 4 (2012) 581–585
http://dx.doi.org/10.1016/j.ccep.2012.08.020
1877-9182/12/$ – see front matter

positive in lead V_1. There was 3:1 atrioventricular conduction with morphology of an incomplete right bundle branch block.

ELECTROPHYSIOLOGY STUDY

The presenting rhythm was an atrial arrhythmia with a regular atrial cycle length of 270 milliseconds and variable atrioventricular conduction. The surface leads showed the same pattern of flutter waves as that seen on the preprocedure electrocardiogram. A transesophageal electrode catheter was inserted and was used for a reference electrogram. A duodecapolar electrode catheter was placed around the tricuspid valve annulus with the distal pole at the lateral tricuspid valve annulus and the proximal pole along the septal tricuspid valve annulus. During attempts to cannulate the coronary sinus with the distal tip of a duodecapolar catheter, long-duration, early, and fractionated atrial electrograms were observed near the ostium of the coronary sinus. These complex electrograms had durations of 130 milliseconds, nearly half of the tachycardia cycle length; they were 75 milliseconds early to a reference esophageal electrogram. Pacing performed at that site resulted in concealed entrainment. Evaluation of the postpacing interval revealed that the septal cavotricuspid isthmus (CTI) was within the tachycardia circuit (**Fig. 1**). Electroanatomic mapping (NavX; St Jude Medical, Minneapolis, MN) was performed, and a propagation map demonstrated a counterclockwise activation pattern around the tricuspid valve annulus with the earliest activation at the septal CTI (**Fig. 2**). Radiofrequency ablation applications at the septal CTI site with a 7F 8-mm tip catheter resulted in a change in the tachycardia cycle length and activation sequence within 10 seconds. The new tachycardia had a cycle length of 350 milliseconds, and an activation sequence that suggested typical CTI-dependent atrial flutter. This finding was confirmed by entrainment pacing performed along the CTI (**Fig. 3**). A linear set of radiofrequency ablation lesions between the inferior vena cava (IVC) and tricuspid valve annulus resulted in termination of the tachycardia. With the ablation catheter at the lateral CTI, pacing from the lateral tricuspid valve annulus (T1) resulted in a conduction time of 190 milliseconds to the ablation catheter. The ablation catheter was then moved to the medial CTI. Pacing from the lateral tricuspid valve annulus (T1) showed a delay in the conduction time to the ablation catheter of 285 milliseconds. This finding confirmed that a line of conduction block had been achieved at the CTI (**Fig. 4**). No

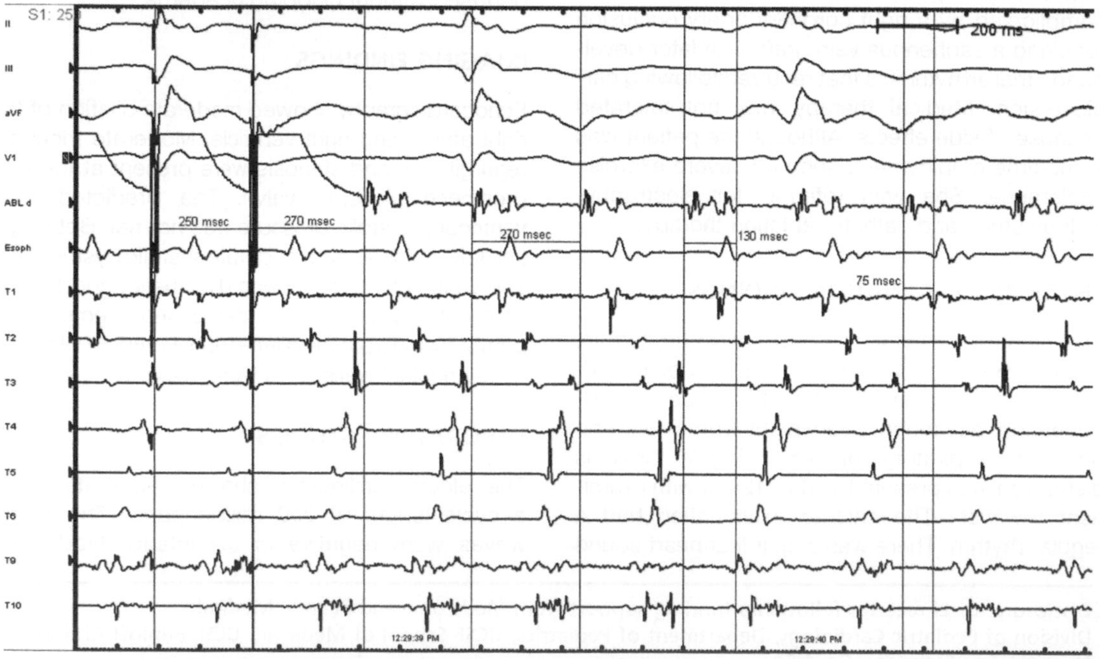

Fig. 1. Concealed entrainment of the clinical atrial arrhythmia. Electrograms were recorded from the surface electrocardiogram, distal ablation catheter (ABL d), esophageal electrode catheter (Esoph), and duodecapolar electrode catheter (T1, distal; T10, proximal). The postpacing interval is shown to be equal to the tachycardia cycle length. The ablation catheter electrogram is approximately half (130 milliseconds) of the tachycardia cycle length. The ablation catheter electrogram occurs during atrial diastole and is early relative to the other recorded atrial electrograms.

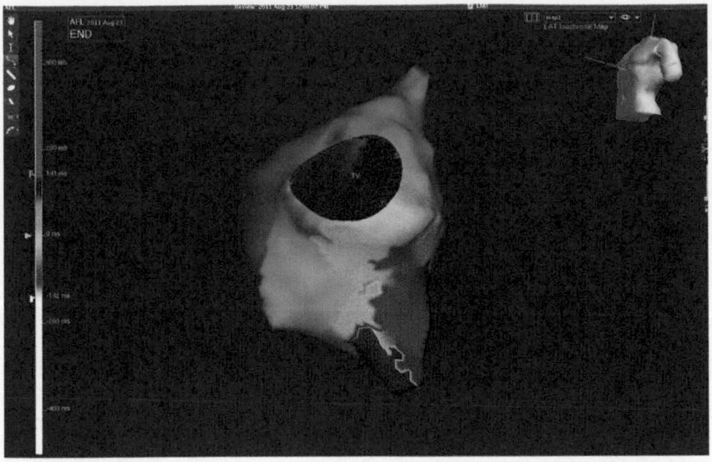

Fig. 2. Right atrial activation map during the clinical atrial arrhythmia. Electroanatomic map is shown from a lateral projection with caudal and anterior angulation. The activation sequence is color-coded: white, red, yellow, aqua, blue, and purple represent progressive transition of the local atrial electrogram timing relative to the esophageal reference electrode, with white and purple representing the earliest and latest activation, respectively.

arrhythmias were induced during postablation testing.

DISCUSSION

Ebstein anomaly of the tricuspid valve was first described in 1866.[1] It is a malformation of the tricuspid valve and right ventricle that typically involves apical displacement of the tricuspid valve leaflets and resultant incompetence of the valve apparatus. This displacement results in varying degrees of dilation and hypertrophy of the right ventricle and dilation of the right atrium.[2] Manifest accessory pathways are common,[3] and often occur as multiple pathways in these patients.[4] Other arrhythmia substrates are also common in these patients, including atrial flutter and atrial tachycardia. These other substrates are often more directly related to prior surgical procedures and chronic hemodynamic abnormalities that result in dilation and hypertrophy of the right atrium and right ventricle. Adults with Ebstein anomaly may develop supraventricular tachycardia owing to ectopic atrial tachycardia, incisional intra-atrial

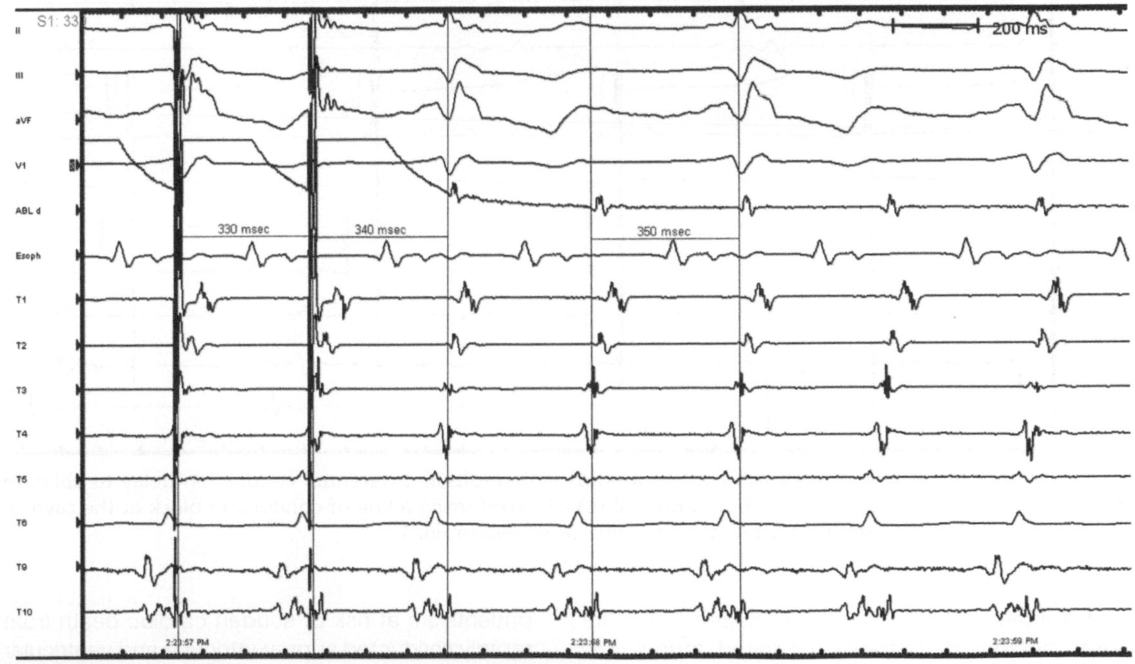

Fig. 3. Concealed entrainment of cavotricuspid isthmus (CTI)-dependent atrial flutter. The postpacing interval indicates that the CTI is within the tachycardia circuit. Electrograms presented are the same as shown in **Fig. 1**.

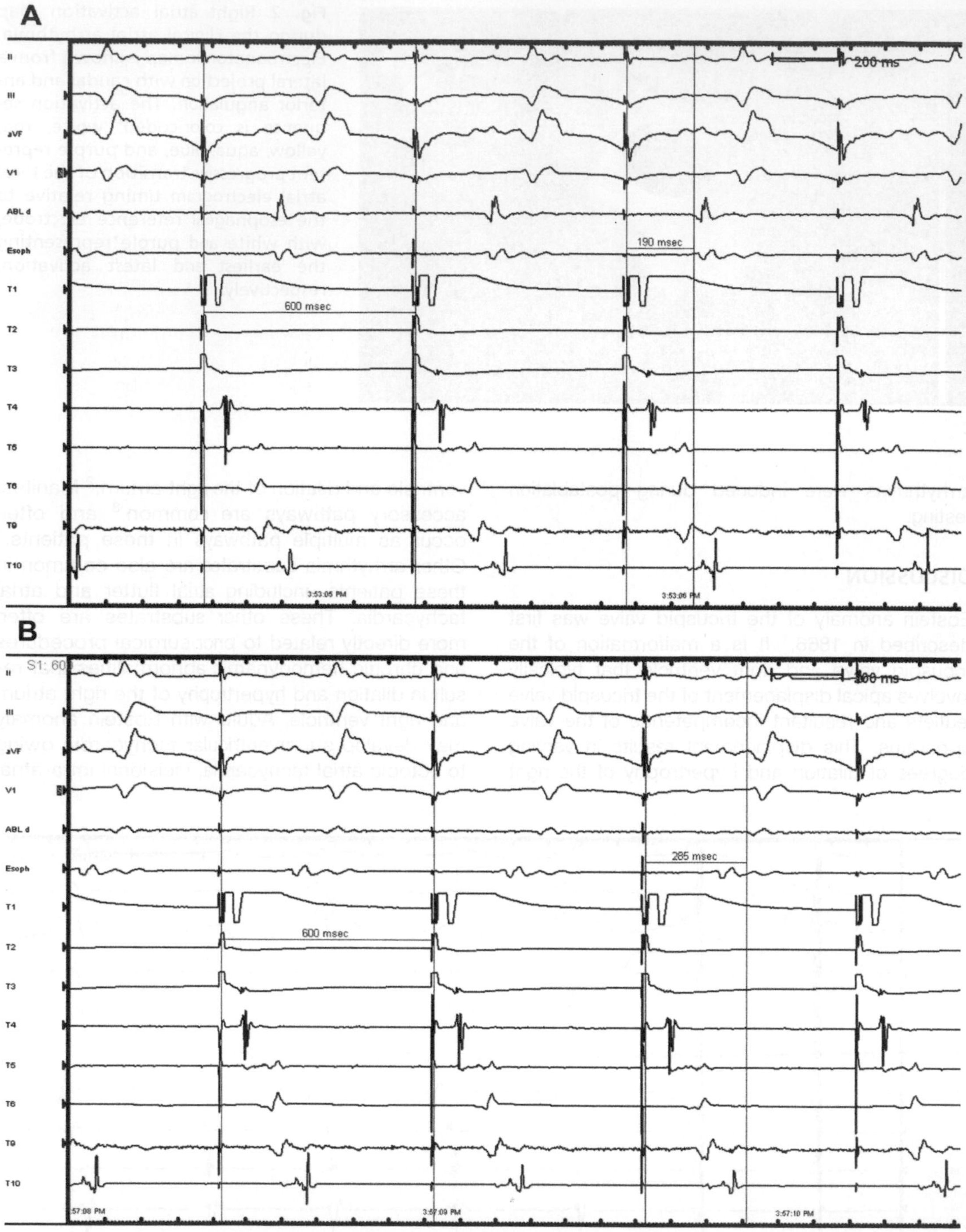

Fig. 4. Pacing from the lateral tricuspid valve annulus (T1) results in differential conduction delay to ablation catheter (ABL d) sites at the lateral (*A*) and medial (*B*) CTI, confirming a line of conduction block at the cavotricuspid isthmus. Electrograms presented are the same as shown in **Fig. 1**.

reentrant tachycardia, typical CTI-dependent atrial flutter, accessory pathway-mediated atrioventricular reciprocating tachycardia, or atrioventricular nodal reentrant tachycardia.[5] In addition, these patients are at risk of sudden cardiac death from rapidly conducted supraventricular and ventricular tachycardia.[6] Arrhythmia recurrences after acutely successful catheter ablation[7] and surgical Maze[8] procedures are common, and add to the complexity of these interventions.

Sophisticated techniques are often necessary to map tachycardia substrates in adults with Ebstein anomaly. A duodecapolar electrode catheter may be helpful when placed around the tricuspid valve annulus to characterize the activation pattern of intra-atrial reentrant tachycardia. In this patient, the enlarged right atrium precluded the usual catheter position. The distal tip of the duodecapolar electrode catheter was placed at the lateral tricuspid valve annulus with the proximal pole at the septal tricuspid valve annulus. Given the abnormal anatomy and possibility of multiple arrhythmia substrates, electroanatomic mapping was used for further definition of the arrhythmia mechanism. Usually a catheter in the coronary sinus provides a stable reference electrogram for both electroanatomic and entrainment mapping. Prior surgical procedures can make this difficult to achieve, and a transesophageal electrode catheter can sometimes be used as a reference. In this patient, propagation and entrainment mapping showed that the clinical tachycardia originated from the septal CTI. The atrial electrogram at that position had a complex, high-frequency, and fractionated signal. All of these findings suggested the presence of an intraisthmus reentry tachycardia. Ablation at that site resulted in termination of the intraisthmus reentry tachycardia with a change in tachycardia cycle length and activation sequence to one consistent with typical CTI-dependent atrial flutter. This finding confirmed that this patient had 2 different tachycardia substrates. The faster intraisthmus reentry tachycardia near the coronary sinus ostium suppressed the slower typical CTI-dependent atrial flutter until the elimination of the former unmasked the latter. A linear set of ablation lesions between the tricuspid valve annulus and the IVC terminated the tachycardia.

Recurrence of tachycardia following an apparently successful ablation is common in adults with congenital heart disease. Proof of a successful ablation is essential and can be demonstrated with differential pacing.[9] However, conventional techniques using typical catheter positions are often difficult in patients with unusual anatomy and repaired congenital heart disease. Success is demonstrated with persistent conduction delay between 2 points on either side of a line of conduction block. Finally, comprehensive stimulation protocols should be performed to assess for additional intra-atrial reentrant tachycardia circuits and other arrhythmia substrates, such as an accessory pathway or atrioventricular nodal reentrant tachycardia.

SUMMARY

Adults with both unrepaired and palliated Ebstein anomaly of the tricuspid valve can have complex arrhythmias. Detailed mapping with electroanatomic and entrainment techniques may be necessary to achieve procedural success. Multiple tachycardia substrates are often observed in the same patient.

REFERENCES

1. van Son JA, Konstantinov IE, Zimmermann V. Wilhelm Ebstein and Ebstein's malformation. Eur J Cardiothorac Surg 2001;20:1082–5.
2. Attenhofer Jost CH, Connolly HM, Dearani JA, et al. Ebstein's anomaly. Circulation 2007;115:277–85.
3. Danielson GK, Driscoll DJ, Mair DD, et al. Operative treatment of Ebstein's anomaly. J Thorac Cardiovasc Surg 1992;104:1195–202.
4. Roten L, Lukac P, de Groot N, et al. Catheter ablation of arrhythmias in Ebstein's anomaly: a multicenter study. J Cardiovasc Electrophysiol 2011;22:1391–6.
5. Hebe J. Ebstein's anomaly in adults. Arrhythmias: diagnosis and therapeutic approach. Thorac Cardiovasc Surg 2000;48:214–9.
6. Tanel RE. Preventing sudden death in the adult with congenital heart disease. Curr Cardiol Rep 2011;13: 327–35.
7. Reich JD, Auld D, Hulse E, et al. The Pediatric Radiofrequency Ablation Registry's experience with Ebstein's anomaly. Pediatric Electrophysiology Society. J Cardiovasc Electrophysiol 1998;9:1370–7.
8. Khositseth A, Danielson GK, Dearani JA, et al. Supraventricular tachyarrhythmias in Ebstein anomaly: management and outcome. J Thorac Cardiovasc Surg 2004;128:826–33.
9. Shah D, Haïssaguerre M, Takahashi A, et al. Differential pacing for distinguishing block from persistent conduction through an ablation line. Circulation 2000;102:1517–22.

Atrial Flutter 23 Years After Classic Fontan

Kurt S. Hoffmayer, PharmD, MD*, Nitish Badhwar, MBBS

KEYWORDS

• Catheter ablation • Atrial flutter • Fontan

KEY POINTS

- Atrial arrhythmias are one of the most common late complications of the Fontan operation.
- Postoperative right atrial dilation in addition to the previous surgical suture lines creates an ideal substrate for the development of macro-reentrant tachycardias.
- The macro-reentrant tachycardia in the majority of patients depends on anatomic or iatrogenic central obstacles of conduction block that are separate from the cavotricuspid isthmus.
- Electroanatomic 3-dimensional mapping and entrainment pacing is helpful in elucidating the mechanism as well as sites for successful ablation.

CLINICAL PRESENTATION

A 25-year-old man with tricuspid atresia treated with Blalock-Taussig shunt at 6 months and subsequent Fontan at 2 years presented with atrial flutter with 1:1 conduction at a heart rate of 240 beats/min. The surface electrocardiogram is shown in **Fig. 1**. Magnetic resonance (MR) imaging revealed a classic Fontan with right and left pulmonary arteries anastomosed to the superomedial right atrium (**Fig. 2**A). The patient was initially treated with adenosine and metoprolol, and referred for electrophysiology study and catheter ablation.

ELECTROPHYSIOLOGY STUDY AND CATHETER ABLATION

The patient presented to the electrophysiology laboratory in atrial flutter. Electrophysiology study was performed using a decapolar catheter positioned in the coronary sinus, a quadripolar catheter in the His bundle region, a duodecapolar placed in the right atrium along the tricuspid annulus, and a 3.5-mm open irrigated catheter for mapping and ablation. The tachycardia had a cycle length of 260 milliseconds. An electroanatomic map (CARTO system; Biosense Webster, Inc, Diamond Bar, CA, USA) was created during the tachycardia (**Fig. 2**B). Entrainment mapping from the medial and lateral isthmus and inferior vena cava was "out" of the circuit (post pacing interval [PPI] – tachycardia cycle length [TCL] >30 milliseconds). Entrainment mapping from the mid superior right atrium inferior and lateral to the base of the Fontan conduit is shown in **Fig. 3**.

QUESTIONS

What is the most likely mechanism of the tachycardia?

What is your primary approach to ablation?

DISCUSSION

At clinical presentation, the most likely diagnosis is macro-reentrant atrial tachycardia (atrial flutter). The Fontan operation, first described in 1971, has been a critical contribution to congenital heart

Section of Electrophysiology, Division of Cardiology, University of California San Francisco, 500 Parnassus Avenue, MUE-434, Box 1354, San Francisco, CA 94143, USA
* Corresponding author.
E-mail address: kurt.hoffmayer@ucsf.edu

Card Electrophysiol Clin 4 (2012) 587–590
http://dx.doi.org/10.1016/j.ccep.2012.08.021
1877-9182/12/$ – see front matter

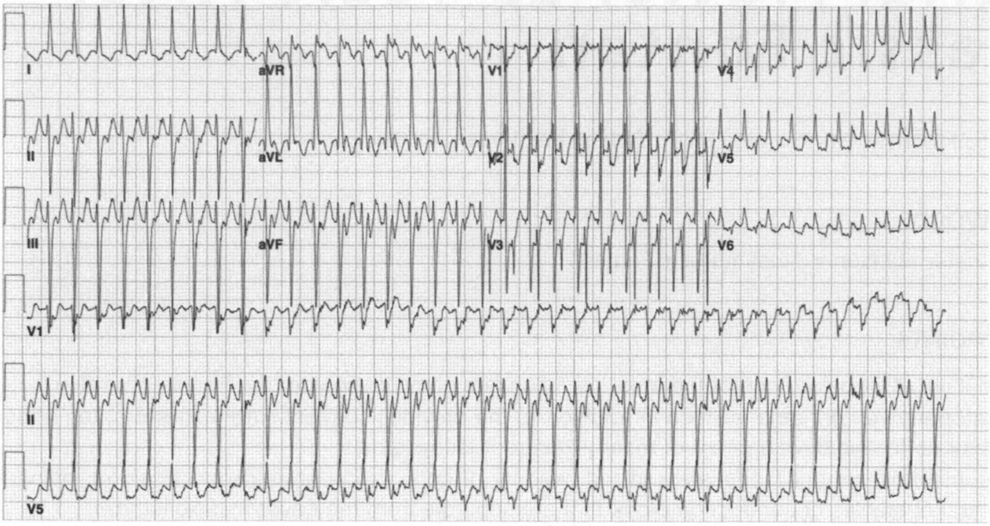

Fig. 1. Twelve-lead electrocardiogram of the clinical tachycardia.

surgery and the care of patients with univentricle physiology.[1,2] There have been several modifications of the Fontan operation; in the classic Fontan the right atrium remains within the systemic venous circulation and acts as the major subpulmonic chamber.[1–3] Atrial arrhythmias have been recognized in more than 50% of post-Fontan patients, and continue to be one of the most common late complications.[4–6]

In the atriopulmonary Fontan, severe right atrial dilation in addition to the previous surgical suture lines create an ideal substrate for the development of macro-reentrant tachycardias.[3] The macro-reentrant tachycardia in the majority of patients depends on anatomic or iatrogenic central obstacles of conduction block that are separate from the cavotricuspid isthmus.[3] Electroanatomic 3-dimensional mapping and entrainment pacing is helpful

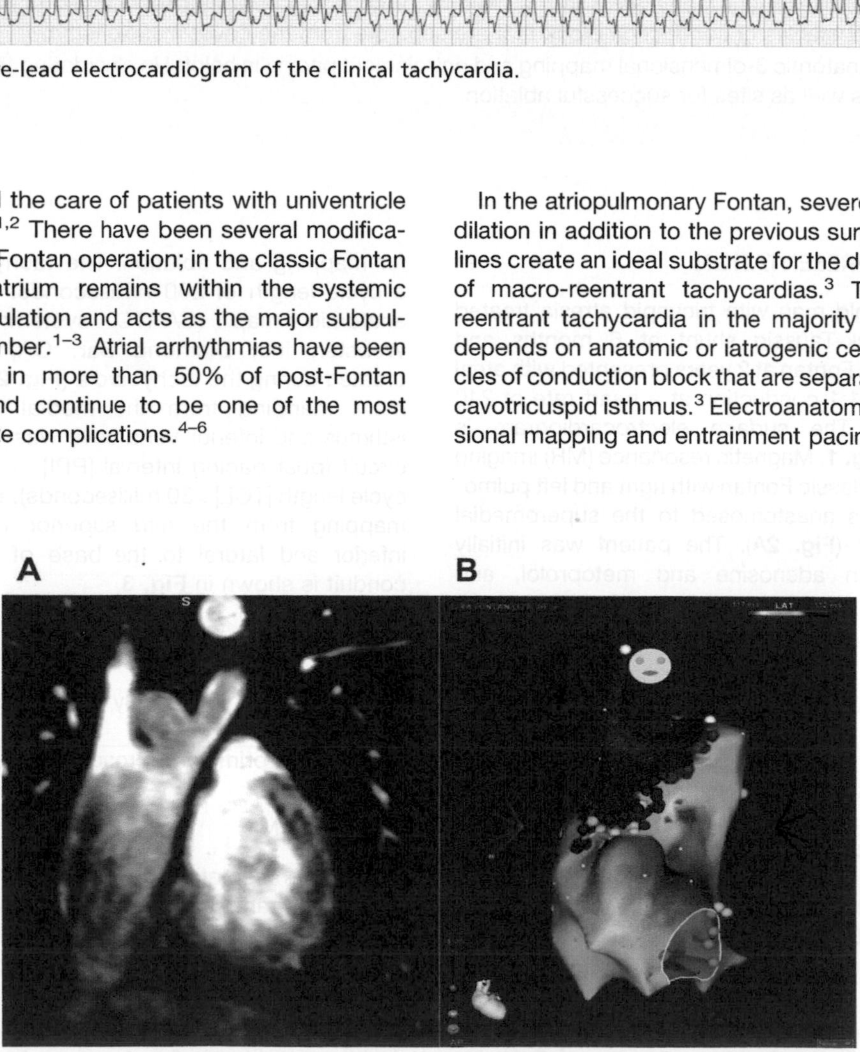

Fig. 2. Comparison of a magnetic resonance (MR) image (*A*) and CARTO electroanatomic map (*B*). (*Left*) Anterior-posterior view of an MR image showing patient's classic Fontan, with right and left pulmonary arteries anastomosed to the superomedial right atrium. (*Right*) Three-dimensional electroanatomic map showing the tachycardia activation pattern as well as the radiofrequency ablation lesions (*red dots*) and scar (*gray dots*). See **Fig. 4** for further discussion.

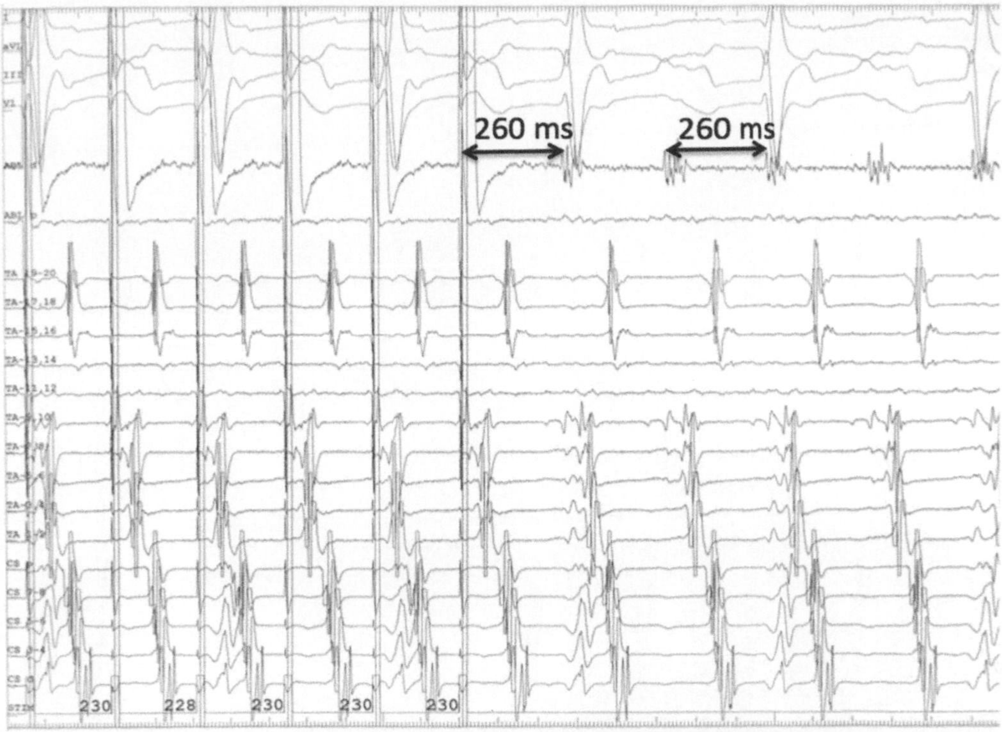

Fig. 3. Entrainment pacing from an area of fractionated electrograms via the distal ablation catheter (ABL d) positioned at the superomedial right atrium at a cycle length of 30 milliseconds faster than the tachycardia cycle length (TCL). The postpacing interval (PPI) is 260 milliseconds and the TCL is 260 milliseconds, with resultant PPI minus TCL of 0 milliseconds, demonstrating that the superomedial right atrium is in the circuit.

in elucidating the mechanism as well as sites for successful ablation. Fractionated diastolic potentials, entrainment with concealed fusion, and PPI = TCL both inside and outside of protected channels, may be identified using a combination of electroanatomic mapping and simultaneous entrainment.[7]

This case exemplifies these findings. The original electroanatomic map is consistent with a macro-reentrant atrial flutter, with an early-meets-late configuration. Long fractionated potentials are seen in the mid superior right atrium (**Fig. 4**). Entrainment mapping from these areas confirms concealed fusion with PPI = TCL. Entrainment mapping from lateral and mid cavotricuspid isthmus were out of the circuit. Electroanatomic mapping revealed areas of low-amplitude recordings (scar) in the superior medial right atrium, corresponding to the area of the Fontan conduit seen on the MR image (see **Fig. 2**). Ablation in the area of the fractionated potentials where the entrainment mapping revealed concealed fusion with PPI = TCL terminated the tachycardia (see **Fig. 3**; **Fig. 5**). A line was created, with further ablation lesions connecting

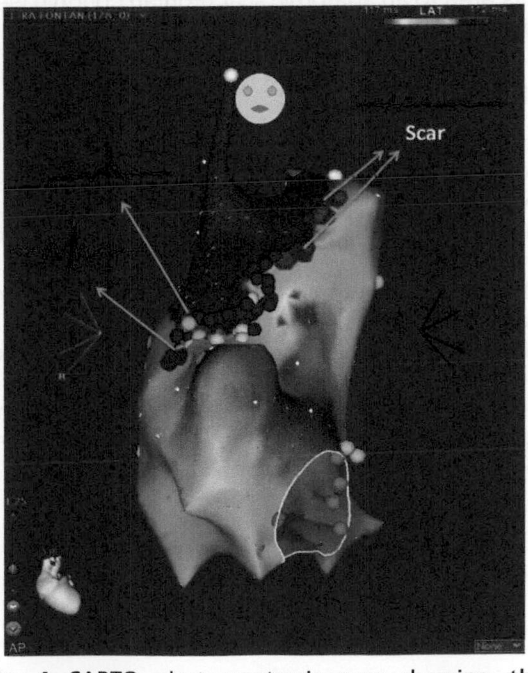

Fig. 4. CARTO electroanatomic map showing the tachycardia activation pattern as well as the radiofrequency ablation lesions (*red dots*) and scar (*gray dots*). The local electrograms of the corresponding regions are shown (*arrows*).

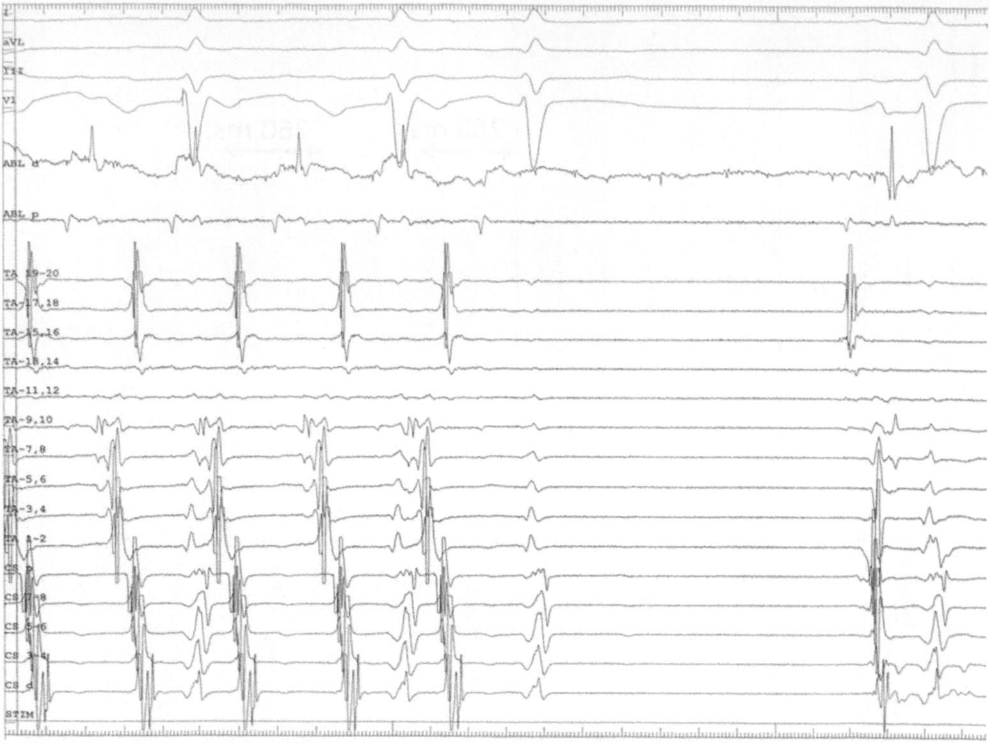

Fig. 5. Termination of the tachycardia with radiofrequency ablation, with catheter positioned at the superomedial right atrium at the area of fractionated potentials where entrainment mapping demonstrated PPI = TCL.

this area to an anatomic scar (Fontan conduit) (see **Fig. 4**).

SUMMARY

Atrial arrhythmias are one of the most common late complications of the Fontan operation. Postoperative right atrial dilation in addition to the previous surgical suture lines creates an ideal substrate for the development of macro-reentrant tachycardias. The macro-reentrant tachycardia in the majority of patients depends on anatomic or iatrogenic central obstacles of conduction block that are distinct from the cavotricuspid isthmus. Electroanatomic 3-dimensional mapping and entrainment pacing is helpful in elucidating the mechanism as well as sites for successful ablation.

REFERENCES

1. Fontan F, Baudet E. Surgical repair of tricuspid atresia. Thorax 1971;26(3):240–8.
2. Kreutzer G, Galindez E, Bono H, et al. An operation for the correction of tricuspid atresia. J Thorac Cardiovasc Surg 1973;66(4):613–21.
3. Abrams D, Schilling R. Mechanism and mapping of atrial arrhythmia in the modified Fontan circulation. Heart Rhythm 2005;2(10):1138–44.
4. Ghai A, Harris L, Harrison DA, et al. Outcomes of late atrial tachyarrhythmias in adults after the Fontan operation. J Am Coll Cardiol 2001;37(2):585–92.
5. Gewillig M, Wyse RK, de Leval MR, et al. Early and late arrhythmias after the Fontan operation: predisposing factors and clinical consequences. Br Heart J 1992;67(1):72–9.
6. Weber HS, Hellenbrand WE, Kleinman CS, et al. Predictors of rhythm disturbances and subsequent morbidity after the Fontan operation. Am J Cardiol 1989;64(12):762–7.
7. Nakagawa H, Shah N, Matsudaira K, et al. Characterization of reentrant circuit in macroreentrant right atrial tachycardia after surgical repair of congenital heart disease: isolated channels between scars allow "focal" ablation. Circulation 2001;103(5):699–709.

Ablation of Atrial Flutter in Complex Congenital Heart Disease

Marwan M. Refaat, MD, Edward P. Gerstenfeld, MD*

KEYWORDS

- Transposition of the great arteries • Atrial switch • Mustard procedure • Electrophysiology
- Radiofrequency ablation

KEY POINTS

- Even in patients with complex congenital heart disease, typical atrial flutter remains the most common supraventricular arrhythmia.
- The flutter circuit in Mustard patients is nearly always in the pulmonary venous atrium.
- Proof of block in the flutter isthmus is critical to achieving long term success.
- Knowledge of the underlying anatomy is critical for guiding mapping and ablation in adult congenital heart disease patients.

CLINICAL PRESENTATION

A 38-year-old man who had a history of D-transposition of the great arteries (D-TGA) status post Mustard atrial switch procedure and a dual-chamber pacemaker for sinus node dysfunction presented with palpitations. His electrocardiogram (ECG) showed a narrow-complex tachycardia at 198 beats/min (**Fig. 1**). After slowing of the ventricular rate, the underlying rhythm was consistent with an atrial flutter. He was treated with diltiazem and flecainide but continued to have episodes of palpitations, chest pain, fatigue, and decreased exercise tolerance. He was thus referred for electrophysiology study and possible ablation.

ELECTROPHYSIOLOGY STUDY

A contrast injection into the systemic venous atrium via a 6F pigtail catheter was first performed to exclude baffle obstruction and delineate the atrial anatomy. A 7F deflectable decapolar catheter was placed in the high systemic venous atrium (HSVA), a 5F quadripolar catheter was placed in the low SVA (LSVA), and a 5F deflectable quadripolar catheter was placed in the morphologic left ventricular apex (LVA) via the right femoral vein. A detailed 3-dimensional electroanatomic map (CARTO3; Biosense Webster, Diamond Bar, CA) (**Fig. 2**A) of the systemic venous atrium during the tachycardia was acquired using a 3.5-mm open-irrigated mapping/ablation catheter (Thermocool; Biosense Webster). Bipolar electrograms (30–500 Hz) were displayed and stored using a digital recording system (EP MedSystems, West Berlin, NJ).

Mapping of the systemic venous atrium revealed a pattern of high to low activation. The response to overdrive ventricular pacing at the site of earliest activation is shown in **Fig. 2**B. Is the origin of the tachycardia in the SVA?

Entrainment of the tachycardia shows a post-pacing interval (PPI) more than 30 milliseconds longer than the tachycardia cycle length (TCL). Therefore, the SVA is not part of the tachycardia circuit. Femoral arterial access was obtained and a retrograde aortic approach to access the pulmonary venous atrium (PVA) was performed. Detailed activation mapping of the SVA and PVA is shown

Conflict of interest: None.
Cardiology Division, Department of Medicine, University of California San Francisco, 500 Parnassus Avenue, MUE-434, Box 1354, San Francisco, CA 94143-1354, USA
* Corresponding author.
E-mail address: EGerstenfeld@medicine.ucsf.edu

Card Electrophysiol Clin 4 (2012) 591–596
http://dx.doi.org/10.1016/j.ccep.2012.08.040
1877-9182/12/$ – see front matter

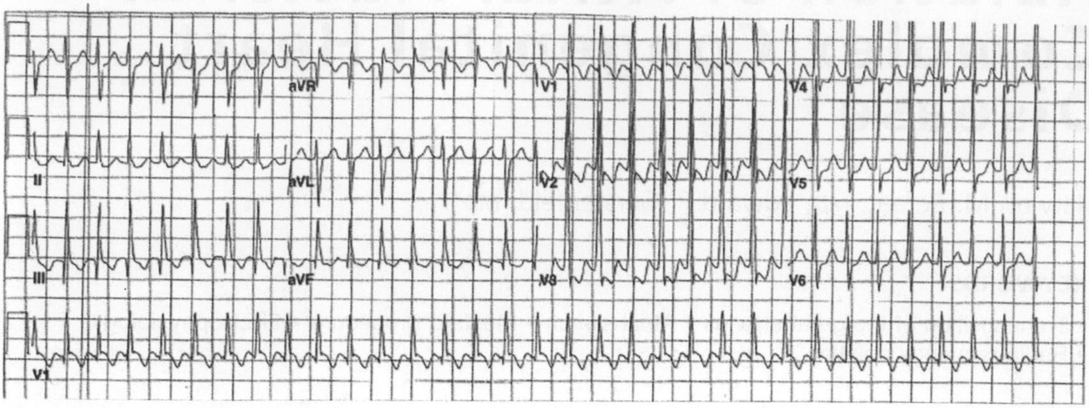

Fig. 1. The patient's electrocardiogram (ECG) shows a narrow-complex supraventricular tachycardia at a rate of 198 beats/min. One cannot discern the mechanism of the tachycardia from the ECG; however in a patient status post Mustard procedure, a slow atrial flutter with 1:1 atrioventricular conduction is the most likely diagnosis.

in **Fig. 3**A. Overdrive pacing from the inferior PVA at the level of the inferior tricuspid valve revealed the response shown in **Fig. 3**B. Is the circuit in the PVA?

The electroanatomic map reveals a reentrant atrial flutter circuit around the pulmonary venous atrioventricular (tricuspid) valve encompassing 95% of the TCL. The response to entrainment shows concealed fusion with a PPI within 10 milliseconds of the TCL. Additional sites within the tachycardia circuit included the high PVA, the posterior PVA, the lateral tricuspid annulus, and the medial tricuspid annulus. This map proves that the tricuspid annulus is part of the tachycardia circuit and that the atrial activation sequence is consistent with a clockwise atrial flutter using the cavotricuspid isthmus with 2-to-1 atrioventricular (AV) conduction.

ABLATION OF THE ATRIAL FLUTTER CIRCUIT

Ablation was performed in the PVA in a linear fashion, starting at approximately 6 o'clock in the left anterior oblique projection (see **Fig. 3**A), from the inferoposterior baffle to the anterior tricuspid annulus, with termination of the tachycardia (**Fig. 4**). Evidence of block across the line was confirmed by pacing the lateral tricuspid annulus (**Fig. 5**) and demonstrating high to low activation of the SVA. Additional lesions were delivered in the systemic venous atrium from inside the baffle to the inferior vena cava.

At the end of the procedure, atrial flutter was no longer inducible. With programmed stimulation, another tachycardia was induced with programmed stimulation. Because it was not the clinical tachycardia and the anatomy suggested a higher risk of heart block, slow-pathway modification was not performed. The patient has remained free of arrhythmias during 6 months of follow-up.

DISCUSSION

Although patients with surgically repaired D-TGA have complex anatomy, typical atrial flutter remains the most common supraventricular tachycardia. The onset usually occurs long after surgical correction.[1–4] The mechanisms predisposing to atrial flutter include altered hemodynamics and surgical scarring.[4,5] Because patients with Mustard repair have normal AV nodal conduction and the flutter cycle length is often slow owing to surgical scarring, 1:1 AV conduction with a rapid ventricular rate is not uncommon. Therefore, catheter ablation is often the preferred therapy.

The typical atrial flutter circuit around the tricuspid valve is not easily accessible from the PVA, as illustrated in this patient. The two options for ablation are retrograde aortic access to the PVA or transbaffle puncture.[6,7] Retrograde aortic access was chosen for this patient. Electroanatomic mapping and entrainment proved that the arrhythmia was typical atrial flutter. Linear ablation from the posterior baffle scar to the tricuspid annulus will typically terminate the tachycardia; however, this does not prove that conduction block has been achieved. After additional ablation, pacing the low lateral PVA revealed high to low activation of the SVA followed by activation of the low septal SVA (see **Fig. 5**). This proves lateral to medial block across the flutter line. Conduction across the isthmus would activate the low septal SVA before the high SVA. The patient is doing well after 6 months, with no recurrent arrhythmia.

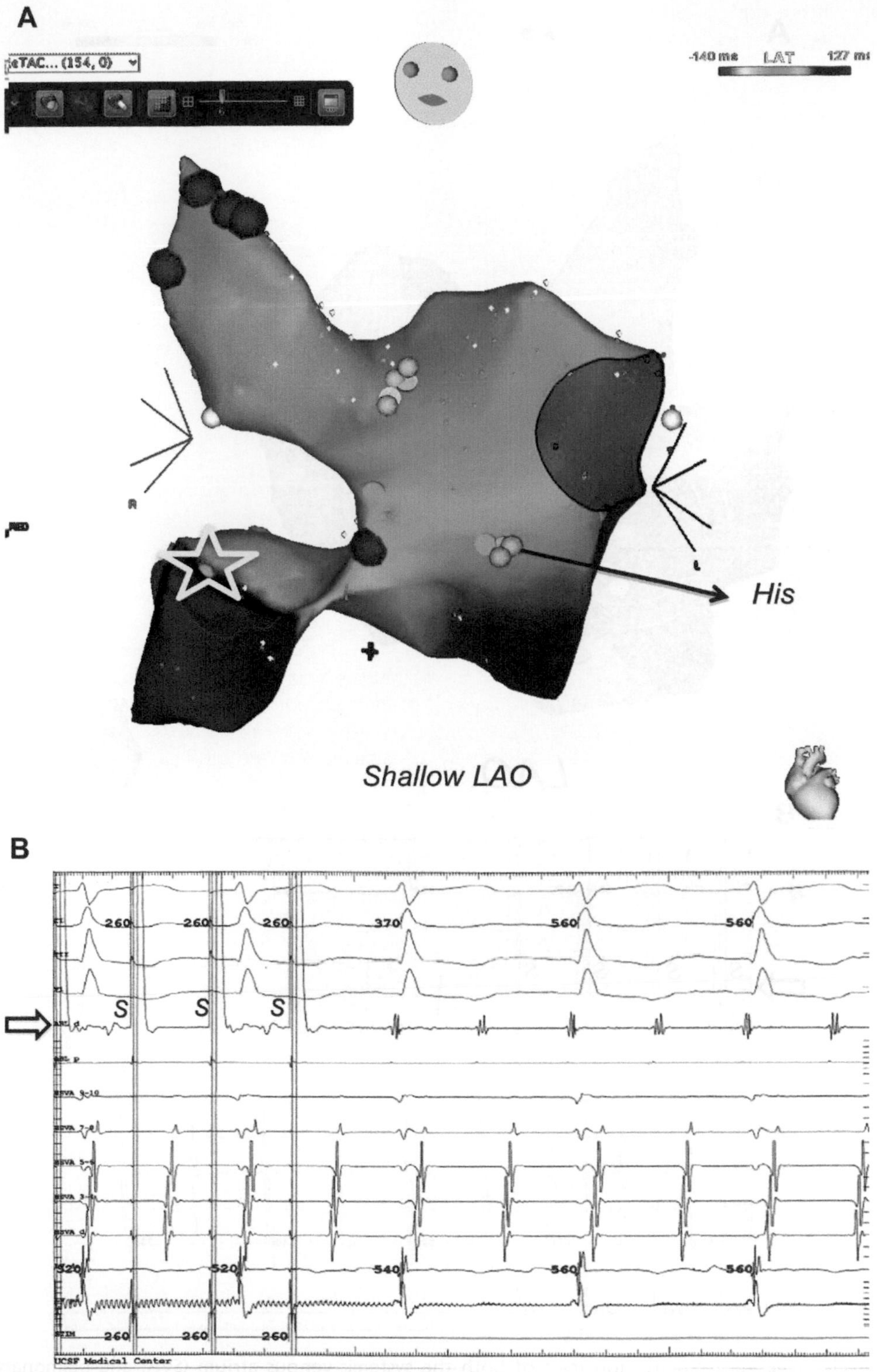

Fig. 2. (*A*) Electroanatomic activation map of the systemic venous atrium. The activation pattern appears passive. Entrainment from the area marked with the star is shown in *B*. (*B*) Entrainment from the systemic venous atrium site. *S*, pacing stimulus.

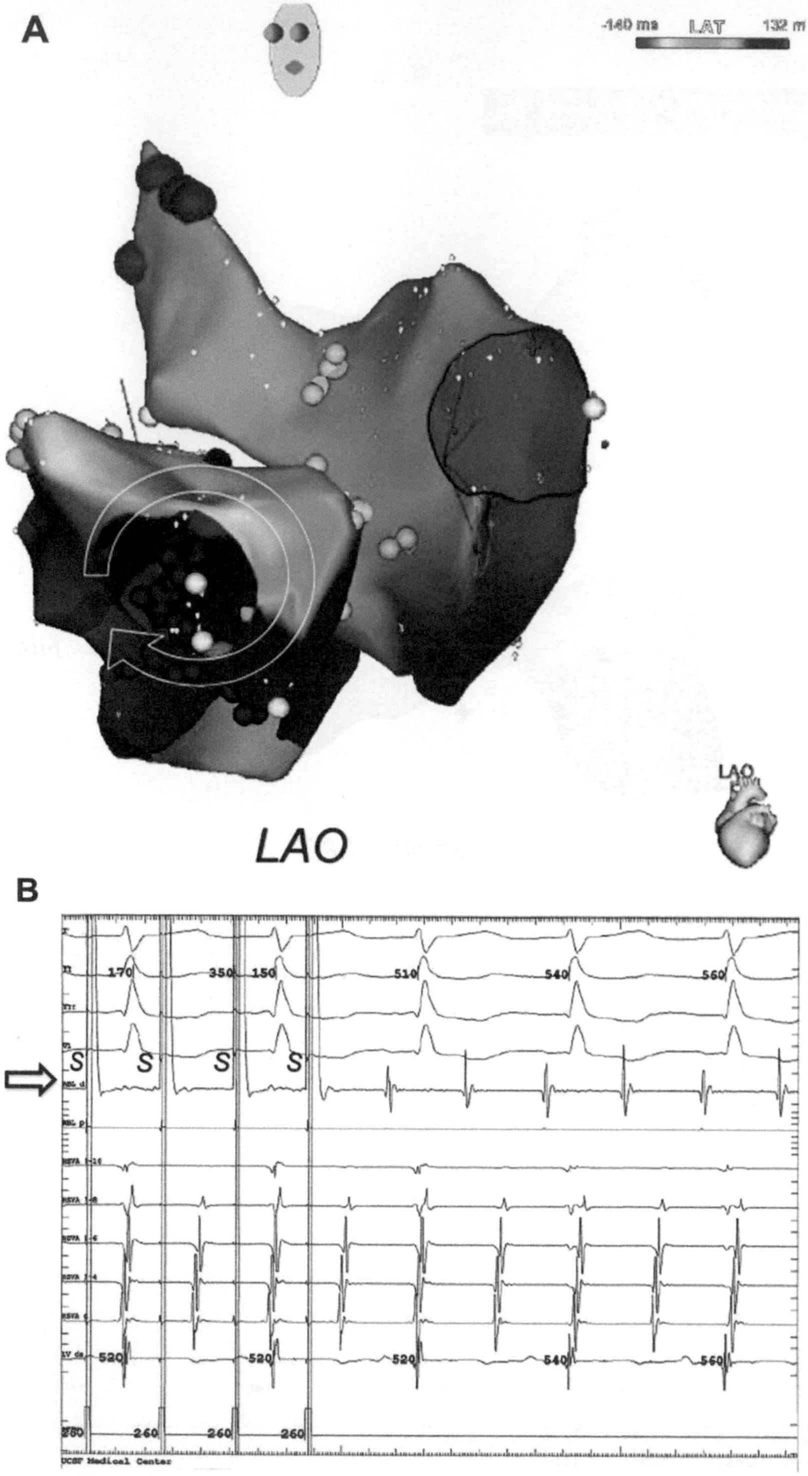

Fig. 3. (*A*) Electroanatomic activation map of both the systemic venous atrium (SVA) and pulmonary venous atrium (PVA) in a left anterior oblique (LAO) projection. The pink circles denote sites with fractionated signals, the light blue circles are sites with double potentials, the dark blue circles are sites where entrainment of the tachycardia yielded a postpacing interval less than 20 milliseconds longer than the tachycardia cycle length, and the yellow circles represent the His-bundle region. (*B*) Overdrive pacing from the ablation cathether (*arrow*) located at the inferior PVA. *S*, pacing stimulus.

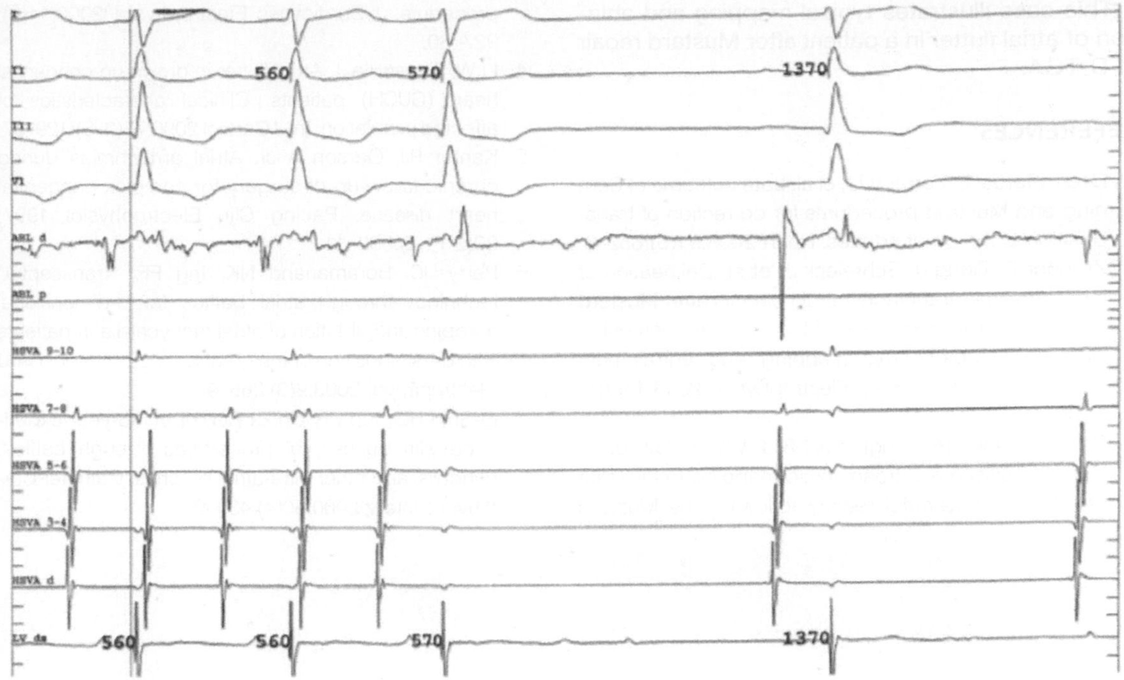

Fig. 4. Termination of the atrial flutter with radiofrequency ablation.

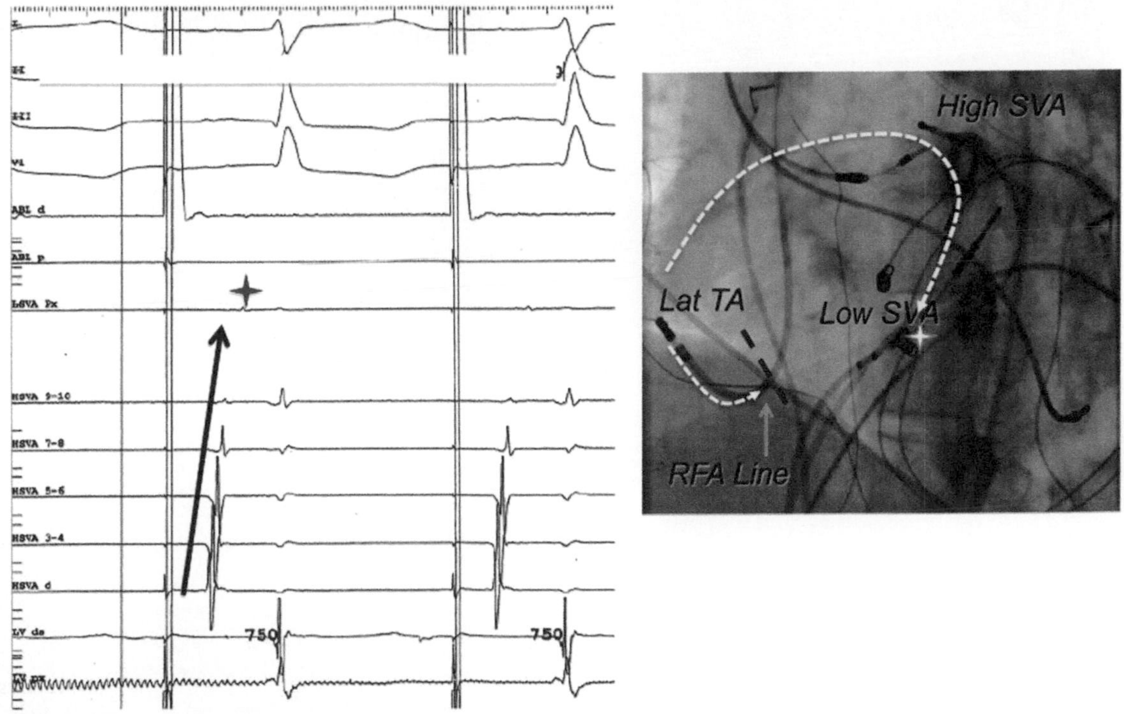

Fig. 5. Pacing the lateral tricuspid annulus (Lat TA) reveals lateral to medial block across the ablation line. Activation proceeds superiorly, activating the high SVA catheter from distal to proximal followed by the low SVA catheter (*blue arrow* on electrograms, *yellow arrows* on fluoroscopy). If there was conduction through the ablation line, the low SVA catheter would be activated before the proximal high SVA catheter, however the low SVA is activated last (*red star*). RFA, radiofrequency ablation.

This case illustrates typical mapping and ablation of atrial flutter in a patient after Mustard repair of D-TGA.

REFERENCES

1. Dos L, Teruel L, Ferreira IJ, et al. Late outcome of Senning and Mustard procedures for correction of transposition of the great arteries. Heart 2005;91(5):652–6.
2. Zrenner B, Dong J, Schreieck J, et al. Delineation of intra-atrial reentrant tachycardia circuits after Mustard operation for transposition of the great arteries using biatrial electroanatomic mapping and entrainment mapping. J Cardiovasc Electrophysiol 2003;14(12): 1302–10.
3. Sokoloski MC, Pennington JC 3rd, Winton GJ, et al. Use of multisite electroanatomic mapping to facilitate ablation of intra-atrial reentry following the Mustard procedure. J Cardiovasc Electrophysiol 2000;11(8): 927–30.
4. Li W, Somerville J. Atrial flutter in grown-up congenital heart (GUCH) patients. Clinical characteristics of affected population. Int J Cardiol 2000;75(2–3):129–37.
5. Kanter RJ, Garson A Jr. Atrial arrhythmias during chronic follow-up of surgery for complex congenital heart disease. Pacing Clin Electrophysiol 1997; 20(2 Pt 2):502–11.
6. Perry JC, Boramanand NK, Ing FF. "Transseptal" technique through atrial baffles for 3-dimensional mapping and ablation of atrial tachycardia in patients with d-transposition of the great arteries. J Interv Card Electrophysiol 2003;9(3):365–9.
7. El-Said HG, Ing FF, Grifka RG, et al. 18-year experience with transseptal procedures through baffles, conduits, and other intra-atrial patches. Catheter Cardiovasc Interv 2000;50(4):434–9.

Sustained Ventricular Tachycardia in a Patient with Tetralogy of Fallot—with a "Twist"

Robert W. Rho, MD, FHRS, FACC

KEYWORDS

• Tetralogy of Fallot • Ventricular tachycardia • Implantable cardioverter-defibrillator
• Ventricular septal defect

KEY POINTS

- There are common and uncommon associated conditions that may accompany patients with tetralogy of Fallot (TOF). These associated conditions may significantly complicate surgical or percutaneous treatment of patients with TOF.
- Arrhythmias are often the result of hemodynamic compromise in TOF. Most commonly this is due to progressive right ventricular dilatation secondary to chronic pulmonary valve regurgitation. Evaluation of arrhythmias should always be preceded by an evaluation of the patient's surgical repair (valves, conduits, ventricular septal defect) and hemodynamics.
- Surgical pulmonary valve replacement has been demonstrated to reduce the risk of ventricular tachycardia in patients with severe pulmonary regurgitation and RV enlargement.
- Among patients who present with ventricular tachycardia in the absence of a correctable lesion or hemodynamic compromise, an electrophysiologic study and radiofrequency ablation may be an effective option for the treatment of ventricular tachycardia.
- Although clinical risk factors associated with ventricular arrhythmias and sudden death have been identified, appropriate selection of patients who would benefit from an implantable cardioverter-defibrillator (ICD) for primary or even secondary prevention of sudden death remains a clinical challenge.
- Preliminary data have demonstrated that appropriate ICD shocks occur frequently among patients who have an ICD implanted, but inappropriate shocks and immediate and long-term complications are frequent in the population, and should be weighed carefully when considering ICD implantation.
- Current guidelines for ICD implantation endorse implantation of an ICD for secondary prevention, or among patients who experience syncope that is concerning for cardiac arrhythmia and inducible sustained monomorphic ventricular tachycardia at electrophysiologic study.

CASE PRESENTATION

A 19-year-old male college student with a history of tetralogy of Fallot (TOF) and dextrocardia presented to the emergency room complaining of sudden onset of palpitations, fatigue, and dyspnea on exertion while playing basketball. He denied any presyncope or syncope. His history was significant for TOF and dextrocardia with situs inversus. He had surgical repair of his TOF at the age of

Sutter Pacific Medical Foundation, Atrial Fibrillation and Complex Arrhythmia Center, 2100 Webster Street, Suite 110, San Francisco, CA 94115, USA
E-mail address: rhor@sutterhealth.org

Card Electrophysiol Clin 4 (2012) 597–602
http://dx.doi.org/10.1016/j.ccep.2012.08.036
1877-9182/12/$ – see front matter

1 year. The procedure included a pericardial patch repair of the right ventricular outflow tract and a patch repair of his ventricular septal defect. He did well until 1 year previously when he was evaluated for palpitations and heart failure. He underwent a successful pulmonary valve replacement 1 year before presentation.

In the emergency room the patient was awake, alert, and oriented. His blood pressure was 90/50 mm Hg with a heart rate of 200 beats/min (12-lead electrocardiogram, **Fig. 1**A). His room air oxygen saturation was 96%. He was sedated and underwent DC cardioversion to sinus rhythm (**Fig. 1**B).

He was admitted to the telemetry unit for further workup. Echocardiogram showed dextrocardia, repaired TOF with no residual ventricular septal defect (VSD), mild pulmonary regurgitation, mildly enlarged right ventricle, and decreased right ventricular (RV) function. His left ventricle was of normal size and his left ventricular (LV) ejection fraction was 50%. Cardiac magnetic resonance angiography (**Fig. 2**) demonstrated dextrocardia with situs inversus, stenotic pulmonary valve

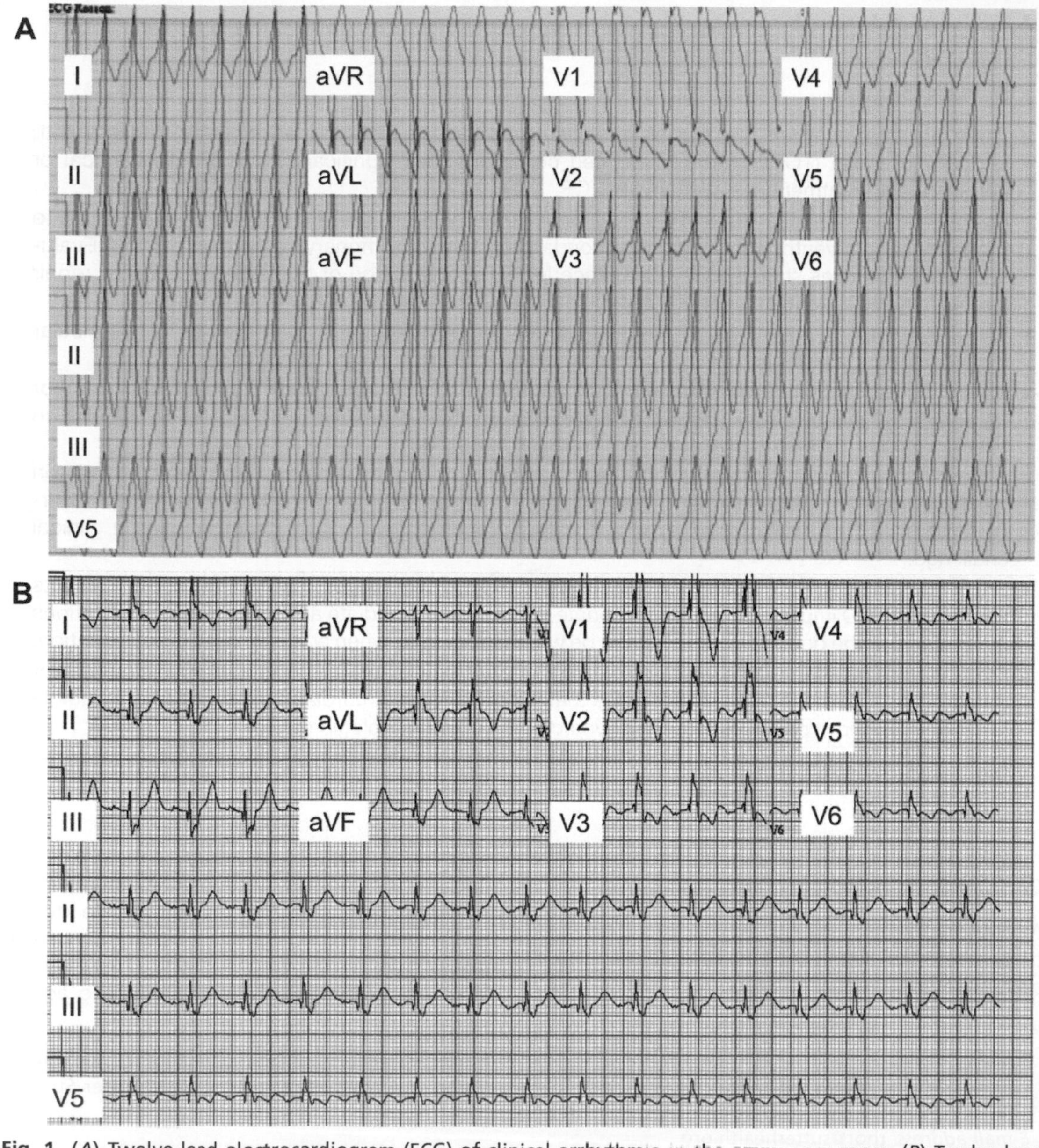

Fig. 1. (*A*) Twelve-lead electrocardiogram (ECG) of clinical arrhythmia in the emergency room. (*B*) Twelve-lead ECG after DC cardioversion in the emergency room.

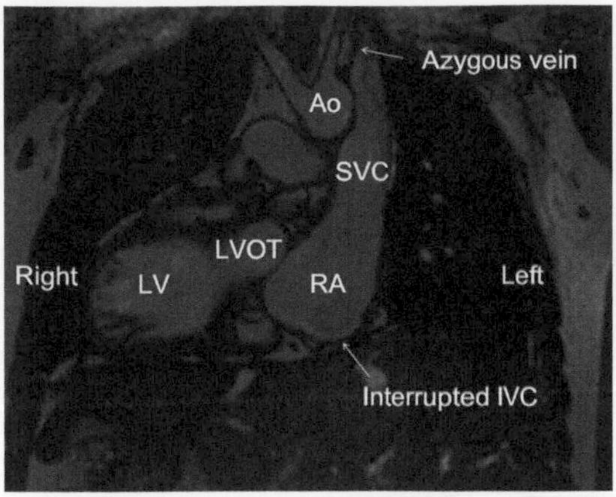

Fig. 2. Magnetic resonance angiography of coronal section, demonstrating dextrocardia with situs inversus and interrupted inferior vena cava.

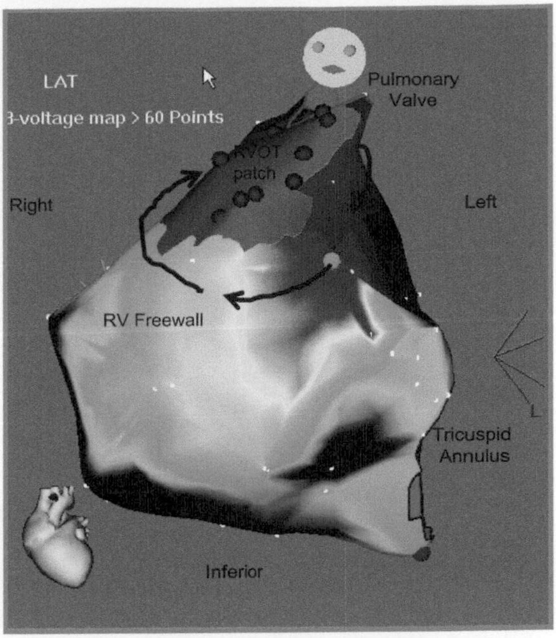

Fig. 3. Three-dimensional electroanatomic activation map of ventricular tachycardia.

prosthesis with mild pulmonary regurgitation, moderately reduced RV function (ejection fraction 32%), moderate RV hypertrophy, and mildly increased RV volume (end-diastolic volume = 109 mL/m^2). LV size was normal with mildly reduced function, and he had no coronary anomalies.

The patient was then taken to electrophysiologic study, with mapping and possible ablation of his ventricular tachycardia.

ELECTROPHYSIOLOGIC STUDY

Access was obtained in the right femoral vein. A mapping catheter was advanced via the right femoral vein, which continued as the azygous vein and entered the right atrium and right ventricle via the superior vena cava. The patient's clinical ventricular tachycardia was easily induced with programmed electrical stimulation in the right ventricle.

The patient was stable during ventricular tachycardia, and an activation map of the right ventricle was created. The 3-dimensional electroanatomic activation map (**Fig. 3**) was consistent with reentry around the RV outflow tract (RVOT) annular pericardial patch (characterized by no recorded electrograms and shown in gray on the map). Activation proceeded around the patch clockwise, from red to yellow to blue to purple and back to red, where the earliest signal (red) meets the latest (purple). The entire cycle length of the ventricular tachycardia was accounted for in this anatomic region. Entrainment of the ventricular tachycardia at 2 points at opposite sides of the patch confirmed reentry around the patch.

ABLATION STRATEGY

To enhance tissue contact, access was obtained in the right subclavian vein, and the ablation catheter was passed via the right subclavian vein into the right ventricle. A series of point-by-point radiofrequency lesions was delivered, starting from the middle of the RVOT patch along the anterior free wall to the tricuspid annulus (**Fig. 4**A). This linear lesion resulted in termination of the ventricular tachycardia (**Fig. 4**B). Programmed stimulation was performed with double and triple extrastimuli at 3 sites in the right ventricle. Ventricular tachycardia was noninducible during the remainder of the procedure.

The patient tolerated the procedure well and without complications. The option of implantation of an implantable cardioverter-defibrillator (ICD) for sustained ventricular tachycardia was discussed with the patient. He declined ICD implantation and was discharged home on no medication.

QUESTIONS AND DISCUSSION

1. What is the general prognosis and quality of life of adults with TOF who have undergone corrective repair?

Many adult patients with repaired TOF can expect excellent long-term survival with excellent functional capacity. In a European survey of 811 patients who had surgical repair of TOF (mean age 26 years), 5-year mortality was 1.3%. The majority of patients report little or no symptoms, with 93% of patients with New York Heart Association Class I or II.[1] The patient in this case report

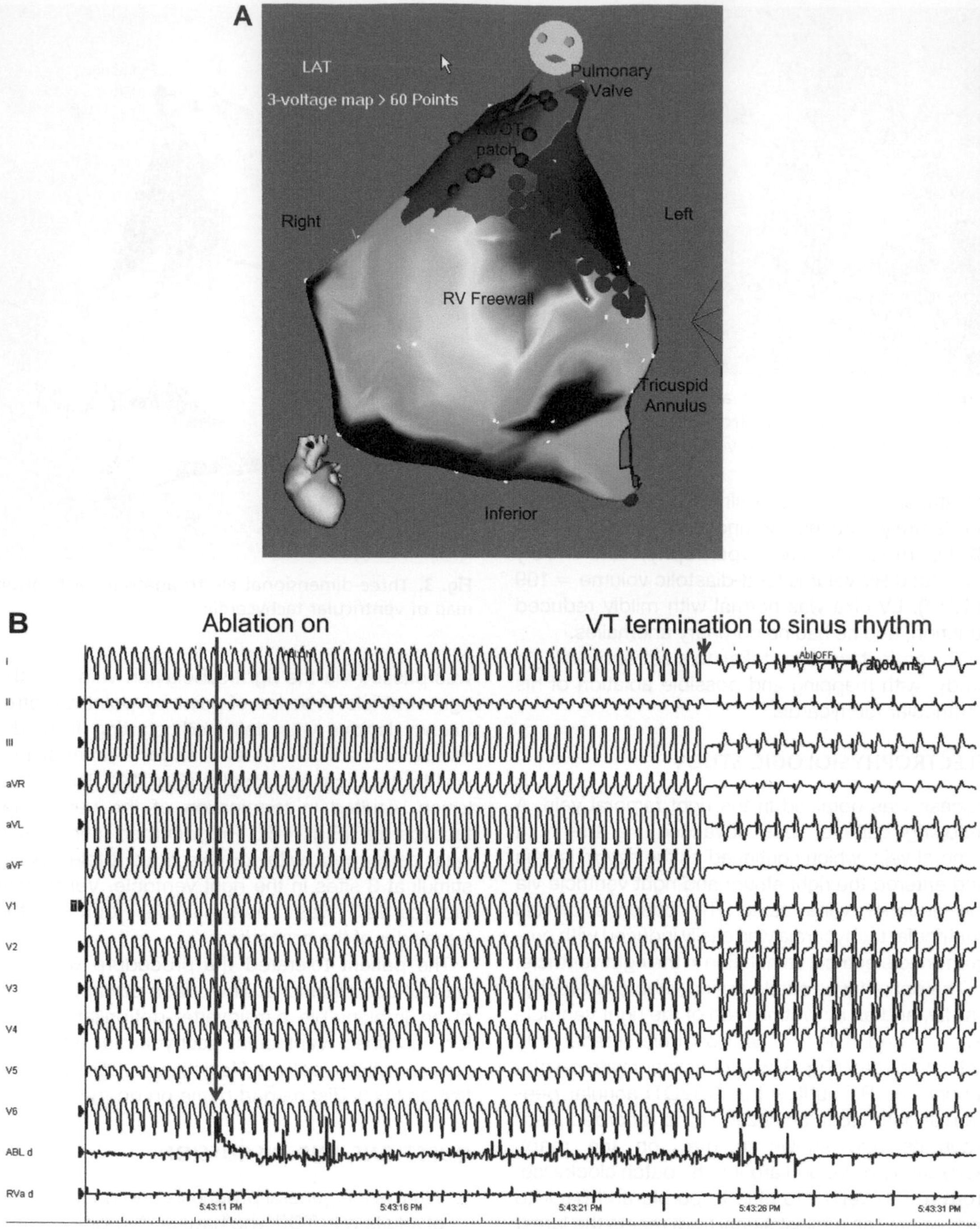

Fig. 4. (*A*) 3D electroanatomic activation map of ablation lesions performed for termination of ventricular tachycardia. (*B*) Intracardiac electrograms demonstrating termination of ventricular tachycardia during application of radiofrequency energy.

enjoyed excellent functional capacity until 1 year before his initial presentation. His functional decline was due to pulmonary valve dysfunction and progressive RV dilatation. He underwent successful replacement of his pulmonary valve with a bioprosthesis. Following corrective surgery, he enjoyed excellent functional capacity, and his QRS duration and RV function and size remained stable over 7 years of follow-up.

2. What associated congenital anomalies may be seen in association with TOF?

Associated conditions found in patients with TOF include atrial septal defect, patent ductus arteriosis, a right-sided aortic arch, and anomalous coronary arteries (9% of patients have an anomalous left anterior descending artery from proximal right coronary artery).[1,2] TOF associated with dextrocardia and situs inversus is rare but has been reported. The patient in this case had an intact atrial septum, a left-sided aortic arch, and normal coronary anatomy. To the best of the author's knowledge, this is the first reported case of TOF with dextrocardia, situs inversus, and interrupted inferior vena cava (IVC) with azygous continuation. Mapping and ablation of ventricular tachycardia in a patient with TOF, interrupted IVC with azygous continuation, and dextrocardia have not previously been reported.

3. What is the most common cause of late mortality in this patient population?

Sudden cardiac death and congestive heart failure are the most common causes of death among adults with TOF.[1,3]

4. How frequently are arrhythmias encountered in adult patients with TOF?

Approximately 40% of adult patients with TOF will encounter atrial or ventricular arrhythmias. Intra-atrial reentry tachycardia and atrial fibrillation occur in one-third of patients, and cause significant morbidity. Ventricular tachycardia occurs in approximately 15% of patients with repaired TOF. Patients with a history of sustained ventricular tachycardia or sudden cardiac death are at high risk of a subsequent event. Risk factors for ventricular tachycardia or sudden cardiac death in the absence of a prior event include an elevated LV end-diastolic pressure, nonsustained ventricular tachycardia, QRS duration longer than 180 milliseconds, inducible monomorphic ventricular tachycardia at electrophysiologic study, and a history of a palliative shunt.[3] Atrial or ventricular arrhythmias are usually a consequence of decompensated hemodynamics. A careful evaluation of the patient's anatomy and hemodynamics is an essential part of the initial assessment of a patient encountering new-onset arrhythmias.

5. What is the mechanism of ventricular tachycardia in patients with TOF?

Most ventricular tachycardia in this population is due to reentry around anatomic obstacles resulting from the surgical repair. Patients who have had a patch repair of the RVOT commonly have ventricular tachycardia from reentry around the patch, as seen in this case. Other reentry circuits have been described involving the VSD patch or ventriculotomy incisions.[4] RV dilatation and remodeling often from pulmonary regurgitation or obstructions in the RVOT, conduits, or branch pulmonary arteries may also provide substrates for reentry. In retrospect, it is likely that this patient would not have experienced ventricular tachycardia 1 year following his pulmonary valve replacement if he had undergone an adjunctive arrhythmia procedure. Because he did not present with ventricular tachycardia at the time he underwent his pulmonary valve replacement, an adjunctive arrhythmia procedure was not performed. The role of a presurgical electrophysiologic study with programmed stimulation to take an "inventory" of potential arrhythmias to guide surgical ablation, electrophysiologic study, and radiofrequency ablation before or following surgery, and even the role of performing empiric lesions during surgery, are under debate.

6. What long-term treatment options are available for managing ventricular tachycardia in adult patients with TOF?

Patients with severe pulmonary regurgitation or outflow-tract obstruction and a dilated right ventricle should undergo pulmonary valve replacement with consideration for adjunctive arrhythmia surgery directed at eliminating ventricular tachycardia circuits.[5] Electrophysiologic study with radiofrequency ablation is an effective treatment option for patients without any indication for surgery.

7. What is the incidence of sudden death among adults with repaired TOF?

Sudden death occurs in up to 0.5% of patients per year and is the cause of death in up to half of adult patients with TOF. Patients are at increased risk if they have a history of aborted sudden death, sustained ventricular tachycardia, or syncope. Additional risks factors in asymptomatic patients with TOF include an elevated LV end-diastolic pressure, nonsustained ventricular tachycardia, a QRS duration longer than 180 milliseconds, history of a ventriculotomy, severe RV enlargement/dysfunction (usually from severe pulmonary valve regurgitation), and LV dysfunction.[3]

8. What is the role of the ICD in lowering the risk of sudden death in this population?

Clinical trial data on ICDs among adult patients with TOF are limited. Observational studies of patients with TOF who have implantable defibrillators report a high number of appropriate shocks. It is not clear how many of these appropriate shocks were necessary (shocks occurring for what would have been nonsustained ventricular tachycardia). A concerning observation is the high rate of inappropriate shocks and complications associated with ICDs in this population.[6] Implantation of an ICD is appropriate among patients with TOF who are successfully resuscitated after an episode of sudden death or experience sustained ventricular tachycardia. The role of an ICD for primary prevention of sudden cardiac death is less clear. Whether successful ablation of clinical sustained ventricular tachycardia adequately protects patients from future sudden cardiac death is also unclear.

LONG-TERM FOLLOW-UP

After a follow-up period of 7 years since his ablation procedure, the patient has had no recurrence of ventricular tachycardia. His pulmonary valve and right ventricular size and function have remained stable. He completed dual degrees at the University and is currently working as a software engineer. He remains active with minimal symptoms.

This case exemplifies some of the challenges encountered in the treatment and risk assessment of recurrent ventricular tachycardia among patients with TOF.

SUMMARY

TOF is the most common form of cyanotic congenital heart disease. Patients who undergo surgical repair of TOF have an excellent prognosis, and the majority live well into adulthood with excellent functional capacity and quality of life. The new natural history following surgical repair of TOF is usually related to pulmonary regurgitation and RV dysfunction, which is accompanied by a high incidence of cardiac arrhythmias. Ventricular tachycardia occurs in 15% of patients with TOF and usually involves reentry around an anatomic obstacle left behind after the repair. RV enlargement from chronic pulmonary valve regurgitation is an important risk factor for ventricular tachycardia and sudden death. Pulmonary valve replacement may lead to a significant reduction in recurrent ventricular tachycardia. However, patients who undergo concomitant arrhythmia surgery are more likely to remain arrhythmia-free. In the absence of hemodynamic compromise requiring surgical correction, electrophysiologic study with radiofrequency ablation is an effective treatment option. Current guidelines for ICD implantation endorse implantation of an ICD for secondary prevention, or among patients who experience syncope that is concerning for cardiac arrhythmia and inducible sustained monomorphic ventricular tachycardia at electrophysiologic study. Although clinical risk factors associated with ventricular arrhythmias and sudden death have been identified, appropriate selection of patients who would benefit from an ICD for primary or even secondary prevention of sudden death remains a clinical challenge. This case illustrates some of the difficulties of accurately predicting the risk of ventricular arrhythmias in patients with TOF.

REFERENCES

1. Engelfriet P, Boersma E, Oechslin E, et al. The spectrum of adult congenital heart disease in Europe: morbidity and mortality in a 5 year follow-up period. The Euro Heart Survey on adult congenital heart disease. Eur Heart J 2005;26(21):2325.
2. Dabizzi RP, Caprioli G, Aiazzi L, et al. Distribution and anomalies of coronary arteries in tetralogy of Fallot. Circulation 1980;61(1):95.
3. Gatzoulis MA, Balaji S, Webber SA, et al. Risk factors for arrhythmia and sudden death late after repair of tetralogy of Fallot: a multicenter study. Lancet 2000; 356:975–81.
4. Zeppenfeld K, Schalij MJ, Bartelings MM, et al. Catheter ablation of ventricular tachycardia after repair of congenital heart disease: electroanatomic identification of the critical right ventricular isthmus. Circulation 2007;116:2241–52.
5. Therrien J, Siu SC, Harris L, et al. Impact of pulmonary valve replacement on arrhythmia propensity late after repair of tetralogy of Fallot. Circulation 2001;103:2489–94.
6. Khairy P, Harris L, Landzberg MJ, et al. Implantable cardioverter-defibrillators in tetralogy of Fallot. Circulation 2008;117:363–70.

Introduction to Ventricular Tachycardia

Edward P. Gerstenfeld, MD

KEYWORDS

• Ventricular tachycardia • Electrocardiography • Entrainment mapping • Cardiomyopathy

KEY POINTS

- Knowledge of the underlying substrate is critical for planning the ventricular tachycardia (VT) mapping strategy.
- Understanding the surface ECG morphology is useful for anticipating the VT exit site.
- Conventional entrainment mapping remains the most useful strategy for localizing the critical isthmus of a reentrant VT circuit.

Mapping and ablation of ventricular tachycardia (VT) has become a critical skill for practicing electrophysiologists. Three general types of VT can be encountered: idiopathic VT occurring in structurally normal hearts, VT associated with cardiomyopathy caused by myocardial infarction, and VT associated with nonischemic cardiomyopathy. Each poses its own unique challenges. Idiopathic VT typically occurs in stereotypical anatomic locations, with the most common including the right or left ventricular outflow tract. Recognition that idiopathic VT can originate from cardiac muscle fibers within or near the aortic root is important for those performing catheter ablation.

In this section, Heath and colleagues present an interesting case of a patient with two distinct VTs that appear to have the same focal origin with different exit sites in the aortic root. This case highlights the importance of recognition of the electrocardiographic morphology of VT originating from the aortic root, and the use of electroanatomic mapping and intracardiac echocardiography to localize the site of origin.

Bala presents a patient with recurrent VT that developed more than 10 years after a large anteroseptal myocardial infarction. Why such VT often occurs years after the index infarction remains a mystery. This case demonstrates some important aspects of entrainment mapping and the utility of entrainment mapping for locating the VT isthmus in patients with a mappable VT.

Tzou presents a case of an incessant VT of right bundle branch morphology in a patient with nonischemic cardiomyopathy after surgery for aortic valve replacement. This common form of incessant VT was easily mapped and ablated, and may often be missed by clinicians who do not recognize the pathognomonic signs.

Finally, Deyall and Garcia present a complex case of recurrent VT in a patient with nonischemic cardiomyopathy undergoing epicardial and endocardial ablation. Epicardial mapping is now commonly performed in patients with nonischemic cardiomyopathy. Unlike patients with ischemic cardiomyopathy whereby the scar and VT circuits are nearly always endocardial, patients with nonischemic cardiomyopathy often have midmyocardial or epicardial scar. In this case, combined endocardial and epicardial mapping revealed an unusual finding about the location of the VT circuit.

These thought-provoking cases highlight several important points about mapping and ablation of VT. First, knowledge of the underlying substrate is critical for planning the mapping strategy. Second, understanding the surface ECG morphology is useful for anticipating the VT exit site. Third, conventional entrainment mapping remains the most useful strategy for localizing the critical isthmus of a reentrant VT circuit. It is hoped that these cases stimulate the reader's interest in mapping and catheter ablation of VT.

Cardiac Electrophysiology, University of California, 500 Parnassus Avenue, MU4-East, San Francisco, CA 94143, USA
E-mail address: egerstenfeld@medicine.ucsf.edu

Card Electrophysiol Clin 4 (2012) 603
http://dx.doi.org/10.1016/j.ccep.2012.08.018
1877-9182/12/$ – see front matter

Bicuspid Ventricular Tachycardia in a Patient with Syncope and a Structurally Normal Heart

Russell R. Heath, MD, Duy Thai Nguyen, MD, Wendy S. Tzou, MD, William H. Sauer, MD*

KEYWORDS

• Ventricular tachycardia • Aortic cusp • Pace mapping

KEY POINTS

- A common origin of ventricular tachycardia (VT) in patients with structurally normal hearts is the aortic root.
- Left bundle inferior-axis VT with an early precordial transition (<V3) commonly originates from the left ventricular outflow tract.
- Patients may have a single VT with multiple exit sites yielding different electrocardiographic morphologies.
- Intracardiac echocardiography is useful to guide mapping of VT originating from the aortic cusps.

CLINICAL HISTORY

A 63-year-old man with a structurally normal heart and a history of prior failed left ventricular outflow tract ventricular tachycardia (VT) ablation presented to the hospital with sustained monomorphic VT requiring lidocaine and procainamide drips for suppression. The prior ablation attempt localized an easily inducible VT to the right coronary cusp. Review of the single-lead telemetry monitor recording revealed an inferiorly directed VT. A baseline electrocardiogram (ECG) in normal sinus rhythm demonstrated right bundle branch block (RBBB) and left anterior fascicular block (LAFB). Cardiac imaging studies demonstrated a structurally normal heart with normal valves, with normal cardiac chamber size and function. The patient was then transferred to the authors' care for management All antiarrhythmics were discontinued, and the patient was taken to the electrophysiology laboratory for mapping and ablation.

ELECTROPHYSIOLOGY STUDY AND TREATMENT

The patient was brought to the electrophysiology laboratory in sinus rhythm (SR). Arterial and venous access was obtained. A quadripolar catheter (St Jude Medical) was advanced to the right ventricle and used to perform programmed stimulation in an attempt to induce VT. Two distinct sustained VTs were easily inducible with ventricular extra-stimuli with the administration of isoproterenol. VT1 was a left bundle, left

Section of Cardiac Electrophysiology, Division of Cardiology, University of Colorado School of Medicine, 12401 East 17th Avenue, B-136, Aurora, CO 80045, USA
* Corresponding author.
E-mail address: William.Sauer@ucdenver.edu

Card Electrophysiol Clin 4 (2012) 605–610
http://dx.doi.org/10.1016/j.ccep.2012.08.013
1877-9182/12/$ – see front matter

cardiacEP.theclinics.com

inferior morphology at a tachycardia cycle length (TCL) of 420 milliseconds (**Fig. 1**). This VT was morphologically distinct from the VT targeted during the prior ablation session. Based on the VT morphology, a left ventricular outflow tract origin was suspected and therefore an intracardiac echocardiography catheter (SoundStar; Biosense Webster, Bar Diamond, CA) was advanced to the right ventricle just across the tricuspid valve to obtain a cross-sectional view of the aortic valve (**Fig. 2**). Anatomic contour data from the aortic cusps were collected and merged with a limited electroanatomic map. Arterial access was obtained, and an externally irrigated ablation catheter (Thermocool; Biosense Webster) was placed at the aortic root.

Repeat programmed stimulation resulted in a morphologically distinct VT (VT2; **Fig. 3**). VT2 was mapped and localized to the right coronary cusp with activation mapping (see **Fig. 2**). Radiofrequency energy titrated to 50 W was delivered at the site of earliest activation, and resulted in termination of VT2 (**Fig. 4**). Worthy of note is the interesting pre-QRS signal on the ablation catheter just before ablation. Following ablation of VT2, an attempt to reinduce VT1 was not successful. Therefore, an attempt was made to localize the site of origin of VT1 using pace mapping at sites in the left ventricular outflow tract, including the aortic cusps. A site at the left coronary cusp distant from the right cusp revealed an exact pace-map match to VT2. Of interest, there was a dramatic change in morphology with higher output pacing, such that both VT1 and VT2 were evoked from the same site (**Fig. 5**). In addition, a possible late potential was observed at this pacing site, suggesting the presence of fibrosis and scarring with delayed activation (**Fig. 6**). Given these findings, additional ablation lesions were delivered to the left coronary cusp greater than 1 cm from the left main ostium as judged by intracardiac echocardiography. After a 30-minute waiting period, programmed stimulation was performed without evidence of any further inducible VT. The patient has remained arrhythmia free off of all medications for more than 1 year since the ablation.

DISCUSSION

This case describes the presentation of a patient with 2 VTs originating from the right and left

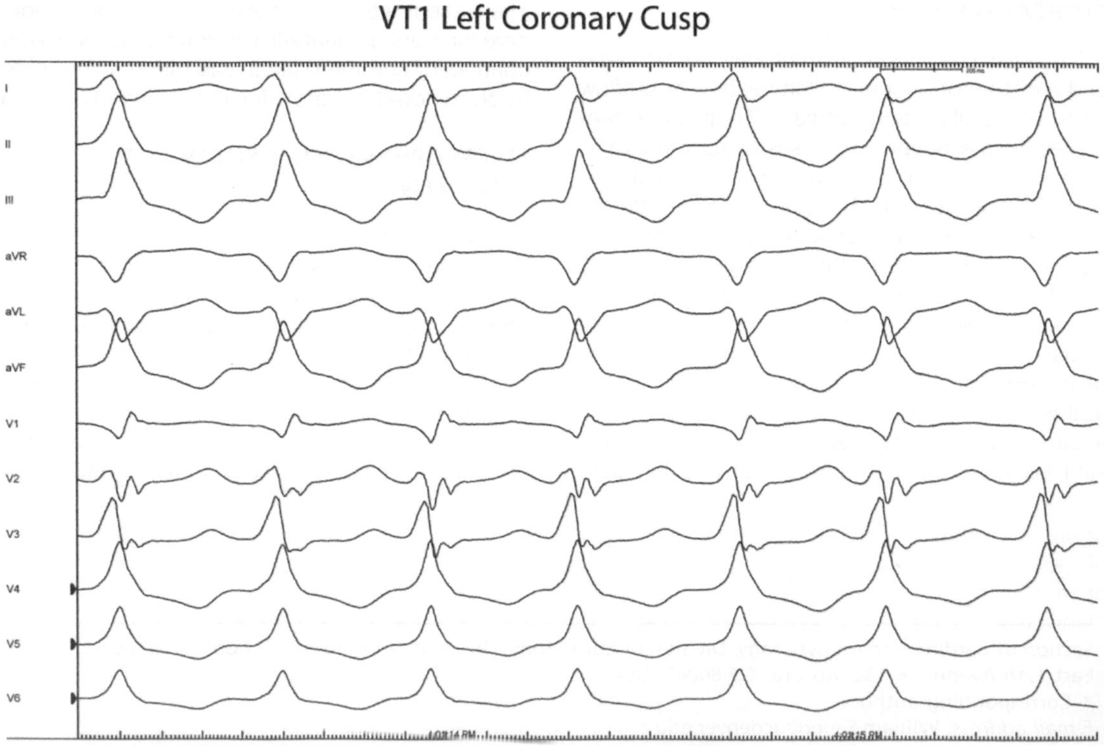

Fig. 1. Twelve-lead electrocardiogram (ECG) of VT1 arising from the left coronary cusp.

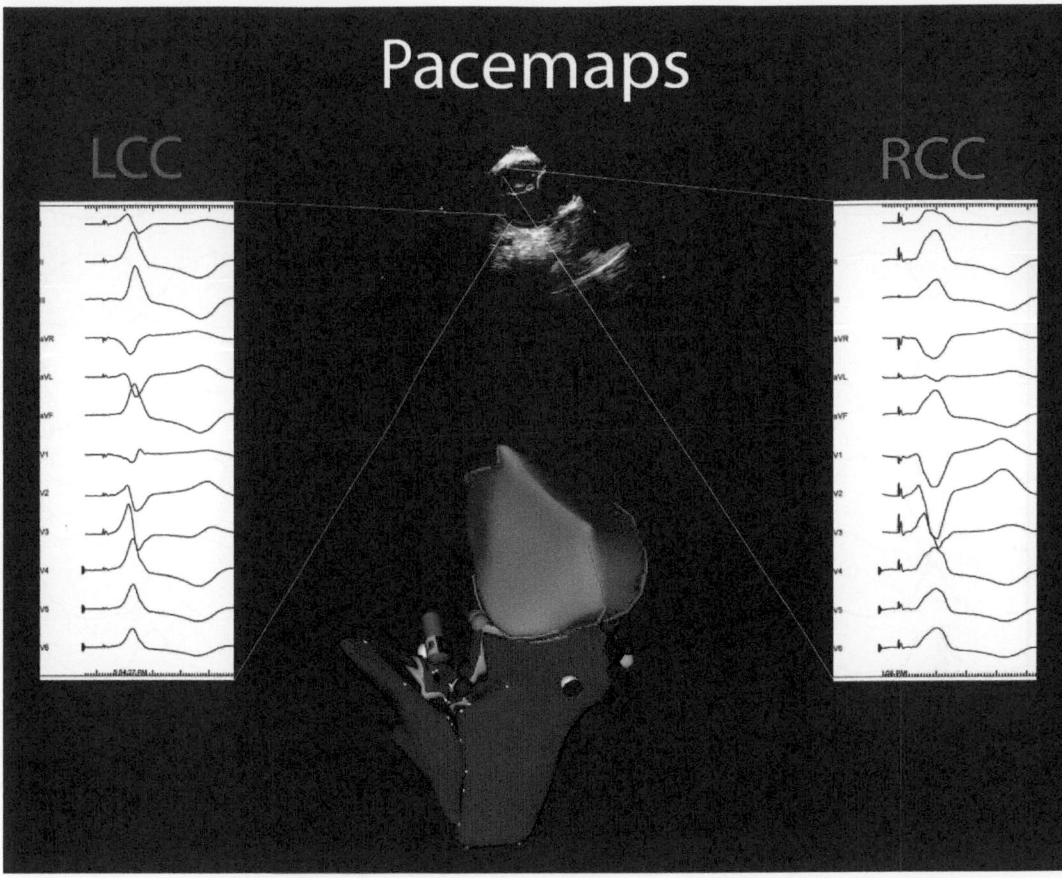

Fig. 2. Intracardiac echocardiography cross-sectional view of the aortic cups with corresponding pace maps. Blue denotes the left coronary cusp (LCC), orange the right coronary cusp (RCC), and yellow the noncoronary cusp. (*Bottom center*) CARTO (Biosense Webster) 3-dimensional electroanatomic map showing earliest activation of VT2 from the right coronary cusp and ablation lesions (*red circles*) at both cusps.

coronary cusps. The presence of these morphologically distinct VTs with similar rates suggests a common mechanism for development of cusp-related VT. In addition, the finding that pace mapping from the left coronary cusp led to a VT morphology that was mapped to the right coronary cusp further supports a common origin for this patient's VT.

Outflow tract VTs are most likely caused by calcium-dependent triggered activity. This group of relatively common idiopathic VTs occurs in patients without structural heart disease. Because of this, ECG localization can be more reproducible and precise than typical scar-mediated VT whereby the 12-lead morphology can be heavily influenced by preexisting scar.[1]

In this case, the 2 different VTs are typical for right and left coronary cusp origins. Both are markedly positive in the inferior leads and both are initially positive in lead I. VT2, arising from the right coronary cusp, is more positive in lead I than VT1 from the left coronary cusp. These differences are consistent with the more posterior position of the right coronary cusp in comparison with the left coronary cusp. The precordial transition is also typical in each example, with a V3 transition for the right coronary cusp VT and a transition at V2 for the left coronary cusp VT, all consistent with the slightly more anterior position of the right coronary cusp as compared with the left coronary cusp.[2,3] Although a common arrhythmia mechanism is suspected given the similar cycle lengths and anatomic proximity of VT1 and VT2 in this case, there is also the possibility of 2 arrhythmic foci, from separate cusps. Another possibility is that the VTs were arising from a common

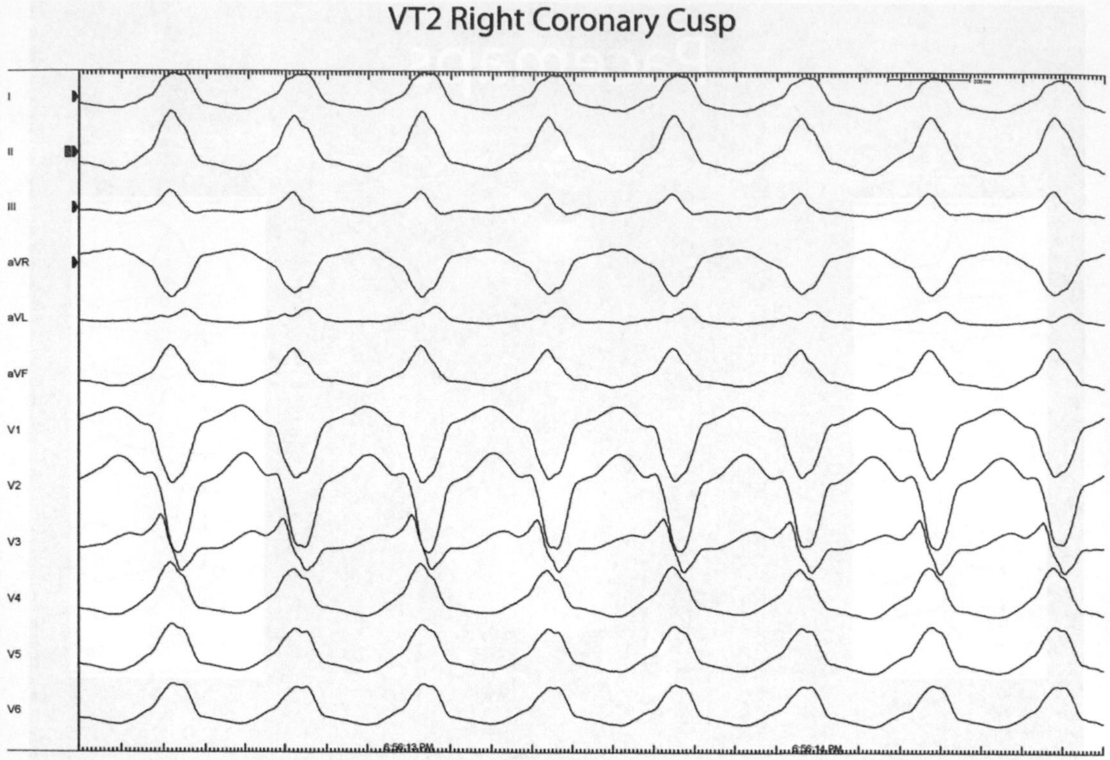

Fig. 3. Twelve-lead ECG of VT2 arising from the right coronary cusp.

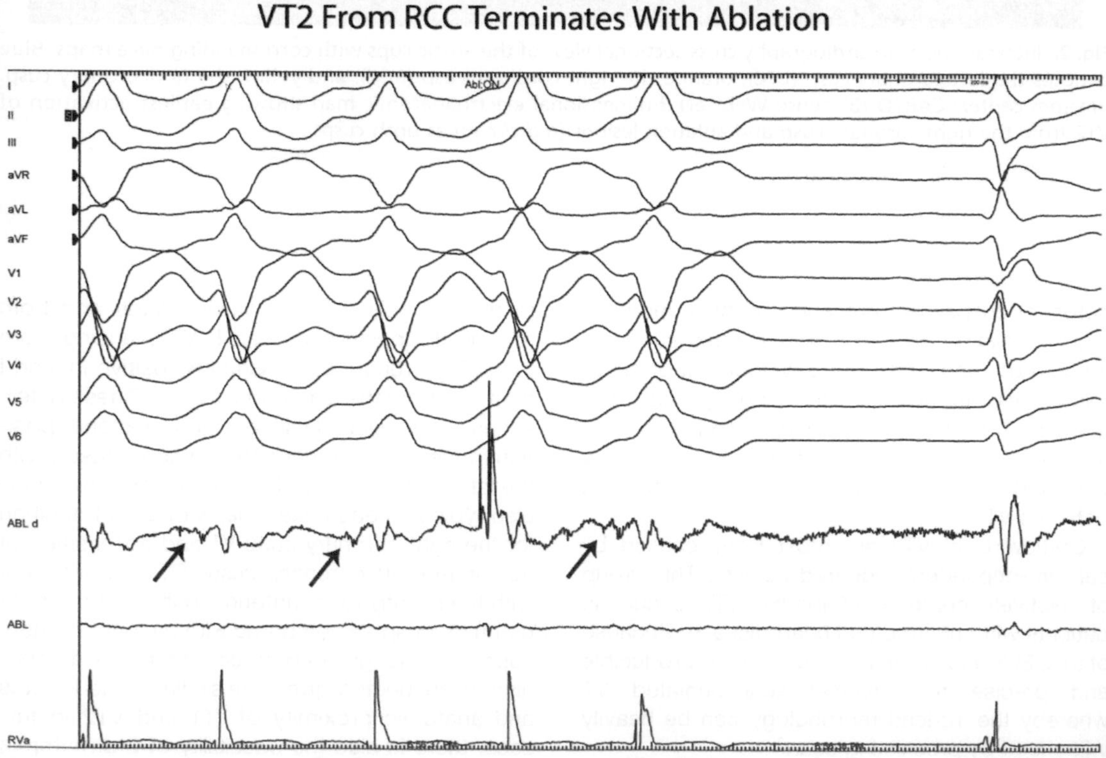

Fig. 4. VT2 from the right coronary cusp terminates with ablation. Note the interesting pre-QRS signal on the ablation catheter (*arrows*) in VT before termination of the tachycardia.

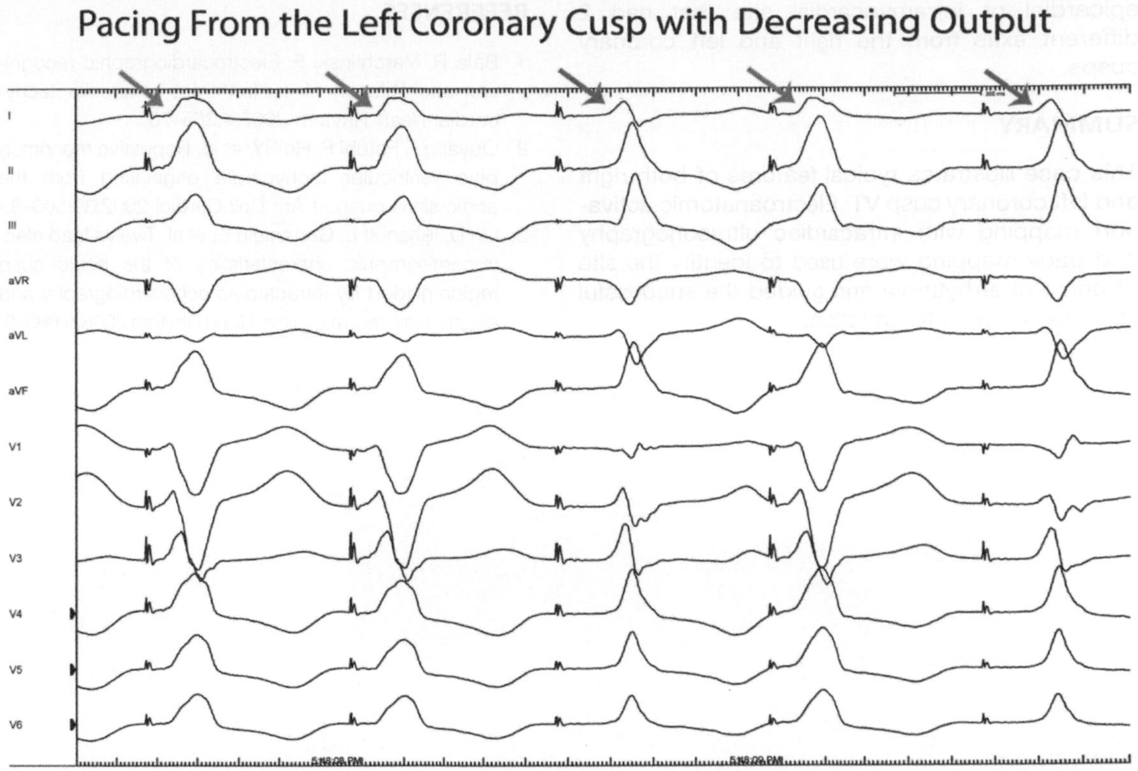

Fig. 5. Pacing from the left coronary cusp with decreasing output. Note how the pace-map morphology changes progressively from right coronary cusp morphology (*orange arrows*) to left coronary cusp morphology (*blue arrows*).

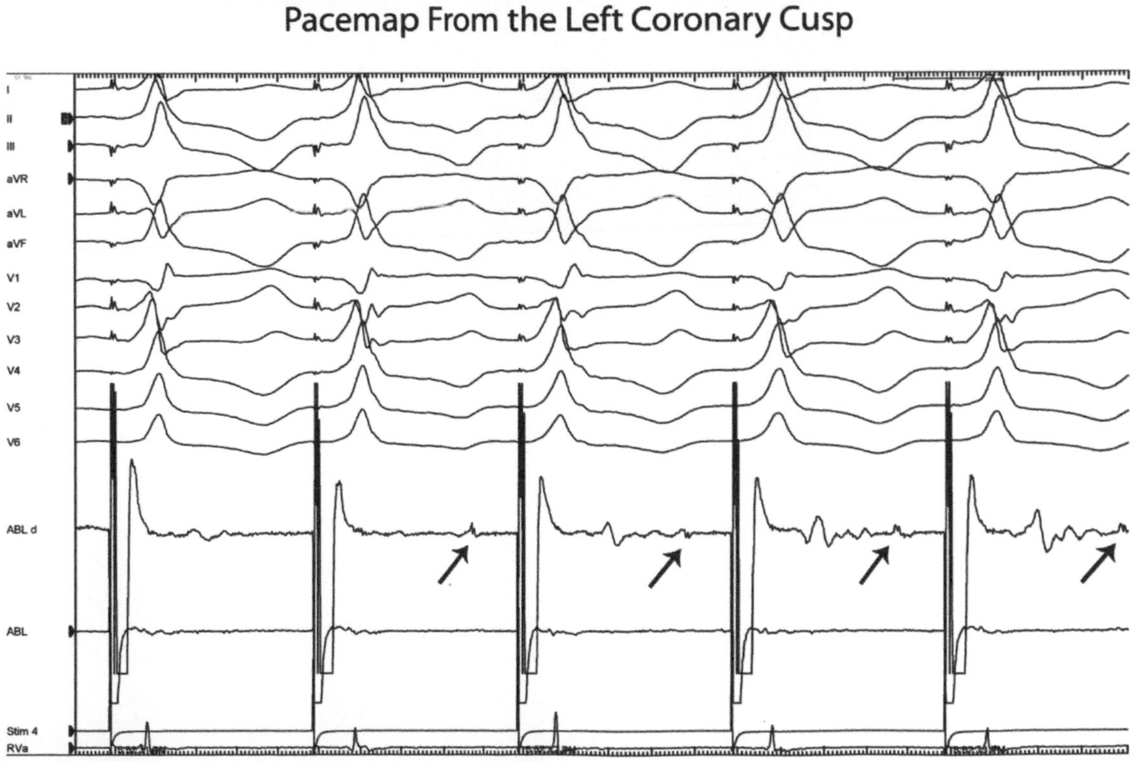

Fig. 6. Pacing from the left coronary cusp before ablation at that site. Note the late potential on the ablation catheter (*arrows*).

epicardial or intramyocardial site that had 2 different exits from the right and left coronary cusps.

SUMMARY

This case illustrates typical features of both right and left coronary cusp VT. Electroanatomic activation mapping with intracardiac ultrasonography and pace mapping were used to identify the site of origin of arrhythmia and guided the successful strategy for catheter ablation.

REFERENCES

1. Bala R, Marchlinski F. Electrocardiographic recognition and ablation of outflow tract ventricular tachycardia. Heart Rhythm 2007;4:365–70.
2. Ouyang F, Fotuhi P, Ho SY, et al. Repetitive monomorphic ventricular tachycardia originating from the aortic sinus cusp. J Am Coll Cardiol 2002;39:500–8.
3. Lin D, Ilkhanoff L, Gertenfeld E, et al. Twelve-lead electrocardiographic characteristics of the aortic cusp region guided by intracardiac echocardiography and electroanatomic mapping. Heart Rhythm 2008;5:663–9.

The Case of the Missing VT Isthmus

Rupa Bala, MD[a,*], Edward P. Gerstenfeld, MD[b]

KEYWORDS

• Ventricular tachycardia • Myocardial infarction • Electroanatomic mapping • Cardiomyopathy

KEY POINTS

- During classic entrainment, the last beat is entrained but not fused.
- Identification of the last entrained beat is critical to interpreting entrainment.
- Termination of ventricular tachycardia (VT) with a nonpropagated stimulus identifies a ciritcal VT isthmus, and ablation at this site typically is successful.
- Mapping of the right ventricular septum may be needed in VT that occurs after anteroseptal myocardial infarction.

CLINICAL HISTORY

A 41-year-old woman presented to the emergency room with presyncope in sustained VT. She had a history of a coronary dissection in her third trimester of pregnancy requiring 2-vessel coronary artery bypass grafting (saphenous vein grafts to obtuse marginal and left anterior descending coronary arteries), resulting in an ischemic cardiomyopathy with a left ventricular ejection fraction of 25%. She did well with New York Heart Association class I–II symptoms for the prior 13 years on metoprolol and lisinopril. In the emergency room she was treated with intravenous amiodarone and cardioverted to sinus rhythm. A coronary angiogram revealed total occlusion of the left anterior descending coronary artery and patent bypass grafts. A dual-chamber implantable cardioverter-defibrillator was implanted and she was started on Tikosyn (500 μg) twice daily. Two weeks later, she presented with implantable cardioverter-defibrillator shocks due to recurrent VT. She was started on IV lidocaine and transferred to the author's institution.

CLINICAL COURSE

Catheter insertion initiated her clinical VT, which had a left bundle, left inferior axis morphology with a cycle-length of 360 ms (**Fig. 1**).

Question 1: What Is the Likely Exit Site of This VT?

The VT has a left bundle, right superior axis morphology; there are Q waves throughout the precordial leads. Although localization in a patient, such as this one, with a large anteroapical scar can be difficult, the morphology suggests an inferoapical septal exit (Josephson site 2). The left bundle branch morphology and positive vector in lead I argue that the exit must be septal rather than lateral apex.[1]

An activation map (Carto, Biosense Webster) of the left ventricle (LV) was acquired during VT with an 8-French, 3.5-mm tip, open-irrigated (Navistar ThermoCool, Biosense Webster) catheter. There was a diffuse area of early activation along the midseptum (**Fig. 2**).

[a] Hospital of the University of Pennsylvania, Division of Electrophysiology, 3400 Spruce Street, 9 Founders, Philadelphia, PA 19104, USA; [b] Cardiology Division, Department of Medicine, University of California at San Francisco, 500 Parnassus Avenue, MUE-434, Box 1354, San Francisco, CA 94143-1354, USA
* Corresponding author.
E-mail address: Rupa.Bala@uphs.upenn.edu

Card Electrophysiol Clin 4 (2012) 611–615
http://dx.doi.org/10.1016/j.ccep.2012.08.011

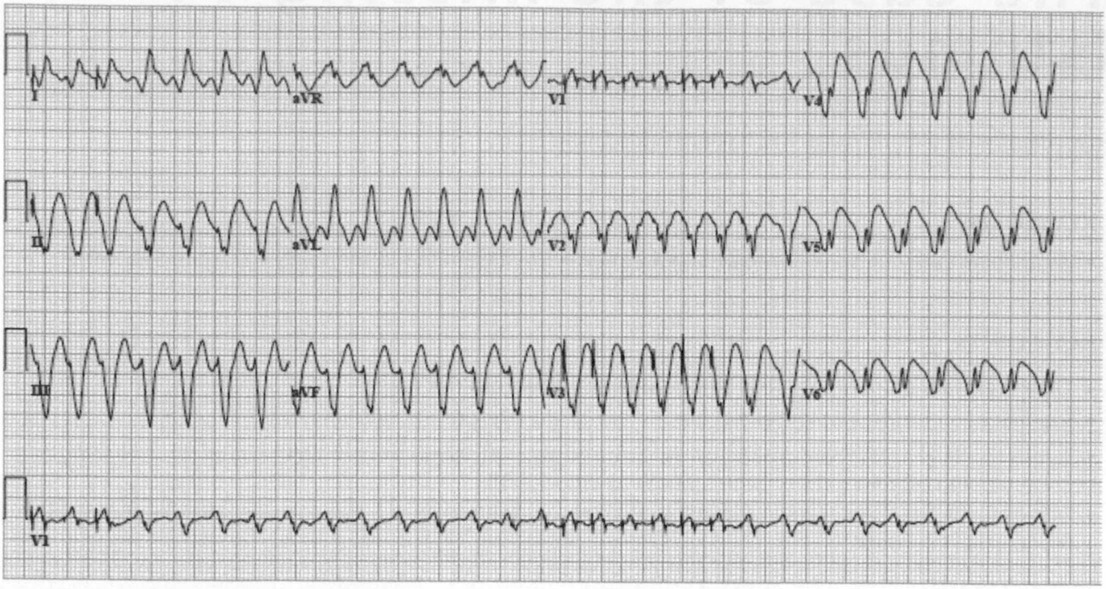

Fig. 1. Clinical VT: left bundle, superior axis. Pacing stimuli can be seen from an implanted defibrillator attempting antitachycardia pacing.

Entrainment mapping was performed at the area of earliest activation in the LV (**Fig. 2**, white tag).

Question 2: How Would This Entrainment Site Be Characterized?

During pacing at 340 ms, 20 ms faster than the tachycardia cycle length, the tachycardia is accelerated to the pacing rate, indicating capture of the ventricle. The pacing stimulus occurs nearly simultaneously with the onset of the QRS (**Fig. 3**).

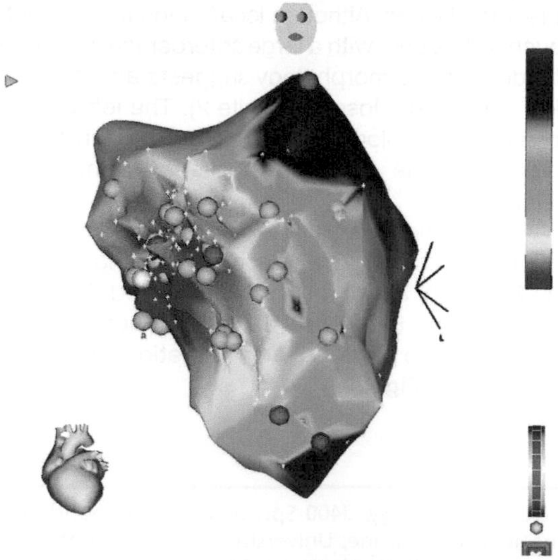

Fig. 2. Activation map of LV. There is an early area of diffuse activation along midseptum. Yellow tags represent pacing sites. The white tag was a site of entrainment with concealed fusion.

Careful measurement of the R-R intervals determines that the pacing stimulus is capturing the following QRS complex (**Fig. 4**).

There is fusion of the surface QRS (seen best in the inferior leads) during entrainment, and the last captured beat is entrained but not fused, consistent with manifest entrainment. Manifest entrainment with a long stimulus to QRS interval characterizes the VT as macroreentrant, even though the reentrant circuit is not readily apparent on the electroanatomic map. The postpacing interval is difficult to ascertain; however, examining the proximal ablation (Carto) catheter bipole, it seems that the second component is the first return beat. The long stimulus to QRS with manifest fusion suggests a site that is an outer loop proximal to the VT isthmus and not part of the protected tachycardia isthmus. Entrainment was performed from multiple LV sites and all revealed some fusion with a long stimulus to QRS interval. Three radiofrequency lesions were applied to the LV outer loop sites with no effect on the clinical VT.

The quadripolar catheter in the right ventricle (RV) was moved, withdrawn to the septum just opposite the outer loop site on the LV septum, and the clinical VT was entrained.

Question 3: How Would This Site Be Characterized?

This site (**Fig. 5**) shows evidence of manifest fusion (examine lead III) on the surface ECG with a postpacing interval approximately equal to tachycardia cycle length and short stimulus to QRS interval.

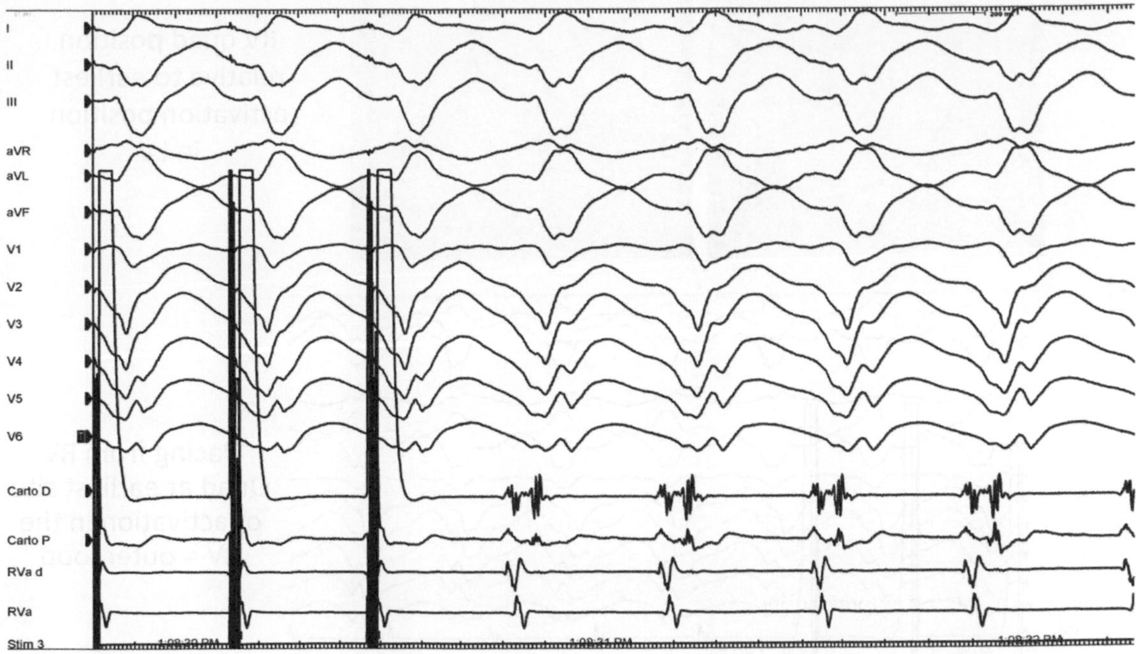

Fig. 3. Entrainment of the VT performed with overdrive pacing 20 ms faster than the VT cycle length from the ablation catheter located at the LV septum.

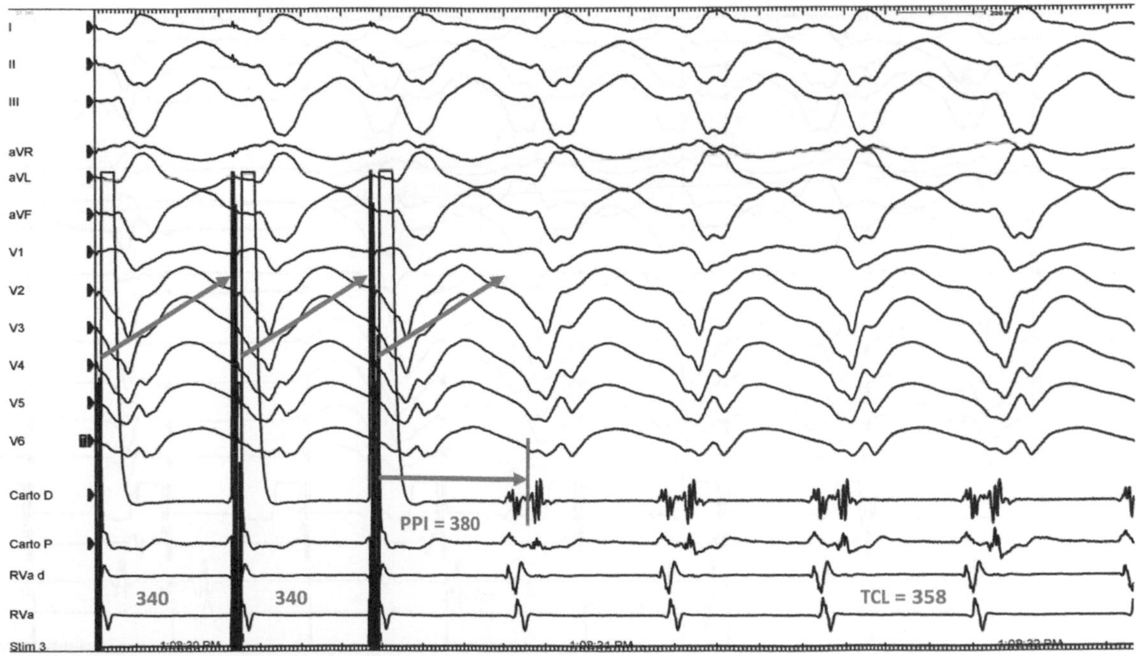

Fig. 4. Entrainment performed from site of earliest activation in the LV (*white tag on activation map*) as shown in **Fig. 2**. Intervals are marked in this figure. Note that the pacing stimulus is capturing the following QRS and that the postpacing interval is measured to the second component of the electrogram on the mapping catheter. The postpacing interval (PPI) is 380 ms. The tachycardia cycle length (TCL) is 358 ms.

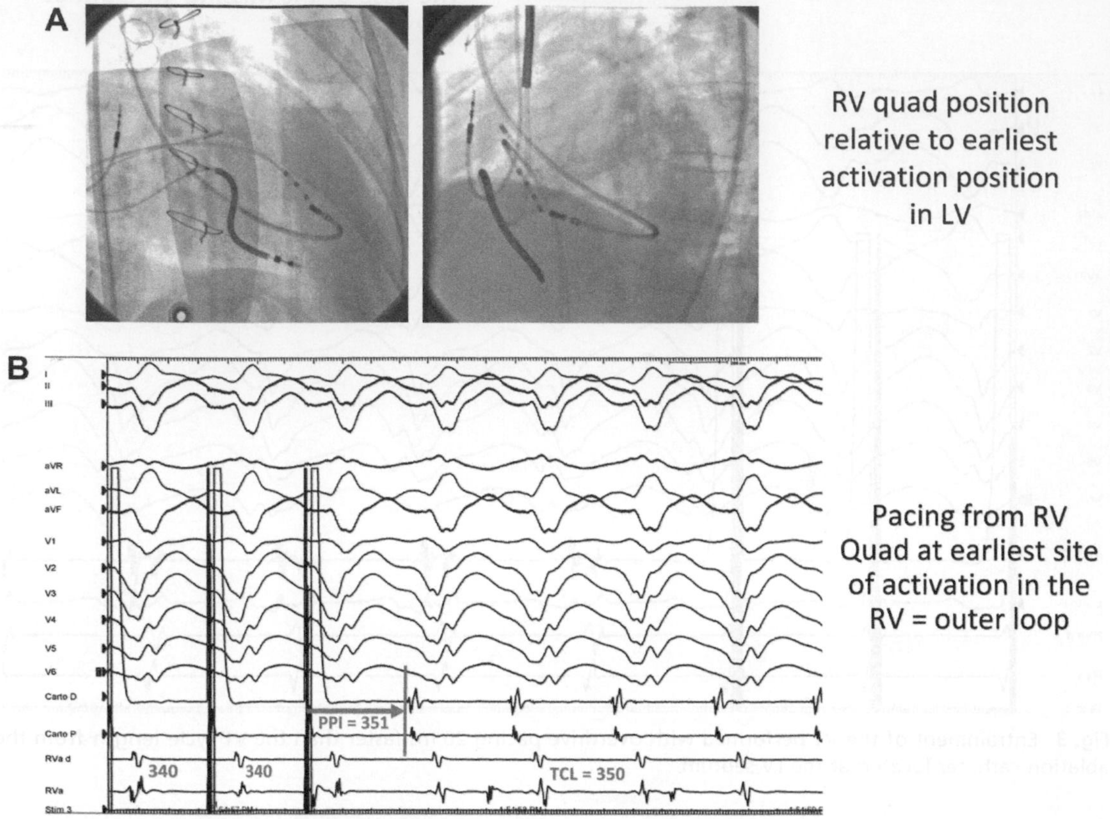

Fig. 5. (*A*) Right anterior oblique (*left panel*) and left anterior oblique (*right panel*) fluoroscopic images of the ablation catheter at the site of earliest activation in the LV relative to the quadripolar catheter on the RV septum. (*B*) The entrainment response with overdrive pacing from the RV catheter. This site was consistent with an outer loop site near the exit of the VT. The postpacing interval (PPI) is 351 ms. The tachycardia cycle length (TCL) is 350 ms.

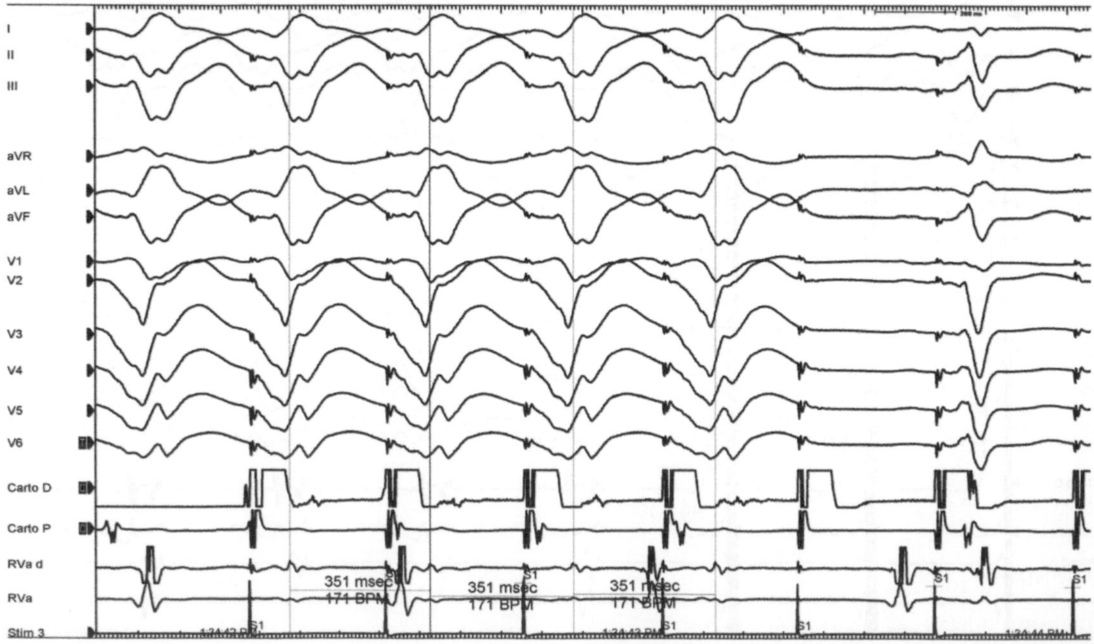

Fig. 6. Pacing is performed from the ablation catheter on the RV septum. During pacing there is termination of the clinical VT with a pacing stimulus that does not result in global capture (fifth pacing stimulus). Sinus rhythm is present after VT termination because the sixth pacing stimulus does not capture the ventricle. The tachycardia cycle length is 351 ms.

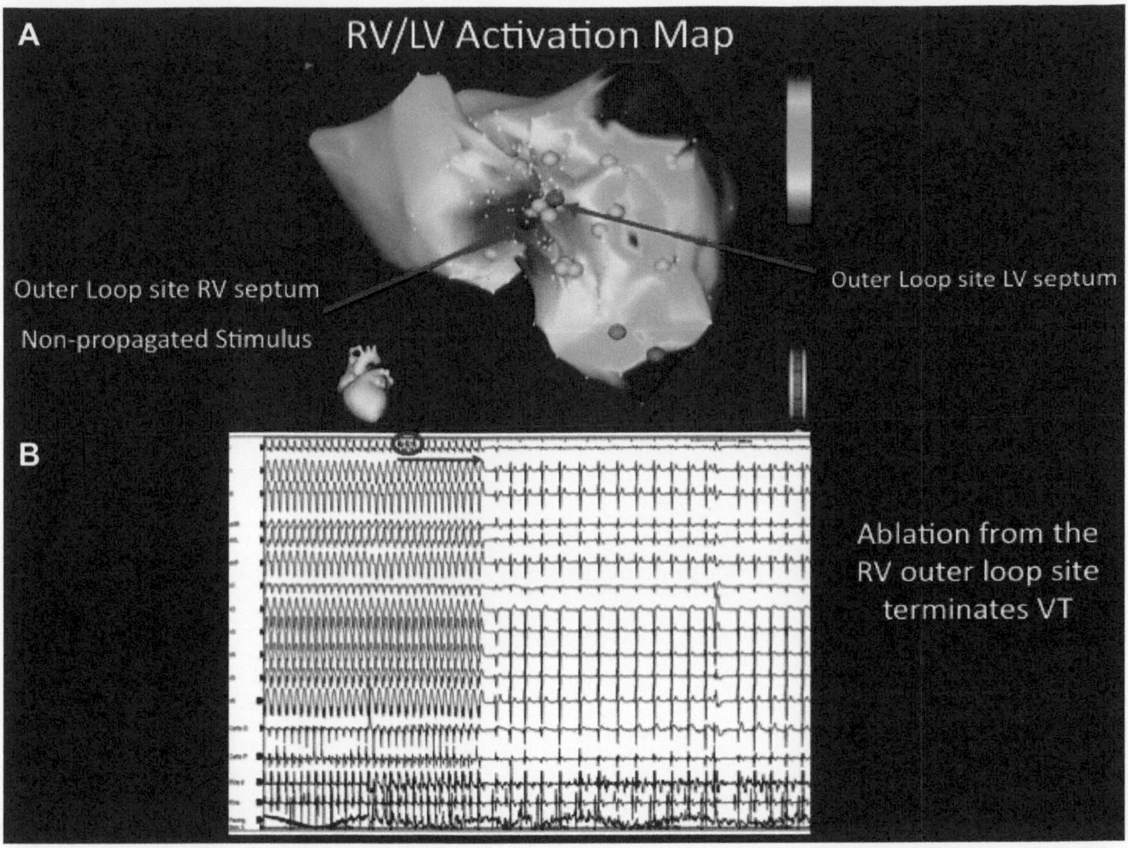

Fig. 7. (*A*) RV and LV activation maps with the RV outer loop/nonpropagated stimulus and LV outer loop site tagged. There is a diffuse area of early activation noted in the midseptum. (*B*) The first RF lesion given on the right ventricular septum at the purple tag in (*A*). This lesion terminated the clinical VT in less than 5 seconds.

This is consistent with an outer loop site near the exit site for the VT. The proximity of the LV and RV septal catheters can be appreciated in the fluoroscopic images.

Further entrainment was performed from the RV septum (shown in **Fig. 6**).

Question 4: What Is the Next Best Step?

In this figure, pacing terminates the VT without global capture. This finding was reproducible and indicated that the pacing catheter is at a critical part of the VT isthmus. Ablation was performed at this site and resulted in termination of the clinical VT in less than 5 seconds. After the first lesion, programmed stimulation was performed, and the clinical VT was no longer inducible (**Fig. 7**).

SUMMARY

This is an unusual case of a patient with an ischemic cardiomyopathy and a chronic anteroapical infarct. She presented with VT 13 years after her left anterior descending coronary artery dissection. As displayed in **Fig. 5**A, the septum was very thin. Activation mapping in the RV and LV revealed diffuse areas of early activation. Entrainment mapping from the left side of the septum revealed outer loop sites proximal to the VT entrance whereas pacing from the right side of the septum revealed outer loop sites near the VT exit, suggesting the isthmus was intramural in the septum. The dense LV scar may have protected the septum from ablation lesions delivered from the LV side; however, ablation from the RV side of the septum at the site of VT termination with a nonpropagated stimulus promptly terminated the VT.

This case highlights the importance of mapping the right side of the septum after anteroseptal infarcts and recognizing termination of the VT with a nonpropagated stimulus as an indication that the pacing catheter is located in a protected isthmus.

REFERENCE

1. Josephson ME, Horowitz LN, Waxman HL, et al. Sustained ventricular tachycardia: role of the 12-lead electrocardiogram in localizing site of origin. Circulation 1981;64(2):257–72.

Fig. 7. (A) RV and LV activation maps with the RV outer loop/nonpropagated stimulus and LV outer loop site tagged. There is a diffuse area of early activation noted in the midseptum. (B) The first RF lesion given on the right ventricular septum at the purple tag in (A). This lesion terminated the clinical VT in less than 5 seconds.

This is consistent with an outer loop site near the exit site for the VT. The proximity of the LV and RV septal catheters can be appreciated in the fluoroscopic images.

Further entrainment was performed from the RV septum (shown in Fig. 6).

Question 4: What Is the Next Best Step?

In this figure, pacing terminates the VT without global capture. This finding was reproducible and indicated that the pacing catheter is at a critical part of the VT isthmus. Ablation was performed at this site and resulted in termination of the clinical VT in less than 5 seconds. After the first lesion, programmed stimulation was performed, and the clinical VT was no longer inducible (Fig. 7).

SUMMARY

This is an unusual case of a patient with an ischemic cardiomyopathy and a chronic anteroapical infarct. She presented with VT 13 years after her left anterior descending coronary artery dissection. As displayed in Fig. 5A, the septum was very thin. Activation mapping in the RV and LV revealed diffuse areas of early activation. Entrainment mapping from the left side of the septum revealed outer loop sites proximal to the VT entrance whereas pacing from the right side of the septum revealed outer loop sites near the VT exit, suggesting the isthmus was intramural in the septum. The dense LV scar may have protected the septum from ablation lesions delivered from the LV side. However, ablation from the RV side of the septum at the site of VT termination with a nonpropagated stimulus promptly terminated the VT.

This case highlights the importance of mapping the right side of the septum after anteroseptal infarcts and recognizing termination of the VT with a nonpropagated stimulus as an indication that the pacing catheter is located in a protected isthmus.

REFERENCE

1. Josephson ME, Horowitz LN, Waxman HL, et al. Sustained ventricular tachycardia: role of the 12-lead electrocardiogram in localizing site of origin. Circulation 1981;64(2):257–72.

Wide Complex Tachycardia Following Cardiac Valve Surgery

Wendy S. Tzou, MD[a,*], Edward P. Gerstenfeld, MD[b]

KEYWORDS

• Ventricular tachycardia • Bundle branch reentry • Catheter ablation

KEY POINTS

- A right bundle branch block pattern on the surface electrocardiogram may represent significant delay rather than a block in the right bundle.
- When ventricular tachycardia (VT) with a right bundle right inferior axis occurs in patients with non-ischemic cardiomyopathy and conduction disease, one should consider antidromic bundle branch reentry.
- A His bundle recording in front of a left bundle branch VT with H-H driving V-V is diagnostic for orthodromic bundle branch reentry.
- Ablation of the right bundle branch is curative for bundle branch reentrant VT.

CLINICAL HISTORY

A 63-year-old man with a history of atrial fibrillation and bicuspid aortic valve with sinus of Valsalva aneurysm underwent complex aortic root replacement, hemiarch repair, pericardial aortic valve replacement, and mitral valve repair. Before surgery, he was in persistent atrial fibrillation with a narrow QRS. Immediately after surgery, he was noted to have developed a new right bundle branch block (RBBB) and first-degree atrioventricular (AV) conduction delay (**Fig. 1**A). His postoperative course was uncomplicated until 1 week later, when he experienced recurrent episodes of sustained, monomorphic ventricular tachycardia (VT) necessitating multiple external cardioversions (**Fig. 1**B). He was treated with intravenous amiodarone and lidocaine, which slowed the rate of the VT from 190 to 130 beats/min; however, the burden increased to the point that the VT became incessant. Because of the extent of his surgery involving the complex aortic valve reconstruction, the patient's cardiothoracic surgeon advised against any systemic anticoagulation or catheter manipulation in the newly reconstructed aortic root. However, after several days of incessant VT despite repeated amiodarone boluses, he was eventually referred for electrophysiology study and VT ablation.

CLINICAL COURSE

The patient's presenting rhythm to the electrophysiology laboratory was a right-bundle, right-axis, inferiorly directed VT with a cycle length of 410 milliseconds. During catheter placement in the apical right ventricle (RV), the VT terminated. Subsequent programmed stimulation or catheter ectopy from the RV reproducibly induced a left-bundle, right-axis, inferiorly directed VT with the same cycle length (CL) as the presenting VT (**Fig. 2**).

Question:

> What is the mechanism of this tachycardia, and the likely mechanism of the presenting tachycardia?

[a] University of Colorado, Anschutz Medical Campus, Cardiology, Electrophysiology Section, 12401 E. 17th Avenue, MS B136, Aurora, CO 80045, USA; [b] Cardiology Division, Department of Medicine, University of California at San Francisco, 500 Parnassus Avenue, MUE-434, Box 1354, San Francisco, CA 94143-1354, USA
* Corresponding author.
E-mail address: wendy.tzou@ucdenver.edu

Card Electrophysiol Clin 4 (2012) 617–621
http://dx.doi.org/10.1016/j.ccep.2012.08.012

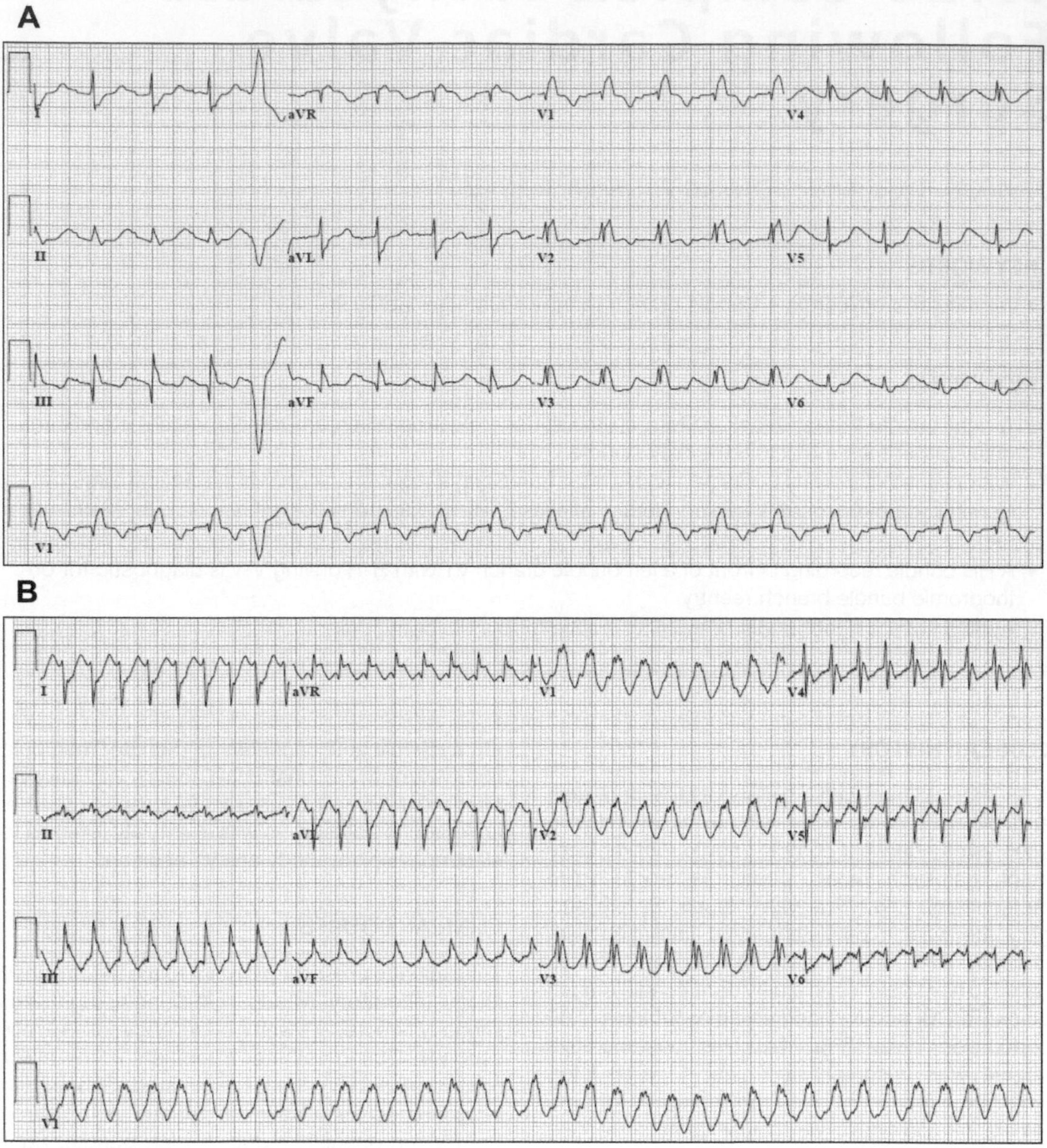

Fig. 1. (*A*) Electrocardiogram (ECG) obtained on postoperative day 1 showing sinus rhythm with prolonged PR interval and new right bundle branch block (RBBB). (*B*) Ventricular tachycardia 1 week following surgery, with RBBB and right inferior axis morphology.

DISCUSSION

The presenting VT had an RBB/right-axis pattern, suggesting an exit from near the left anterior fascicle. Although "apparent" complete RBBB was present in sinus rhythm, the overall vector of the clinical VT was quite similar to the sinus rhythm axis. Termination of the VT with His bundle catheter placement led the surgeon to suspect that the RBB might also be involved in the tachycardia circuit. Ventricular programmed stimulation easily induced a left bundle late transition VT at the exact same CL of the clinical VT. During this VT, RV apical activation occurred before the surface QRS. Placement of a catheter at the His and RBB positions demonstrated that variations in the VT CL were preceded by variations in the His-His interval (**Fig. 3**).[1] Entrainment from a catheter recording an RBB potential demonstrated concealed fusion with a postpacing interval within 10 milliseconds of the tachycardia CL.

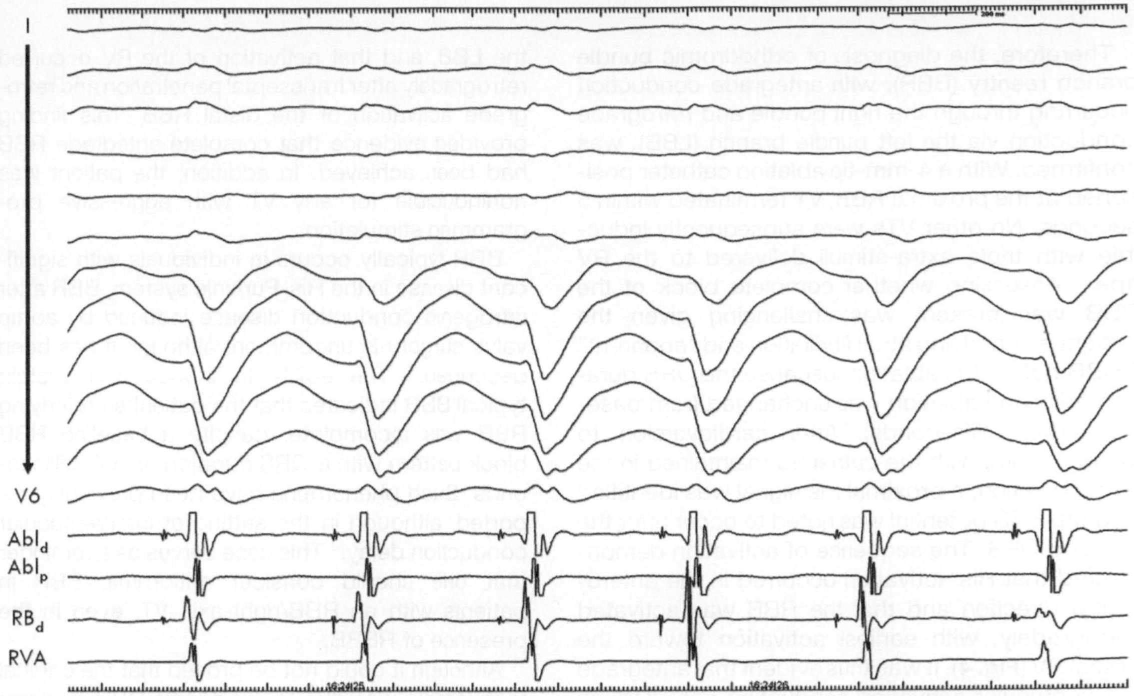

Fig. 2. Surface 12-lead ECG together with intracardiac electrograms recorded from an ablation catheter positioned at the proximal RB (Abl), distal RB, and right ventricular apex. Abl$_d$, distal pole ablation catheter; Abl$_p$, proximal pole ablation catheter; RB, right bundle potential; RB$_d$, catheter positioned at distal right bundle branch; RVA, right ventricular apex catheter; V, ventricular electrogram.

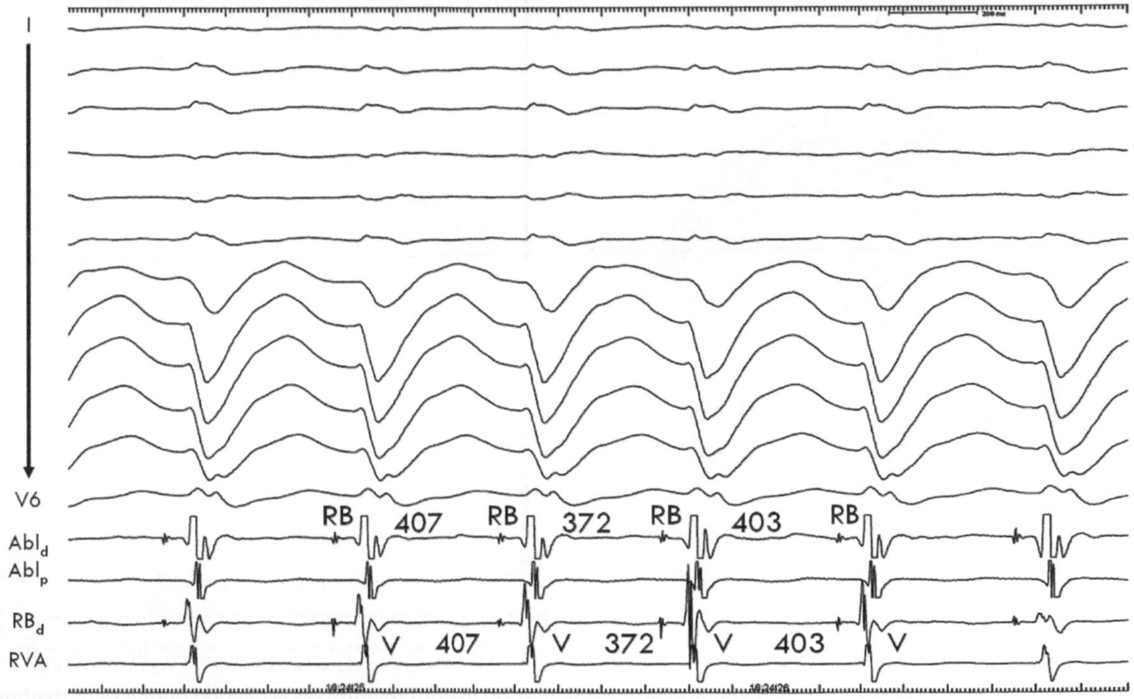

Fig. 3. Surface 12-lead ECG together with intracardiac electrograms recorded from an ablation catheter positioned at the proximal RB (Abl), distal RB, and right ventricular apex. Variations in RB-RB intervals predicted variations in ventricular tachycardia cycle length. Abl$_d$, distal pole ablation catheter; Abl$_p$, proximal pole ablation catheter; RB, right bundle potential; RB$_d$, catheter positioned at distal right bundle branch; RVA, right ventricular apex catheter; V, ventricular electrogram.

Therefore, the diagnosis of orthodromic bundle branch reentry (BBR), with antegrade conduction occurring through the right bundle and retrograde conduction via the left bundle branch (LBB), was confirmed. With a 4-mm-tip ablation catheter positioned at the proximal RBB, VT terminated within 5 seconds. No other VTs were subsequently inducible with triple extra-stimuli delivered to the RV apex. Assessing whether complete block of the RBB was present was challenging given the patient's underlying atrial fibrillation and "apparent" RBBB before the ablation, because the QRS duration following ablation was unchanged from baseline (160 milliseconds). After cardioversion to sinus rhythm, with the catheters maintained in the same position, a proximal His signal was identified and the RBB potential was noted to occur after the ensuing QRS. The sequence of activation demonstrated that His activation occurred in the anterograde direction and that the RBB was activated retrogradely, with earliest activation toward the apical RV (**Fig. 4**). It was thus evident that antegrade left ventricular activation conduction occurred via the LBB, and that activation of the RV occurred retrogradely after transseptal penetration and retrograde activation of the distal RBB. This finding provided evidence that complete antegrade RBB had been achieved. In addition, the patient was noninducible for any VT with aggressive programmed stimulation.

BBR typically occurs in individuals with significant disease in the His-Purkinje system. BBR after iatrogenic conduction disease induced by aortic valve surgery is uncommon, although it has been described.[2] The ability to induce and sustain typical BBR indicates that the patient's underlying RBB was incomplete, despite a baseline RBB block pattern with a QRS duration of 160 milliseconds. Such phenomena have been previously reported, although in the setting of interventricular conduction delay.[3] This case serves as a reminder that one should consider antidromic BBR in patients with an RBB/right-axis VT, even in the presence of RBBB.

Although it could not be proved that the original tachycardia was due to antidromic BBR, findings

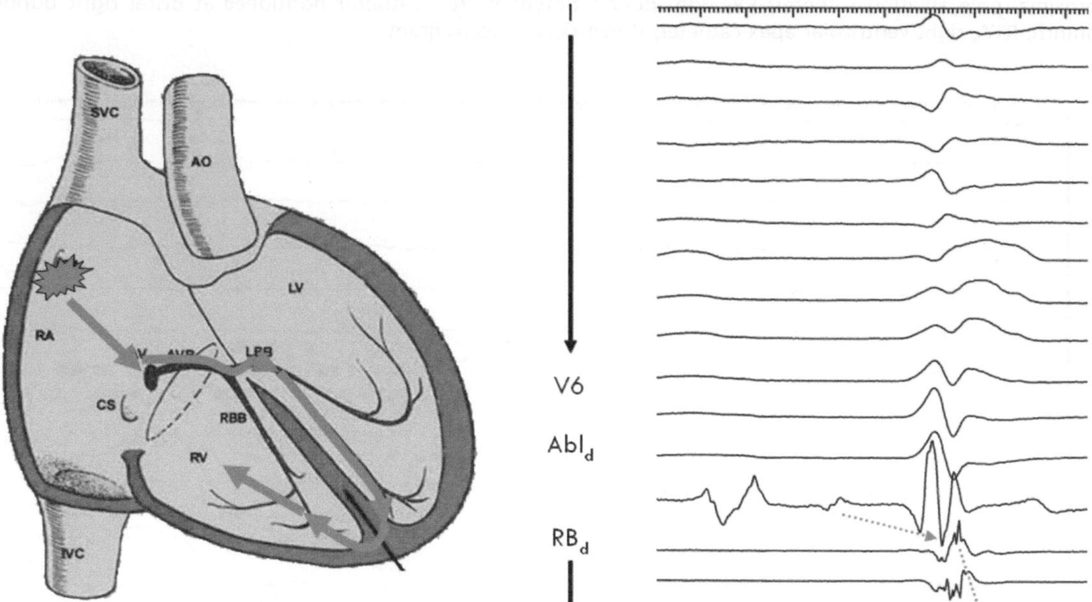

Fig. 4. Following right bundle branch ablation and cardioversion to sinus rhythm, His activation during sinus rhythm is depicted on the left panel (*solid red arrows*). The right panel displays corresponding intracardiac activation (*dotted red arrows*), antegrade via the His bundle (Abl_d), and retrograde right bundle branch/RV activation. Abl_p, proximal pole ablation catheter; AO, aorta; CS, coronary sinus; IVC, inferior vena cava; LBB, left bundle branch; LV, left ventricle; RA, right atrium; RBB, right bundle branch; RB_d, catheter positioned at distal right bundle branch; RV, right ventricle; RVA, right ventricular apex catheter; SVC, superior vena cava.

favoring this diagnosis include: (1) recent valve surgeries with subsequent conduction system disease; (2) similar RBB morphology during baseline AV conduction and the presenting VT; (3) subsequent inducible orthodromic BBR VT with identical CL to the presenting VT; and (4) inability to induce the VT after RBB ablation. In this case, although the complex surgery limited access to the left ventricle to treat an RBB morphology VT, the patient was successfully cured with RBB ablation without the need for systemic anticoagulation and left ventricular access.

Documenting completeness of the RBB following ablation was difficult in the setting of a preexisting RBB pattern. It was possible to record an anterograde His bundle activation during sinus rhythm, and retrograde distal RBB activation, presumably after anterograde conduction down the left fascicle with transseptal retrograde activation of the RBB. Transseptal catheterization to prove this activation sequence was not performed because of the patient's recent surgery.

SUMMARY

This article describes an unusual case of an incessant RBB VT in a patient who developed new RBB after aortic valve surgery. The complex surgery limited access to the left ventricle for mapping, yet the patient's arrhythmia was cured after a diagnosis of antidromic BBR was established. Proof of complete RBB after ablation was obtained using detailed mapping of RBB activation with a multipolar catheter. This case serves as a reminder that BBR should be considered in the case of postoperative VT occurring after apparent surgically induced BBB, even if the VT has an RBB morphology.

REFERENCES

1. Akhtar M, Gilbert C, Wolf FG, et al. Reentry within the His-Purkinje system. Elucidation of reentrant circuit using right bundle branch and his bundle recordings. Circulation 1978;58:295–304.
2. Narasimhan C, Jazayeri M, Sra J, et al. Ventricular tachycardia in valvular heart disease: facilitation of bundle-branch reentry by valve surgery. Circulation 1997;96:4307–13.
3. Mizusawa Y, Sakurada H, Nishizaki M, et al. Characteristics of bundle branch reentrant ventricular tachycardia with a right bundle branch block configuration: feasibility of atrial pacing. Europace 2009;11:1208–13.

Nonischemic Ventricular Tachycardia

Marc W. Deyell, MD, MSC*[,1], Fermin C. Garcia, MD

KEYWORDS

• Ventricular tachycardia • Nonischemic cardiomyopathy • Entrainment • Electroanatomic mapping

KEY POINTS

- Nonischemic cardiomyopathies may have a mid-myocardial or epicardial substrate.
- A unipolar endocardial voltage map may indicate the presence of epicardial scar.
- If no endocardial isthmus sites exist when mapping ventricular tachycardia, consider a mid-myocardial or epicardial isthmus.
- Repeat ablation is sometimes needed for patients with multiple complex ventricular tachycardias.

CLINICAL HISTORY

A 49-year-old man with long-standing left ventricular (LV) nonischemic cardiomyopathy (NICM), in the setting of remote alcohol and stimulant drug abuse, presented with recurrent ventricular tachycardia (VT) and implantable converter-defibrillator (ICD) shocks. His baseline LV ejection fraction was 40% to 45% and his functional status was New York Heart Association Class 1. He underwent implantation of a primary prevention cardiac resynchronization therapy defibrillator (CRTD) (Renewal H210; Boston Scientific, Natick, MA) 4 years prior. His first occurrence of VT was 12 months before his current procedure.

The patient had undergone multiple prior attempts at VT mapping and ablation, including epicardial mapping and ablation. Despite termination of VT with ablation during prior procedures and extensive substrate-based ablation through regions of myocardial scar with pace maps matching the clinical VT morphologies, he continued to experience ICD shocks. He presented with recurrent VT and ICD shocks despite medical therapy with sotalol.

CLINICAL COURSE

He presented to the emergency room after experiencing several ICD shocks; the presenting electrocardiogram (ECG) revealed a VT at a cycle length of 490 milliseconds, matching his prior dominant clinical VT. At electrophysiologic study, the clinical VT was induced with catheter manipulation.

Question 1: Based on the morphology of the VT in **Fig. 1**, what is the most likely exit site?

The VT has a right bundle branch block (RBBB) morphology with a right inferior axis. There is precordial concordance which, in combination with the limb lead axis, places the exit site at the basal superolateral LV wall (Josephson site 10). There is an rS pattern in leads I and AVL, which argues against an epicardial exit because of the absence of a q wave.[1,2] Interval criteria (intrinsicoid deflection in V2 = 71 milliseconds, pseudo-delta 16 milliseconds, maximum deflection index

Electrophysiology Section, Hospital of the University of Pennsylvania, 9 Founder's, 3400 Spruce Street, Philadelphia, PA 19104, USA
[1] Present address: Heart Rhythm Services, St. Paul's Hospital, University of British Columbia, #211 - 1033 Davie Street, Vancouver, British Columbia, Canada V6E 1M7.
* Corresponding author. Holy Family Hospital, Vancouver, BC, Canada.
E-mail address: mdeyell@ProvidenceHealth.bc.ca

Card Electrophysiol Clin 4 (2012) 623–630
http://dx.doi.org/10.1016/j.ccep.2012.08.010
1877-9182/12/$ – see front matter

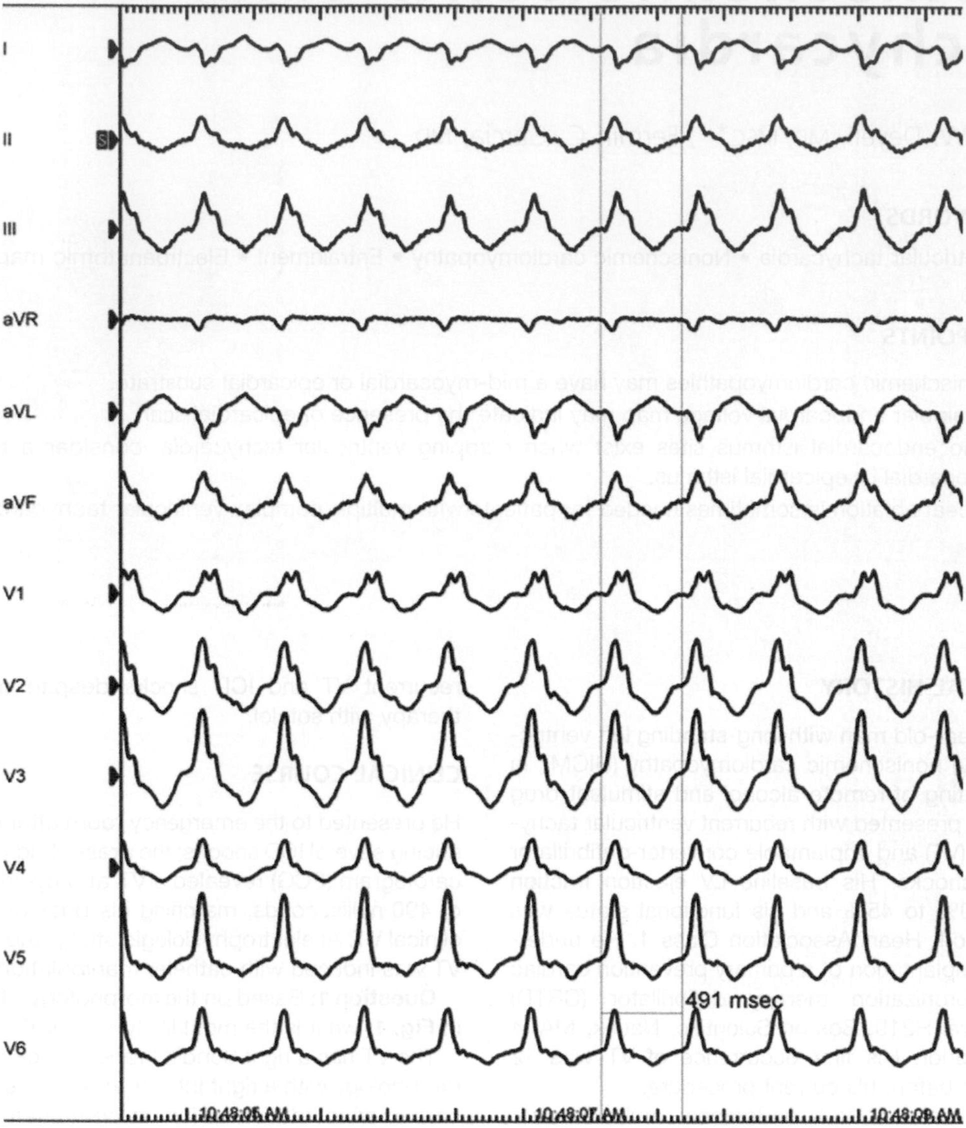

Fig. 1. Clinical VT reinduced in the laboratory.

60 milliseconds/176 milliseconds = 0.34) also favor an endocardial exit site.

Electroanatomic mapping of the LV endocardium revealed extensive basal inferior and lateral bipolar scar (**Fig. 2**A). Note that the bipolar endocardial scar does not extend to the superolateral basal left ventricle, the purported exit site of the clinical VT. The unipolar endocardial voltage map (**Fig. 2**B) shows more extensive abnormality suggestive of a mid-myocardial or epicardial scar. The earliest endocardial diastolic activity during VT was mapped to Josephson site 10. Entrainment at this site is shown in **Fig. 3**.

Question 2: How would you characterize this entrainment site?

Entrainment confirms that the LV endocardial site is an exit site for the VT (entrainment with concealed fusion, postpacing interval ≈ tachycardia cycle length [TCL], stimulus-QRS <30% VT cycle length). Further endocardial entrainment mapping

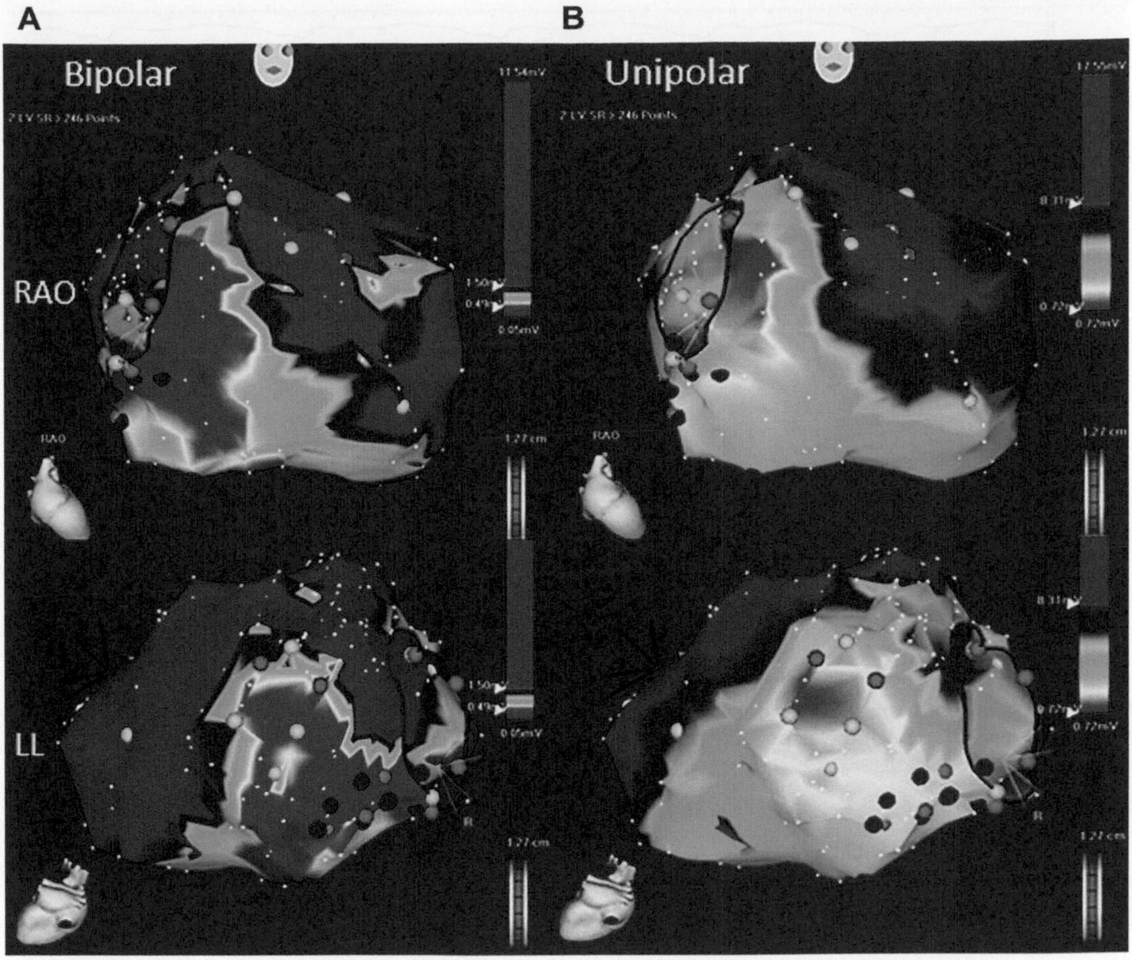

Fig. 2. Left ventricular (LV) endocardial voltage maps. The LV endocardial bipolar (*A*) and unipolar (*B*) electroanatomic maps from the CARTO XP system (Biosense Webster, Diamond Bar, CA) are shown. There is basal LV endocardial scar involving the septal, inferior, and inferolateral walls with extension to the mid cavity. Note the unipolar abnormality is more extensive, suggesting more mid-myocardial or epicardial scar. The black points on the maps indicate areas of fractionated electrograms or late potentials. The fill threshold for all maps is 15 mm. LL, left lateral; RAO, right anterior oblique.

during VT identified no entrance or isthmus sites. Multiple radiofrequency ablation lesions placed at the exit site, delivered at up to 50 W with a 12- to 14-Ω impedance drop, did not slow or terminate the VT.

Question 3: What is your next step?

Because no endocardial isthmus sites could be identified and the unipolar voltage map suggested a large burden of epicardial scar, percutaneous subxyphoid epicardial access was obtained. The epicardial voltage map is shown in **Fig. 4**. Note the more extensive epicardial voltage abnormalities in comparison with the endocardial bipolar abnormalities. Entrainment with high-output pacing (required to obtain capture of the myocardium) within the dense basal lateral scar yielded the response shown in **Fig. 5**.

Question 4: How would you characterize this entrainment site?

Despite maximal gain of the ablation catheter bipolar signal, it is difficult to see the local electrogram (EGM). The only visible EGM is clearly far-field, as it is not captured during overdrive pacing. The absence of an obvious EGM makes

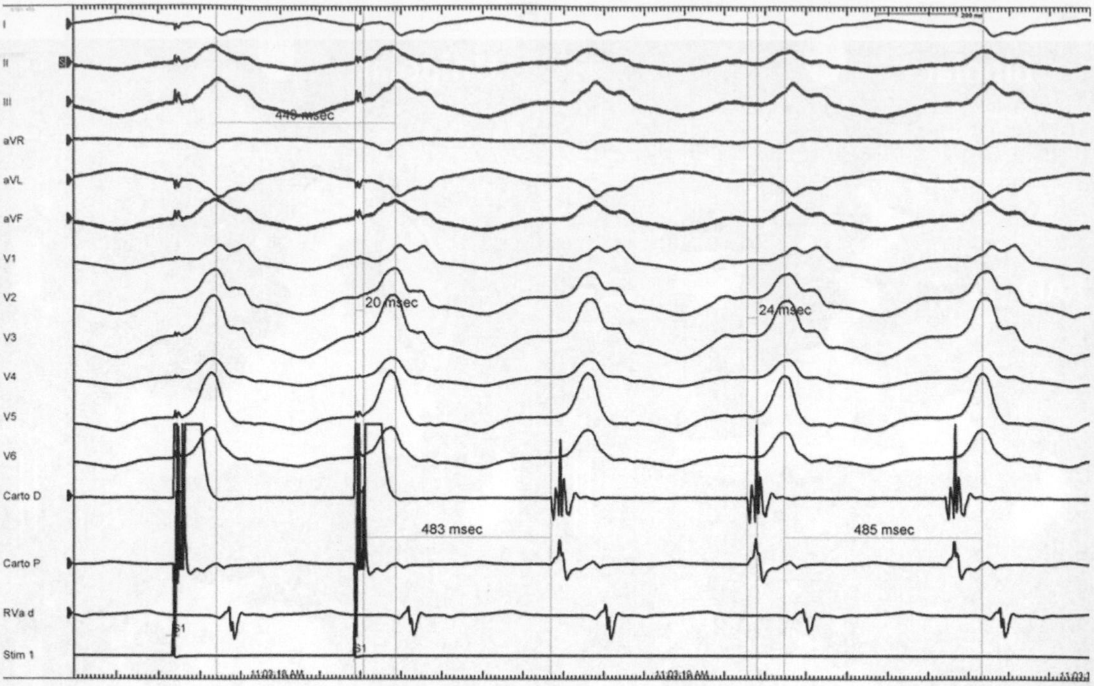

Fig. 3. Entrainment from the LV endocardium at Josephson site 10. The tachycardia cycle length was 485 milliseconds, and overdrive pacing was performed at 450 milliseconds from the distal ablation catheter (CARTO D).

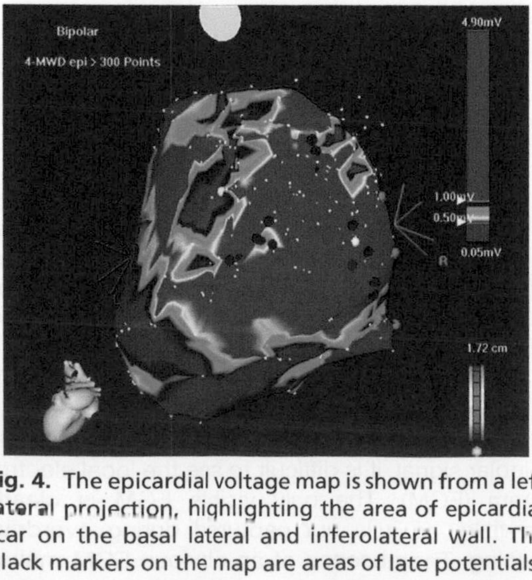

Fig. 4. The epicardial voltage map is shown from a left lateral projection, highlighting the area of epicardial scar on the basal lateral and inferolateral wall. The black markers on the map are areas of late potentials.

interpretation of the entrainment difficult. There is concealed fusion on the surface ECG. While initial review might suggest an exit site similar to **Fig. 4**, careful measurement of the VT cycle length indicates that the each pacing stimulus is leading to the second QRS complex following the pacing stimulus. The stimulus capturing the subsequent QRS complex indicates that the rhythm is macro-reentrant and not automatic. The stimulus to QRS is long and variable, likely representing a bystander site or possibly an inner-loop site. This finding highlights the limitations of entrainment mapping in dense scar at high pacing output.

Further mapping of the epicardium during VT then revealed an area of mid-diastolic potentials on the basal lateral wall at Josephson site 8. Entrainment produced the response shown in **Fig. 6** on numerous occasions.

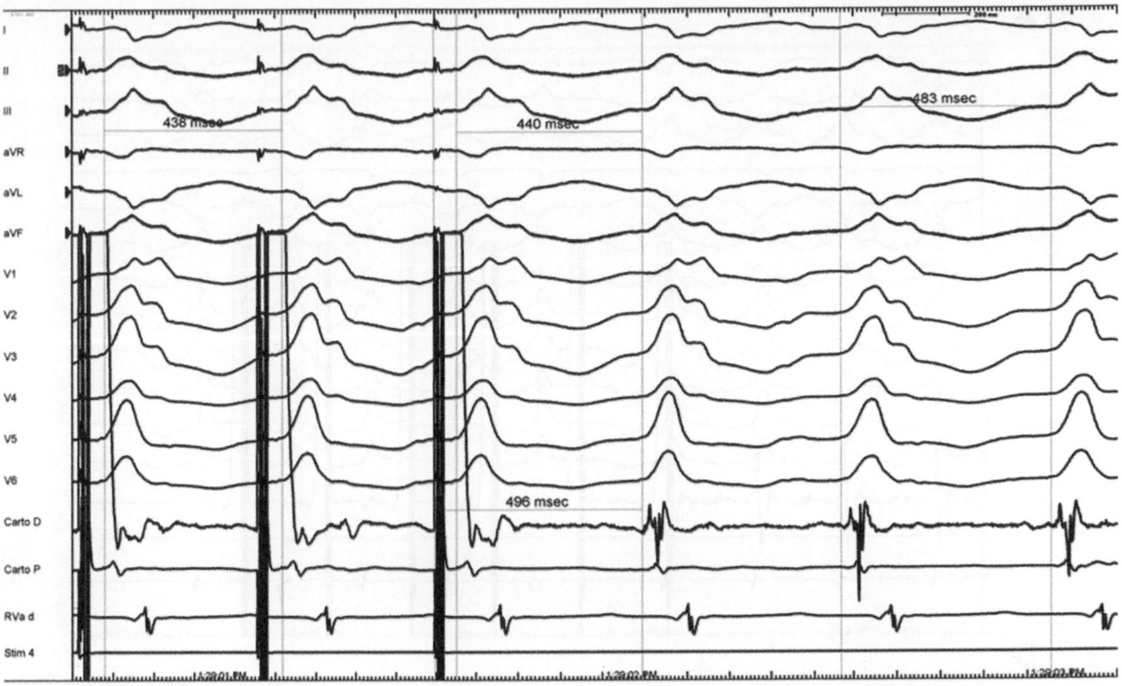

Fig. 5. Entrainment from within the dense scar on the epicardium. The tachycardia cycle length was 480 milliseconds and overdrive pacing was performed at 440 milliseconds using the distal ablation catheter (CARTO D). There is a long stimulus to QRS complex, measured at 496 milliseconds. Note that the dominant EGM on the distal ablation catheter is not being directly captured during the overdrive pacing.

Question 5: What happens during overdrive pacing at this site?

Pacing at this site shows termination of the VT with the first pacing stimulus, but without an accompanying QRS! This feature represents VT termination with a nonpropagated stimulus and indicates that the pacing stimulus has been delivered to a protected isthmus of the VT circuit. Following VT termination, capture can be seen with a pace map matching the clinical VT. This phenomenon was reproducible. Finally, on pacing at 10 milliseconds slower than the TCL at this site, entrainment was possible from this site and is shown in **Fig. 7**. The postpacing interval (PPI) minus the TCL is essentially 0 milliseconds, confirming the site is within the circuit, and the S-QRS is just greater than 50% of the TCL, indicating this is a distal entrance or isthmus site. The presence of an entrance/isthmus site on the epicardium and an exit site on the epicardium indicates that the VT circuit is transmural (**Fig. 8**).

After confirmation that this site was a safe distance from the left circumflex coronary artery after coronary angiography (not shown), and after confirming the absence of phrenic nerve capture with pacing, ablation at the site of VT termination with the nonpropagated stimulus terminated the VT in less than 3 seconds (**Fig. 9**). The patient was noninducible thereafter for the clinical VT or any other slow VTs. With triple extra-stimuli, fast VT/ventricular flutter was induced with RBBB morphology and right inferior axis; therefore, further epicardial substrate ablation was performed targeting the basal lateral scar.

Forty-eight hours after the procedure, the patient underwent noninvasive programmed stimulation under sedation through his ICD. He was noninducible for any VT with triple extra-stimuli at 600- and 400-millisecond drive trains (down to 400/220/210/200). He remains off all antiarrhythmics apart from β-blockade, and has had only one 9-beat run of nonsustained VT at 6 months of follow-up.

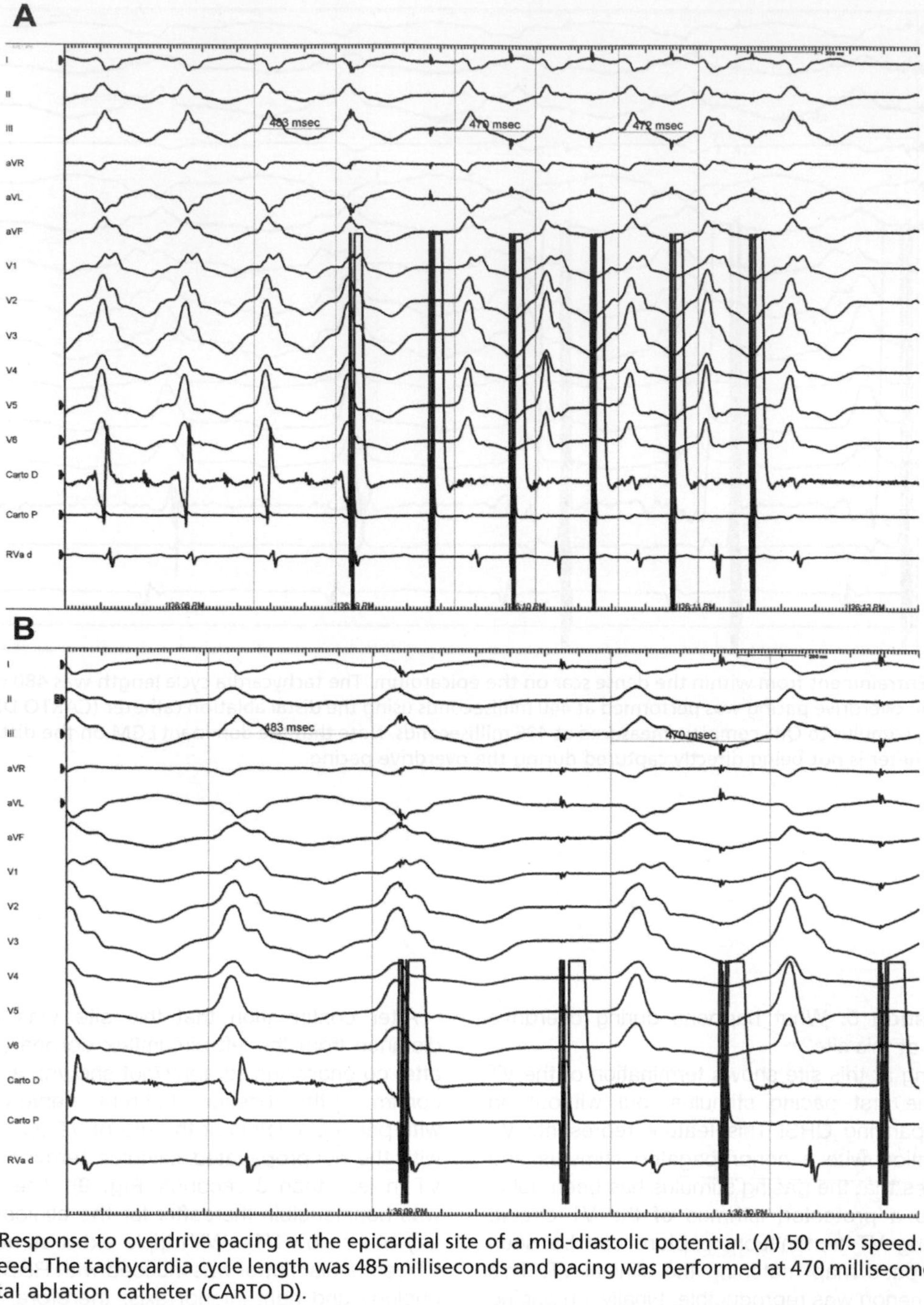

Fig. 6. Response to overdrive pacing at the epicardial site of a mid-diastolic potential. (*A*) 50 cm/s speed. (*B*) 100 cm/s speed. The tachycardia cycle length was 485 milliseconds and pacing was performed at 470 milliseconds from the distal ablation catheter (CARTO D).

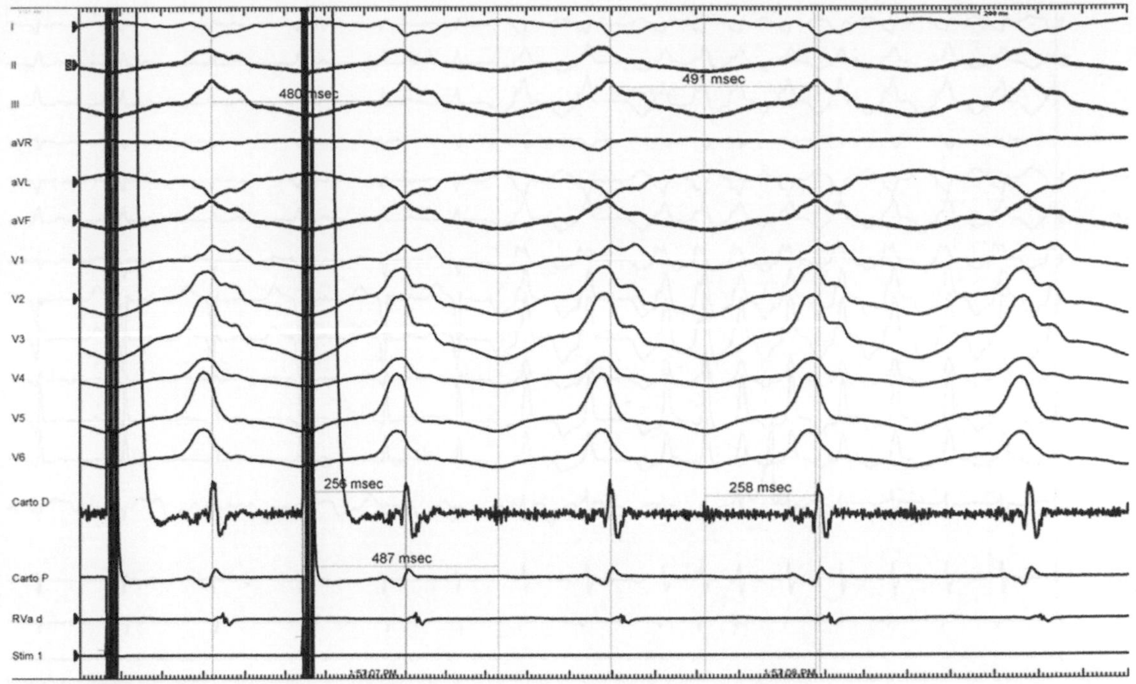

Fig. 7. Entrainment at the site of mid-diastolic potentials. The tachycardia cycle length was 490 milliseconds and pacing was performed at 480 milliseconds from the distal ablation catheter (CARTO D).

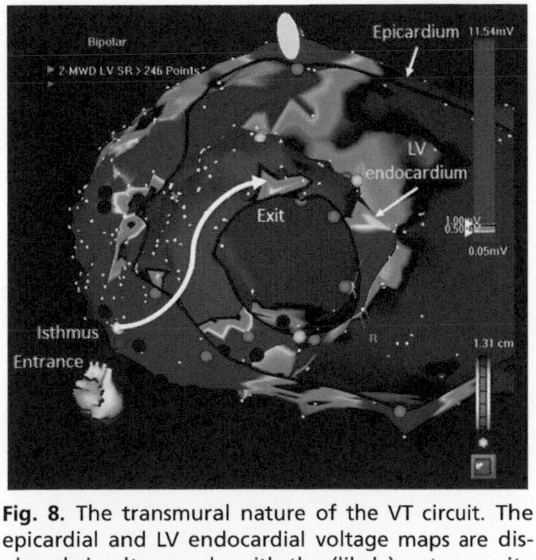

Fig. 8. The transmural nature of the VT circuit. The epicardial and LV endocardial voltage maps are displayed simultaneously with the (likely) entrance site (*blue dot*), isthmus site (*white dot*), and exit sites (*red dots*), as determined by entrainment mapping. A transmural VT circuit is demonstrated.

DISCUSSION

This case highlights the complex nature of the substrate in nonischemic cardiomyopathy. This patient had dense inferolateral and lateral scar of the basal left ventricle on the endocardium, one of the typical patterns seen in NICM, but an even greater distribution on the epicardium. Although the suspicion for epicardial VT circuits is high in NICM, the presenting ECG suggested, correctly, that the exit was endocardial. Despite this, no critical component of the VT circuit could be found on the epicardium, and exit site ablation was unsuccessful. Epicardial mapping confirmed the critical components of the circuit were, at least in part, epicardial. Therefore, this represented a case of a transmural VT circuit. Unlike ischemic VT whereby the circuit usually involves the subendocardium, VT in NICM may involve the endocardium, epicardium, or both. The added degree of complexity of arrhythmia circuits in NICM also

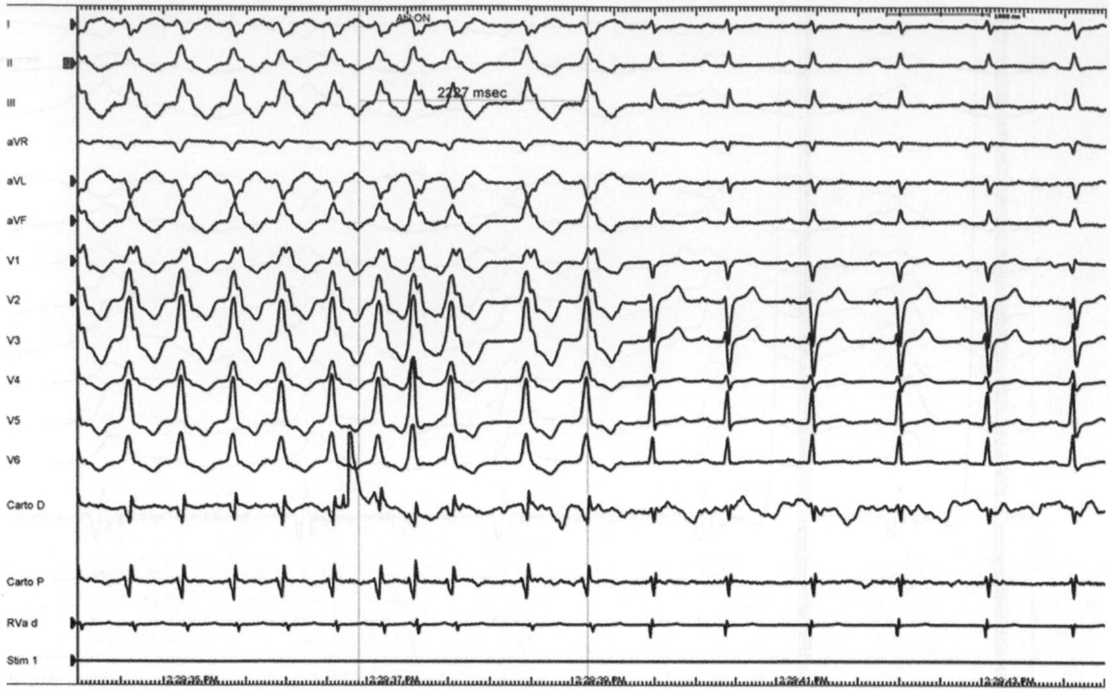

Fig. 9. Ablation at the isthmus site terminates the clinical VT. Radiofrequency ablation terminates the VT in less than 3 seconds.

explains, in part, the lower success rate for VT ablation in this population.[3,4]

REFERENCES

1. Bazan V, Gerstenfeld EP, Garcia FC, et al. Site-specific twelve-lead ECG features to identify an epicardial origin for left ventricular tachycardia in the absence of myocardial infarction. Heart Rhythm 2007;4(11):1403–10.
2. Valles E, Bazan V, Marchlinski FE. ECG criteria to identify epicardial ventricular tachycardia in nonischemic cardiomyopathy. Circ Arrhythm Electrophysiol 2010;3(1):63–71.
3. Soejima K, Stevenson WG, Sapp JL, et al. Endocardial and epicardial radiofrequency ablation of ventricular tachycardia associated with dilated cardiomyopathy: the importance of low-voltage scars. J Am Coll Cardiol 2004;43(10):1834–42.
4. Haqqani HM, Tschabrunn CM, Tzou WS, et al. Isolated septal substrate for ventricular tachycardia in nonischemic dilated cardiomyopathy: incidence, characterization, and implications. Heart Rhythm 2011;8(8):1169–76.

Cardiac Device Troubleshooting

Byron K. Lee, MD

KEYWORDS

• Cardiac devices • Troubleshooting • Cardiac device interrogation

KEY POINTS

- The steps for cardiac device troubleshooting are a careful history, physical examination, and device interrogation.
- Synthesis of data from the history, physical examination, and device typically resolves the problem, allowing the physician to formulate and execute a treatment plan.

Cardiac device troubleshooting should be fun. You can approach it like a mystery that needs to be solved. When a patient presents with a new symptom or device-related issue (such as a shock from his or her implantable cardioverter-defibrillator), your task is to figure out why it is happening. Your steps to solving the mystery are the history, physical examination, and device interrogation.

The evaluation of any new complaint related to a cardiac device should always begin with a careful history, but this is too frequently skipped or glossed over. A poor history may lead to programming changes that could be appropriate, but fail to alleviate the patient's main presenting symptom.

Next, a brief physical examination is frequently helpful. Looking at the device pocket is necessary if the patient has pain or discomfort in that region. Listening to the heart and lungs is important if the patient is complaining of palpitations or shortness of breath.

Last is the actual interrogation of the device. The new devices have many self-diagnostic features that will alert you on interrogation of new problems such as a sudden increase in lead impedance or threshold. The device log and rate histograms can also be helpful to alert you to any new arrhythmias that the patient may be experiencing.

Synthesis of the data from the history, physical examination, and device typically solves the mystery. Eureka! A plan can now be formulated and executed. Only rarely does the mystery remain unsolved after a step-by-step approach. In such situations, further testing may need to be done.

This section includes several cases concerning cardiac devices that illustrate the mystery solving process of device troubleshooting. In each instance, one or more clinical questions arose that needed to be solved. History, physical examination, and device interrogation were the steps taken by the clinician to arrive at the answers.

Cardiac Electrophysiology and Arrhythmia Service, UCSF Medical Center, 500 Parnassus Avenue, Box 1354, San Francisco, CA 94143-1354, USA
E-mail address: leeb@medicine.ucsf.edu

Card Electrophysiol Clin 4 (2012) 631
http://dx.doi.org/10.1016/j.ccep.2012.08.023

Atrial Oversensing and Mode Switching Caused by Lead Polarization Artifact During an Automatic Ventricular Capture Threshold Test

Russell R. Heath, MD, William H. Sauer, MD,
Duy Thai Nguyen, MD, Ryan G. Aleong, MD*

KEYWORDS

• Automatic capture threshold testing • Lead polarization • Dual-chamber pacemaker

KEY POINTS

- Most pacemakers now include an automatic capture threshold testing (ACTT) feature designed to increase battery longevity; however, these algorithms can rarely result in adverse clinical outcomes.
- Lead polarization artifact was a problem with older polished leads but is less often observed with newer porous leads.
- Without careful consideration of the interaction between the ACTT algorithm and previously placed high polarization leads, artifact may be misdiagnosed as atrial fibrillation. Recognition of this potential ACTT problem is important in preventing unnecessary treatment and guiding appropriate device programming.

CLINICAL PRESENTATION

A 41-year-old woman with a dual-chamber pacemaker placed in 1998 for complete heart block and a subsequent recent generator replacement (Boston Scientific 1291 generator; Medtronic 5068 leads) presented to the clinic complaining of palpitations. The sensing, impedance, and capture threshold of each lead was within normal limits and similar to values recorded at generator change. Programming was unchanged and set to DDDR with a lower rate limit of 70 beats/min and a maximum tracking rate of 140 beats/min. Postventricular atrial refractory period was set to dynamic. Mode-switching episodes recorded demonstrated a repeated pattern of atrial sensed events associated with ventricular stimulation during automatic capture threshold testing (ACTT) (**Fig. 1**).

CLINICAL QUESTION

What causes inappropriate mode switching?

CLINICAL COURSE

As shown in **Fig. 1**, for each sinus event there are several A-sensed events followed closely by a V-pace. Normally the autocapture algorithm decreases the AV delay to 60 milliseconds to maximize pacing for the threshold test. The V-pace appears to have a normal evoked response on the ventricular electrogram (EGM); however, it is

Disclosures: None.
University of Colorado, USA
* Corresponding author. Section of Cardiac Electrophysiology, University of Colorado Hospital, 12401 East 17th Avenue, B136, Aurora, CO 80045.
E-mail address: ryan.aleong@ucdenver.edu

Card Electrophysiol Clin 4 (2012) 633–636
http://dx.doi.org/10.1016/j.ccep.2012.08.007

cardiacEP.theclinics.com

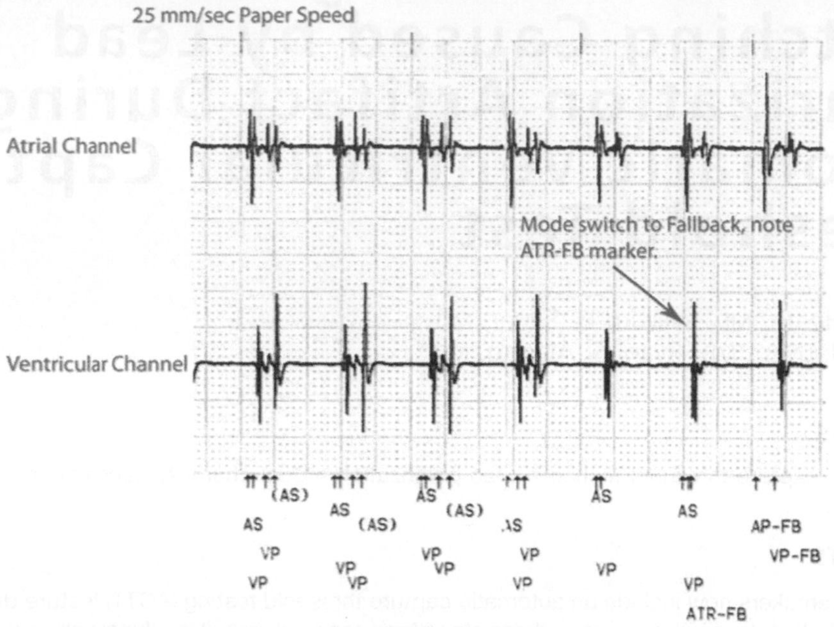

Fig. 1. Frequent episodes of high atrial rate were recorded by the new device, owing to a repeated pattern of signals on the atrial channel during automatic capture threshold testing. Electrogram (EGM) of 25 mm/s paper speed.

followed quickly by a second V-pace, which is again a normal function during the ambulatory automatic threshold testing. This second V-pace is delivered to avoid dropped beats after the auto-capture test drops below threshold. At 100 mm/s paper speed, it appears that the second V-pace represents a backup ventricular pacing stimulus and the third ventricular stimulus corresponds to a polarization artifact (**Fig. 2**). In addition, there are 3 distinct signals on the atrial EGMs for each atrial sensed, ventricularly paced event. The first atrial sensed event is the native p wave, the second is far-field sensing of the backup ventricular pacing stimulus that falls within the blanking period, and the third likely corresponds to a far-field EGM from the polarization artifact on the ventricular lead. It is the third atrial EGM that initiates detection of a high atrial rate and subsequent mode switching. Based on these findings, the Auto Capture feature was programmed to off, which eliminated the second far-field atrial EGM. The patient's pacemaker was interrogated several months later and no further high atrial rates were recorded.

DISCUSSION

Most pacemakers now include an ACTT feature designed to increase battery longevity.[1] However, these algorithms can rarely result in adverse clinical outcomes.[1,2] This is a case of inappropriate classification of an episode of high atrial rate and associated mode switching attributable to atrial oversensing of lead polarization artifact during ACTT.

In this device, the ACTT algorithm temporarily decreases the AV delay to 60 milliseconds until loss of capture is detected, at which point a second higher output backup ventricular pacing stimulus is delivered. Because this patient had older polished Medtronic 5068 leads, the higher output pacing stimulus resulted in a lead polarization artifact. Lead polarization artifact refers to the residual electrical current generated between the lead and tissue that creates a signal after a high-output pacing impulse is delivered. Traditionally this was a problem with older polished leads and is less often observed with newer porous leads.[1] In this case, the artifact was only observed after the high-output stimulation occurred as part of the ACTT algorithm. ACTT algorithms have been designed to differentiate between the myocardial evoked response and the polarization artifact.[3] The pacing stimulus amplitude has been shown to affect the degree of polarization artifact and, therefore, the ACTT algorithm has been recommended with low polarization leads.[4]

Without careful consideration of the interaction between the ACTT algorithm and the previously placed high polarization lead, these episodes

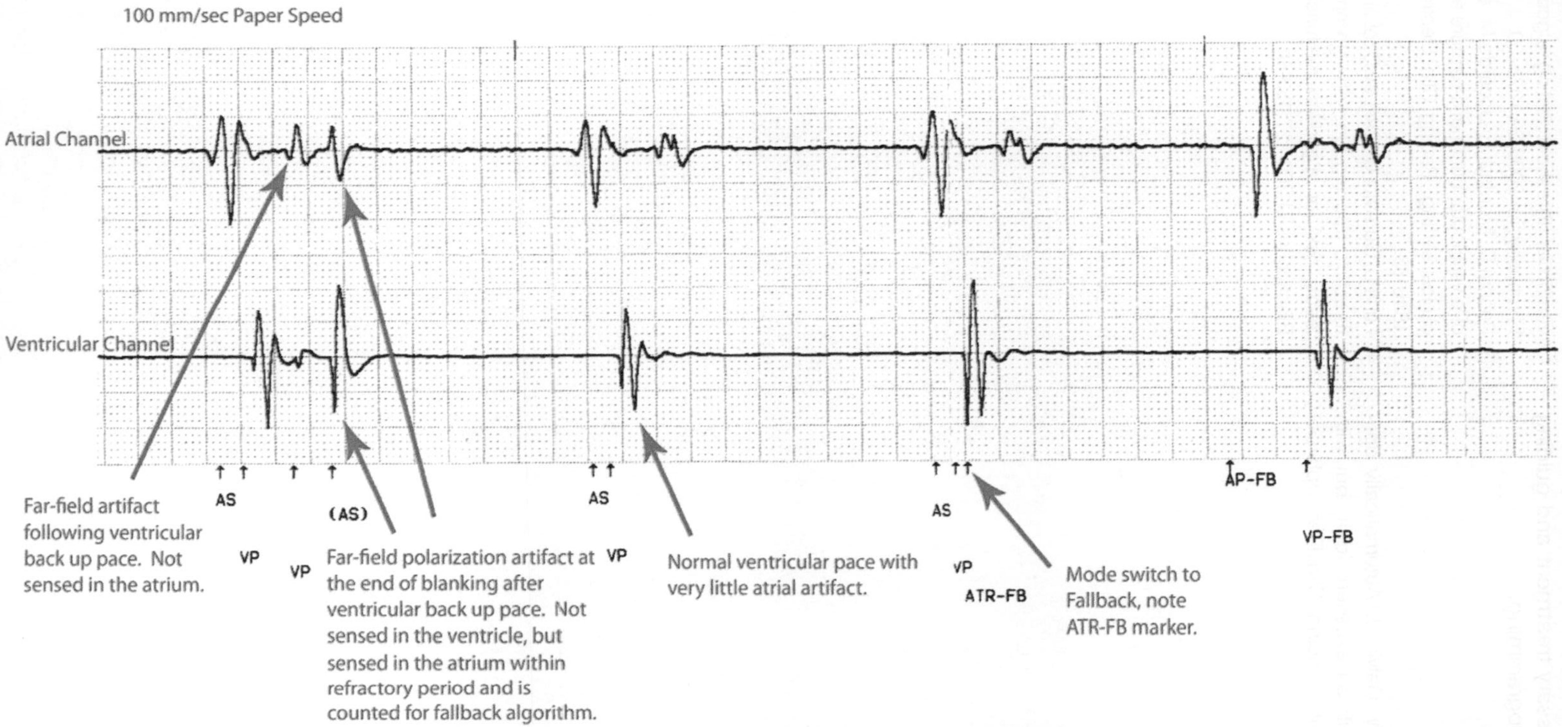

Fig. 2. Polarization artifact is oversensed by the atrial lead, causing inappropriate mode switching. During the initial set of atrial EGMs, the atrial sensed artifact is followed by 2 EGMs that may represent far-field EGMs from the backup ventricular pacing stimulus and polarization artifact. EGM of 100 mm/s paper speed.

may be misdiagnosed as atrial fibrillation. Recognition of this potential ACTT problem is important in preventing unnecessary treatment and guiding appropriate device programming.

REFERENCES

1. Suri R, Harthorne JW, Galvin J. Automatically optimizing pacing output: an excellent idea, but with potentially lethal pitfalls. Pacing Clin Electrophysiol 2001;24:520–3.
2. Sauer WH, Cooper JM, Lai RW, et al. Underestimation of pacing threshold as determined by an automatic ventricular threshold testing algorithm. Pacing Clin Electrophysiol 2006;29:1028–30.
3. Pecora D, Morandi F, Liccardo M, et al. Performance of a ventricular automatic-capture algorithm in a wide clinical setting. Pacing Clin Electrophysiol 2008;31:1546–53.
4. Luria D, Gurevitz O, Bar Lev D, et al. Use of automatic threshold tracking function with non-low polarization leads: risk for algorithm malfunction. Pacing Clin Electrophysiol 2004;27:453–9.

A Tale of Two Tachycardias

Seth R. Bender, MD, Jim W. Cheung, MD*

KEYWORDS

• ICD • Ventricular tachycardia • Atrial fibrillation • Implantable cardioverter-defibrillator

KEY POINTS

- Dual tachycardias in patients with implantable cardioverter-defibrillators (ICDs) are common, and studies have reported that up to 10% of ventricular tachyarrhythmias detected by ICDs are preceded by supraventricular tachycardia.
- It is imperative to distinguish ventricular from supraventricular tachyarrhythmias seen in stored ICD electrograms, as it has significant implications for appropriate ICD programming and use of medical and catheter ablation therapy.

CASE REPORT

A 77-year-old man with a history of paroxysmal atrial fibrillation (AF), coronary artery disease status post coronary artery bypass surgery, and ischemic cardiomyopathy with severely reduced left ventricular function (ejection fraction 15%) was admitted with chest discomfort and a fluttering sensation in his chest. A Medtronic Maximo II DR dual-chamber implantable cardioverter-defibrillator (ICD) was implanted 18 months earlier at an outside institution after he suffered a cardiac arrest in the setting of right lower lobectomy for the treatment of early-stage lung cancer. On admission he was found to be in AF with a rapid ventricular rate. Cardiac enzymes were mildly elevated. He underwent cardiac catheterization, which revealed stable coronary artery disease; hence, no intervention was performed.

Interrogation of the patient's ICD revealed that the device had been programmed with a single zone to detect and treat ventricular tachyarrhythmias at a rate of 200 beats/min or more. Therapy was programmed to deliver high-voltage shocks with antitachycardia pacing during charging. Review of the arrhythmia log was notable for numerous episodes (43) of tachyarrhythmia that were all clustered in a 2-month period before the patient's admission. A representative strip of an episode is shown in **Fig. 1**A. An A-A and V-V interval plot of the episode is shown in **Fig. 1**C. Termination of the arrhythmia with antitachycardia pacing is shown in **Fig. 1**B. Total atrial and ventricular arrhythmia burden during the period before the patient's admission is shown in **Fig. 2**.

CLINICAL QUESTIONS

What is the rhythm problem?
What are the diagnostic and prognostic implications of the scenario described?

DISCUSSION

This patient had multiple episodes of dual tachycardia manifest as recurrent ventricular tachycardia (VT) in the setting of AF. In **Fig. 1**A, the atrial electrograms are consistent with AF. The initial ventricular electrograms in the rhythm strip reveal an irregular ventricular rhythm consistent with conducted AF. The irregular nature of the ventricular cycle length is best illustrated by the interval plot in **Fig. 1**C. With the sixth complex of the ventricular electrogram in **Fig. 1**A, a rapid regular ventricular rhythm is initiated. Close examination of the ventricular electrogram reveals a subtle change in morphology during the rapid rhythm consistent with altered ventricular activation. During this period the atrial

Division of Cardiology, Department of Medicine, Weill Cornell Medical College, New York, NY, USA
* Corresponding author. Cornell University Medical Center, 520 East 70th Street, Starr 4 Pavilion, New York, NY 10021.
E-mail address: jac9029@med.cornell.edu

Card Electrophysiol Clin 4 (2012) 637–640
http://dx.doi.org/10.1016/j.ccep.2012.08.025
1877-9182/12/$ – see front matter

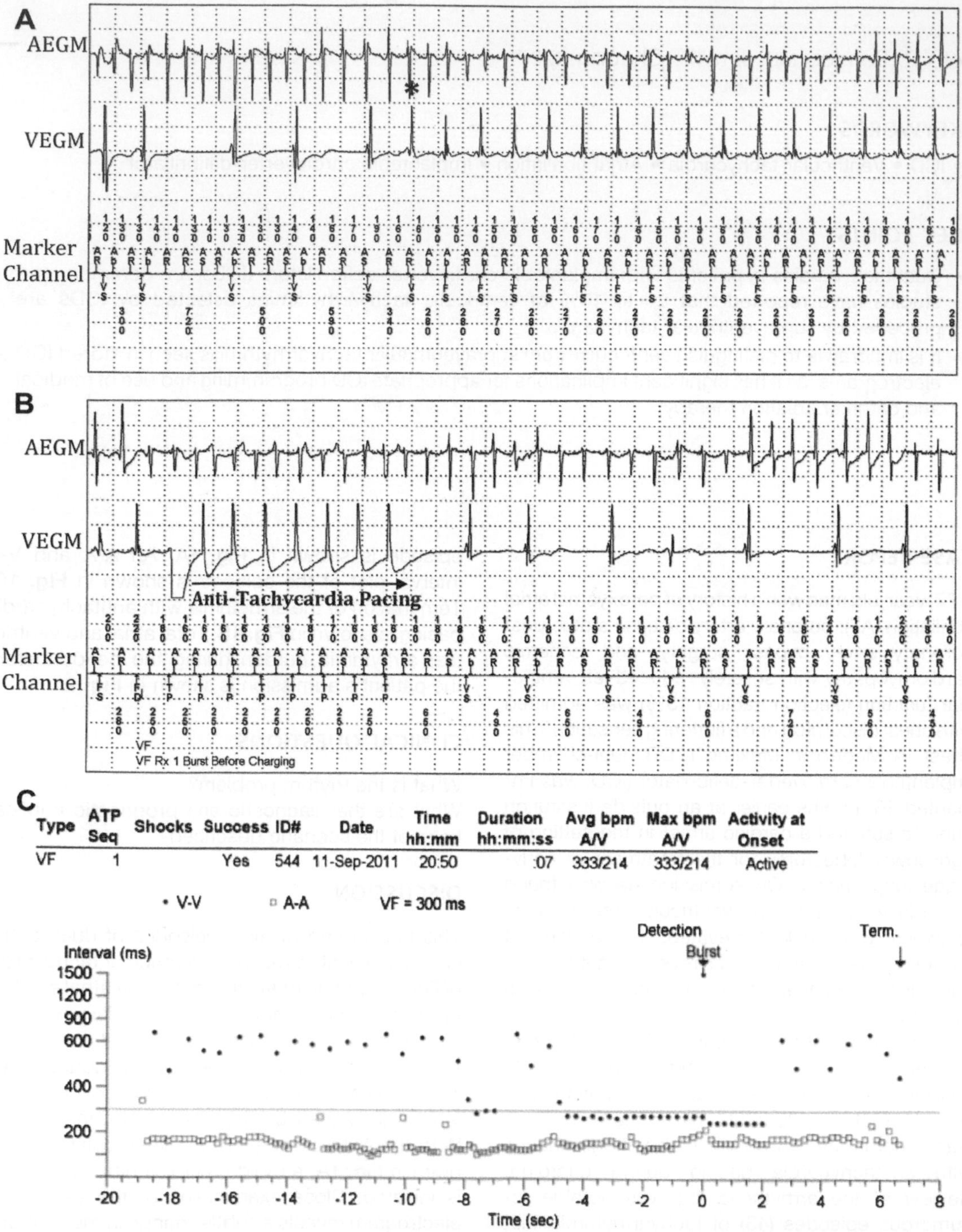

Fig. 1. (*A, B*) Stored electrograms with marker channels from a representative episode of arrhythmia organized as follows: bipolar atrial electrogram (AEGM), bipolar ventricular electrogram (VEGM), marker channel (*bottom*). Initial beat of ventricular tachycardia is noted with an asterisk in *A*. Anti-tachycardia pacing is highlighted by the arrow in *B*. (*C*) A-A (*open dots*) V-V (*closed dots*) interval plot from the representative episode in *A* and *B*. Time (seconds) is shown on the x-axis with detection of arrhythmia at time 0. Beat-to-beat interval (milliseconds) is shown on the y-axis. VF zone was programed to 300 milliseconds. *Arrows* denote arrhythmia detection and termination. The delivery of anti-tachycardia pacing is marked by "Burst." See text for description.

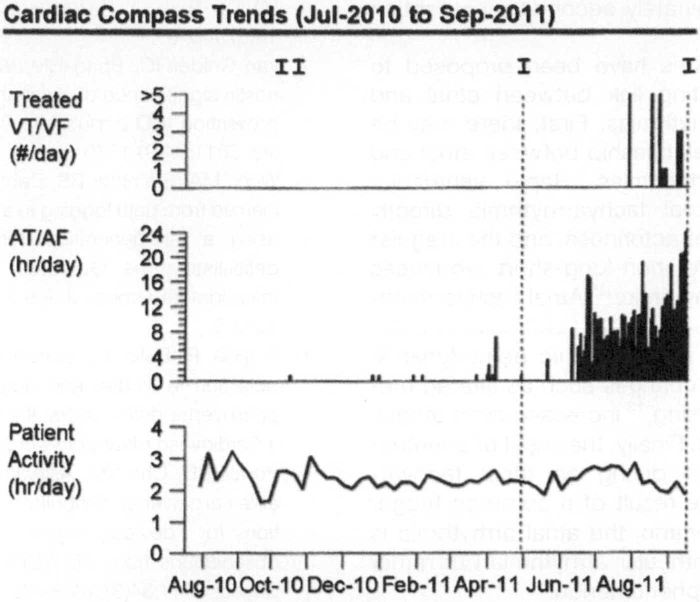

Fig. 2. Trends in arrhythmia burden between time of device implantation to time of hospital admission. A marked increase in detected atrial tachyarrhythmia (*middle plot*) is seen at 3 months before admission, followed by multiple episodes of ventricular tachycardia requiring ICD therapy over a 2-month period before admission. See text for discussion.

rhythm continues unperturbed. The sudden change from an irregular ventricular rhythm to a rapid regular rhythm is consistent with the onset of VT. The device appropriately detects VT, and antitachycardia pacing is delivered (see **Fig.** 1B, C). The pacing therapy successfully terminates VT, and AF with irregular ventricular conduction continues.

Dual tachycardias in patients with ICDs are common.[1,2] Studies have reported that up to 10% of ventricular tachyarrhythmias detected by ICDs are preceded by supraventricular tachycardia (SVT).[1] Unfortunately, inappropriate ICD therapies for supraventricular arrhythmias are even more common.[3–5] Variables used by device algorithms for SVT discrimination include assessments of arrhythmia onset, rate interval variability, and electrogram morphology. Furthermore, the use of dual-chamber sensing has been shown to aid in differentiating supraventricular from ventricular arrhythmias.[6,7] However, even with the use of dual-chamber sensing and SVT discrimination algorithms, the rate of inappropriate ICD shocks remains unacceptably high.[6] Inappropriate ICD shocks have been associated with increased morbidity and mortality.[8,9] It is imperative to distinguish ventricular tachyarrhythmias from SVTs seen in stored ICD electrograms, as this has significant implications for appropriate ICD programming and use of medical and catheter ablation therapy. The case of dual tachycardia presented here further underscores the challenges of accurate adjudication of arrhythmia mechanisms from stored ICD electrograms.

In this case, the onset of recurrent VT in the patient was preceded by a significant increase in the burden of AF (see **Fig. 2**). In the 3 months before the patient's admission, his AF burden increased from less than 10% to more than 33%. This increase was associated with an increase in VT burden over a 2-month period, giving rise to the notion of "AF begetting VT." Several studies suggest that the presence of atrial tachyarrhythmias has been shown to be a potent predictor of VT.[1,2,10,11] In a prospective analysis of 398 dual-chamber ICD recipients, Stein and colleagues[2] found that 8.6% (233 of 2602) of all VT/ventricular fibrillation (VF) episodes were dual tachycardias, with 1 in 5 patients that had VT/VF during follow-up having at least one episode of dual tachycardia. Moreover, when atrial tachyarrhythmia persisted after successful treatment of ventricular tachyarrhythmia, a recurrent episode of ventricular arrhythmia occurred sooner than if the atrial tachycardia had terminated.[2] Similarly, Smit and colleagues[10] found that patients who received primary prophylaxis ICDs who have a history of AF experienced a 7-fold increase in appropriate ICD shocks compared with similar patients in sinus rhythm. In addition, similar findings have been shown in a predominately secondary prevention population.[11]

Several mechanisms have been proposed to explain this interesting link between atrial and ventricular tachyarrhythmias. First, there may be a direct causative relationship between atrial and ventricular tachyarrhythmias. Rapid ventricular rates during an atrial tachyarrhythmia directly reduce ventricular refractoriness, and the irregular rhythm of AF leads to short-long-short sequences that may be proarrhythmic.[12] Atrial tachyarrhythmias also may indirectly affect ventricular electrophysiology through proarrhythmic hemodynamic and neurohormonal changes such as altered mechanoelectrical coupling,[13] increased sympathetic tone,[14] and ischemia. Finally, the onset of a ventricular tachyarrhythmia during an atrial tachyarrhythmia may be the result of a common trigger for both. In this scenario, the atrial arrhythmia is not causative of ventricular arrhythmia but rather is an associated epiphenomenon.

SUMMARY

Patients with ICDs are at risk of not only ventricular arrhythmias but also supraventricular tachyarrhythmias. This case illustrates the diagnostic challenges faced by clinicians in situations whereby two simultaneous tachycardias occur. The case also underscores the effects of increased AF burden on the occurrence of ventricular arrhythmias.

REFERENCES

1. Marchlinski FE, Callans DJ, Gottlieb CD, et al. Benefits and lessons learned from stored electrogram information in implantable defibrillators. J Cardiovasc Electrophysiol 1995;6(10 Pt 1):832–51.
2. Stein KM, Euler DE, Mehra R, et al. Do atrial tachyarrhythmias beget ventricular tachyarrhythmias in defibrillator recipients? J Am Coll Cardiol 2002;40(2): 335–40.
3. Klein RC, Raitt MH, Wilkoff BL, et al. Analysis of implantable cardioverter defibrillator therapy in the Antiarrhythmics Versus Implantable Defibrillators (AVID) Trial. J Cardiovasc Electrophysiol 2003; 14(9):940–8.
4. van Gelder IC, Phan HM, Wilkoff BL, et al. Prognostic significance of atrial arrhythmias in a primary prevention ICD population. Pacing Clin Electrophysiol 2011;34(9):1070–9.
5. Wood MA, Stambler BS, Damiano RJ, et al. Lessons learned from data logging in a multicenter clinical trial using a late-generation implantable cardioverter-defibrillator. The Guardian ATP 4210 Multicenter Investigators Group. J Am Coll Cardiol 1994;24(7): 1692–9.
6. Francia P, Balla C, Uccellini A, et al. Arrhythmia detection in single- and dual-chamber implantable cardioverter defibrillators: the more leads, the better? J Cardiovasc Electrophysiol 2009;20(9):1077–82.
7. Powell BD, Cha YM, Asirvatham SJ, et al. Implantable cardioverter defibrillator electrogram adjudication for device registries: methodology and observations from ALTITUDE. Pacing Clin Electrophysiol 2011;34(8):1003–12.
8. Daubert JP, Zareba W, Cannom DS, et al. Inappropriate implantable cardioverter-defibrillator shocks in MADIT II: frequency, mechanisms, predictors, and survival impact. J Am Coll Cardiol 2008;51(14):1357–65.
9. van Rees JB, Borleffs CJ, de Bie MK, et al. Inappropriate implantable cardioverter-defibrillator shocks: incidence, predictors, and impact on mortality. J Am Coll Cardiol 2011;57(5):556–62.
10. Smit MD, Van Dessel PF, Rienstra M, et al. Atrial fibrillation predicts appropriate shocks in primary prevention implantable cardioverter-defibrillator patients. Europace 2006;8(8):566–72.
11. Klein G, Lissel C, Fuchs AC, et al. Predictors of VT/VF-occurrence in ICD patients: results from the PROFIT-Study. Europace 2006;8(8):618–24.
12. Denker S, Lehmann M, Mahmud R, et al. Facilitation of ventricular tachycardia induction with abrupt changes in ventricular cycle length. Am J Cardiol 1984;53(4):508–15.
13. Lerman BB. Mechanoelectrical feedback: maturation of a concept. J Cardiovasc Electrophysiol 1996;7(1): 17–9.
14. Lown B, Verrier RL. Neural activity and ventricular fibrillation. N Engl J Med 1976;294(21):1165–70.

Difficulties in Implantable Cardioverter-Defibrillator Programming

Walter Li, MD[a,*], Ronn E. Tanel, MD[b]

KEYWORDS

• Implantable cardioverter-defibrillator • Supraventricular tachycardia • Catheter ablation

KEY POINTS

- Interrogation of an implantable cardioverter-defibrillator (ICD) following a device discharge should begin with an evaluation of the current programming, because inappropriate device programming is a common cause of inappropriate shocks.
- One common pitfall is programming the ventricular fibrillation or ventricular tachycardia detection criteria within the physiologic range of the heart rate, particularly in younger patients.

CLINICAL PRESENTATION

A 15-year-old boy had an implantable cardioverter-defibrillator (ICD) implanted for a history of sudden cardiac arrest. During the evaluation for sudden cardiac arrest, he was diagnosed with Wolff-Parkinson-White syndrome. He was treated with catheter ablation therapy, which was acutely successful. However, because the accessory pathway did not have rapid antegrade conduction characteristics during the electrophysiology study to explain the sudden cardiac arrest, an ICD was implanted.

Subsequently the patient presented to the Emergency Department following an ICD discharge while playing basketball. Interrogation of the device showed a single-chamber ICD with stable lead-impedance measurements, electrogram amplitudes, and capture thresholds. The device was programmed with single-tier therapy for ventricular fibrillation (VF) at heart rates greater than 222 beats/min. There was a single event stored by the device that corresponded to the time the patient reported receiving a shock. The electrogram showed a regular tachycardia at a rate of 300 beats/min with a morphology similar to that during sinus rhythm (**Fig. 1**).

CLINICAL QUESTION

Is the device functioning appropriately and is there reprogramming that can avoid therapy delivery in the future for this arrhythmia?

DISCUSSION

Interrogation of an ICD following a device discharge should begin with an evaluation of the current programming. Inappropriate device programming is a common cause of inappropriate shocks. One common pitfall is programming the VF or ventricular tachycardia (VT) detection criteria within the physiologic range of the heart rate, particularly in younger patients. Occasionally, VT zones are inadvertently activated as a result of inaccurate QRS complex counts during T-wave

---

Disclosure: Dr Li receives fellowship funding support from Medtronic and St Jude Medical.
[a] Division of Pediatric Cardiology, Department of Pediatrics, University of California, San Francisco, CA, USA;
[b] Division of Pediatric Cardiology, Department of Pediatrics, UCSF Medical Center, University of California, 521 Parnassus Avenue, Room C-350, Box 0632, San Francisco, CA 94143, USA
* Corresponding author.
E-mail address: walter.li@ucsf.edu

Card Electrophysiol Clin 4 (2012) 641–644
http://dx.doi.org/10.1016/j.ccep.2012.08.026
1877-9182/12/$ – see front matter

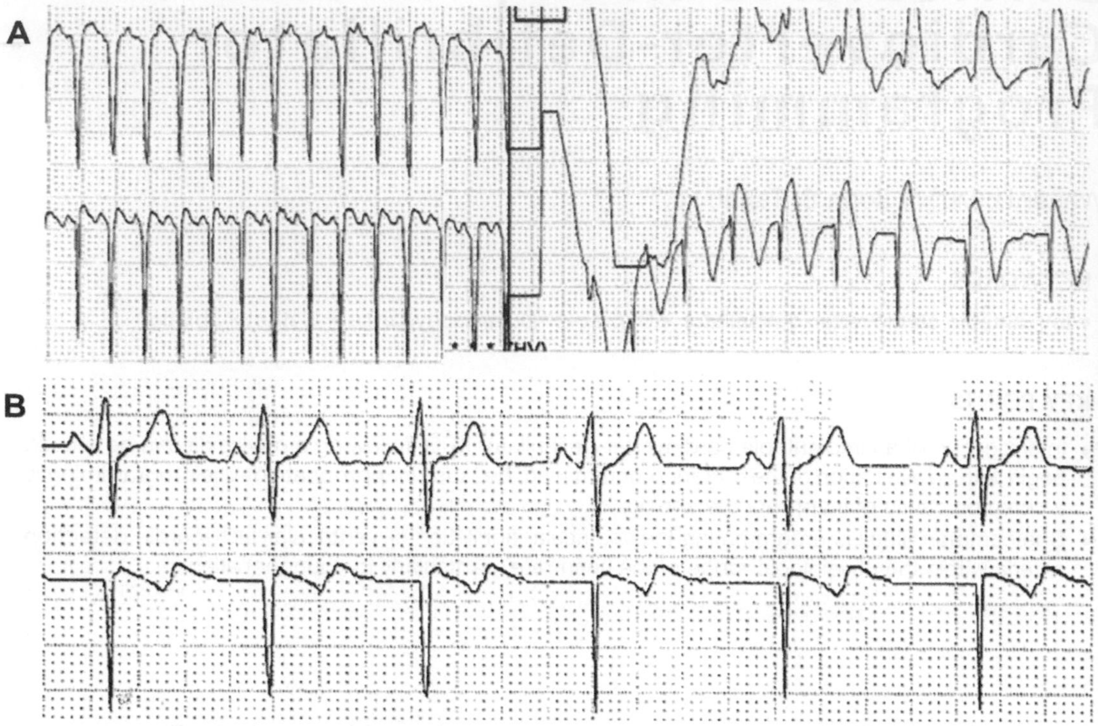

Fig. 1. (*A*) Stored device electrogram of tachycardia at a cycle length of 200 milliseconds meets criteria for ventricular fibrillation and results in an ICD discharge. (*B*) Recording of a surface rhythm strip above and an intracardiac electrogram below, illustrating the similarity between the morphology of the intracardiac ventricular electrogram during tachycardia (*A*) and sinus rhythm (*B*).

oversensing or cumulative counts of isolated ventricular ectopic beats. In this case, the VF zone was appropriately set well above physiologic heart rates, and the VT zone was not enabled. Review of the stored electrogram before the shock showed that the device correctly assessed the ventricular rate. The ICD appropriately delivered a shock according to the programmed parameters. The device and lead were functioning normally. Unfortunately, the patient had an episode of supraventricular tachycardia (SVT) owing to recurrence of accessory pathway conduction, which resulted in a tachycardia rate within the VF detection zone.

ICD discharges caused by rapidly conducted SVT are not uncommon.[1] Although this patient had an acutely successful ablation of a right posteroseptal accessory pathway, antegrade conduction returned during long-term follow-up (**Fig. 2**). Ideally the VF detection cycle length can be programmed short enough to avoid delivering therapies for SVT, but this can only be achieved for relatively slow rates of SVT (slower than the rate expected for a potentially malignant ventricular arrhythmia). For patients with an ICD who also have SVT, SVT discriminator algorithms are often used to differentiate between SVT and VT when their rates overlap.[2] Most algorithms rely on either a QRS morphology match or recognition of atrial to ventricular relationship patterns. These algorithms are usually only applied to the tachyarrhythmias that fall within the VT zone, and therefore would not have been relevant for this patient. The SVT cycle length was so short that it would invariably fall within the programmed VF zone. It is unsafe to program the VF detection cycle length shorter than what was programmed in this case, because this could result in failure to sense a potentially malignant arrhythmia. There is no way to differentiate this patient's SVT from VF based on ventricular rate alone.

Chronic medical therapy may be prescribed to minimize the potential for recurrent SVT. In general, medications that affect atrioventricular nodal conduction, such as digoxin, β-blockers, or calcium-channel blockers, are reasonable options. However, in the patient with preexcitation, digoxin and calcium-channel blockers should generally be avoided. Catheter ablation therapy to eliminate the SVT substrate is often effective in

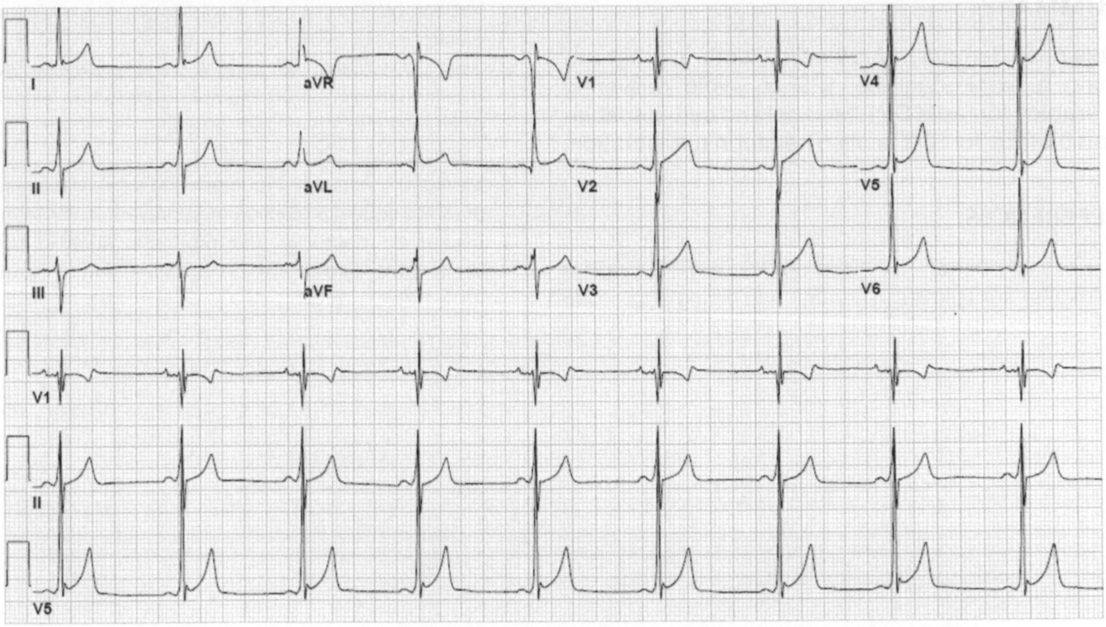

Fig. 2. Electrocardiogram showing return of preexcitation following catheter ablation of a right posteroseptal accessory pathway.

this situation.[3] Ultimately, a second electrophysiology study was performed, and antidromic reciprocating tachycardia was induced at a cycle length similar to the SVT that led to this patient's ICD discharge (**Fig. 3**). The accessory pathway was successfully modified with radiofrequency catheter ablation, and the patient has subsequently remained free of both SVT and ICD discharges.

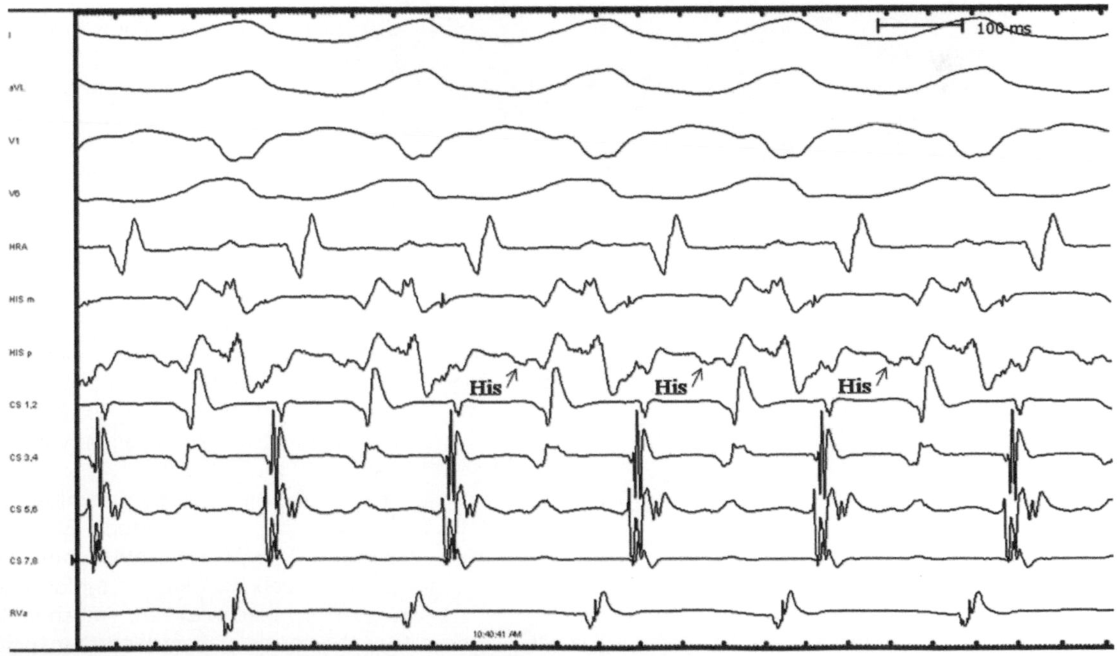

Fig. 3. Antidromic reciprocating tachycardia at a cycle length of 200 milliseconds induced during the electrophysiology study. The His bundle electrogram is indicated by the arrow. CS, coronary sinus; HISm, mid His bundle electrogram; HISp, proximal His bundle electrogram; HRA, high right atrium; RVa, right ventricular apex.

SUMMARY

This case demonstrates the limitations in programming a single-chamber ICD to avoid delivering therapies for rapid SVT. Medical and catheter ablation therapy for SVT is often helpful in this situation.

REFERENCES

1. Love BA, Barrett KS, Alexander ME, et al. Supraventricular arrhythmias in children and young adults with implantable cardioverter defibrillators. J Cardiovasc Electrophysiol 2001;12:1097–101.
2. Klein GJ, Gillberg JM, Tang A, et al. Improving SVT discrimination in single-chamber ICDs: a new electrogram morphology-based algorithm. J Cardiovasc Electrophysiol 2006;17:1310–9.
3. Mainigi SK, Almuti K, Figueredo VM, et al. Usefulness of radiofrequency ablation of supraventricular tachycardia to decrease inappropriate shocks from implantable cardioverter-defibrillators. Am J Cardiol 2012;109:231–7.

Infra-Hisian Atrioventricular Block

Wendy S. Tzou, MD[a,*], Ryan Foley, MD[b],
Duy Thai Nguyen, MD[a], Ryan G. Aleong, MD[a]

KEYWORDS

• Infra-Hisian atrioventricular block • Pacemaker • Bundle branch block

KEY POINTS

- Bundle branch block and aberrancy can involve multiple, dynamic phenomena.
- The presence of acceleration-dependent and phase 4 aberrancy or block are pathologic, and indicate disease of the conduction system.

CLINICAL PRESENTATION

A 72-year-old woman, with a history of hypertension and hyperlipidemia, presented with episodes of presyncope and 2:1 atrioventricular (AV) block, with alternating left bundle branch block (LBBB) and right bundle branch block (RBBB). She was admitted for further management. Twelve-lead electrocardiograms (ECGs) during her initial presentation are shown in **Fig. 1**.

CLINICAL QUESTION

What is the explanation for the alternating BBB?

ELECTROPHYSIOLOGY STUDY AND CLINICAL COURSE

A quadripolar catheter was placed at the His-bundle region. At baseline, the patient was in sinus rhythm with 2:1 AV block with RBBB on conducted beats (see **Fig. 1**A). Intracardiac recordings demonstrated infra-Hisian block with nonconducted beats (**Fig. 2**). Intermittently, 1:1 AV conduction would resume, sometimes, but not always, following a premature atrial contraction (PAC) with RBBB aberrancy, followed by LBBB with the 1:1 conducted beats (see **Fig. 1**B; **Fig. 3**). Note that the conducted beat following a PAC is of differing RBBB morphology than the beats conducted with 2:1 AV block (see **Figs. 1**B and **3**). Note also that PP (and associated His-His [HH]) intervals also correspond with differing patterns of aberrancy: generally with shorter HH intervals, 1:1 AV conduction with LBBB is observed, while with longer HH intervals, RBBB is observed. Finally, the His-ventricular (HV) interval with 2:1 AV block was normal (58 milliseconds, **Fig. 4**). With 1:1 AV conduction and LBBB, marked prolongation in the HV interval (108 milliseconds, see **Fig. 4**) was observed.

The patient met Class I guidelines for pacemaker implantation (advanced second-degree AV block with bradycardia and symptoms),[1] so the quadripolar catheter was advanced to the right ventricle for backup pacing if needed during dual-chamber pacemaker implantation.

DISCUSSION

Type II second-degree AV block is typically infranodal, usually occurring below the level of the His bundle, as was the case for this patient.[2] Symptoms are common in this group of patients, and progression to complete heart block, as well

Disclosure: None of the authors have any conflicts to disclose relevant to this article.

[a] Cardiac Electrophysiology, University of Colorado Anschutz Medical Campus, 12401 East 17th Avenue, Mail Stop B136, Aurora, CO 80045, USA; [b] Department of Medicine, University of Colorado Anschutz Medical Campus, Denver, 12605 East 16th Avenue, Mail Stop B136, Aurora, CO 80045, USA
* Corresponding author.
E-mail address: wendy.tzou@ucdenver.edu

Card Electrophysiol Clin 4 (2012) 645–649
http://dx.doi.org/10.1016/j.ccep.2012.08.039
1877-9182/12/$ – see front matter Published by Elsevier Inc.

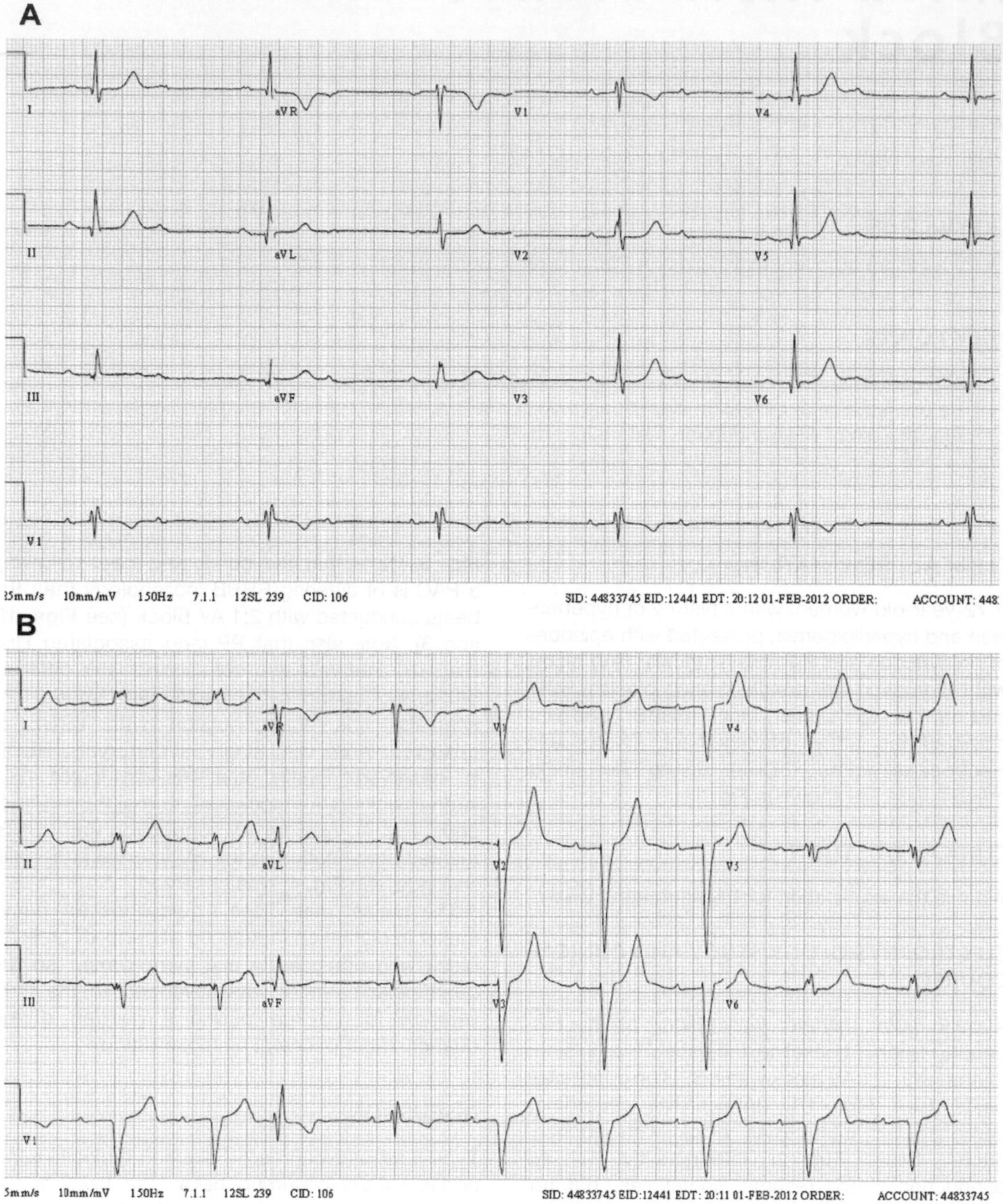

Fig. 1. 12-Lead electrocardiograms (ECGs) of patient's presenting rhythm. (*A*) 2:1 Atrioventricular (AV) block with right bundle branch block (RBBB) on AV conducted beats. (*B*) Alternating bundle branch block during 1:1 AV conduction, with differing RBBB aberrancy noted during ventricular conduction following premature atrial contraction, compared with that observed during 2:1 AV block.

as mortality, is increased in comparison with those without evidence for infranodal disease.[3,4]

Potential mechanisms of conduction block or delay include phase-3 block, acceleration-dependent block, phase-4 (bradycardia-dependent) block, and concealed conduction.[5–8] Phase-3 block occurs when a premature impulse attempts to depolarize His-Purkinje tissue during phase 3 of the action potential, at the time of relative refractoriness, and is a physiologic phenomenon, in contradistinction to acceleration-dependent block whereby conduction delay occurs in response to

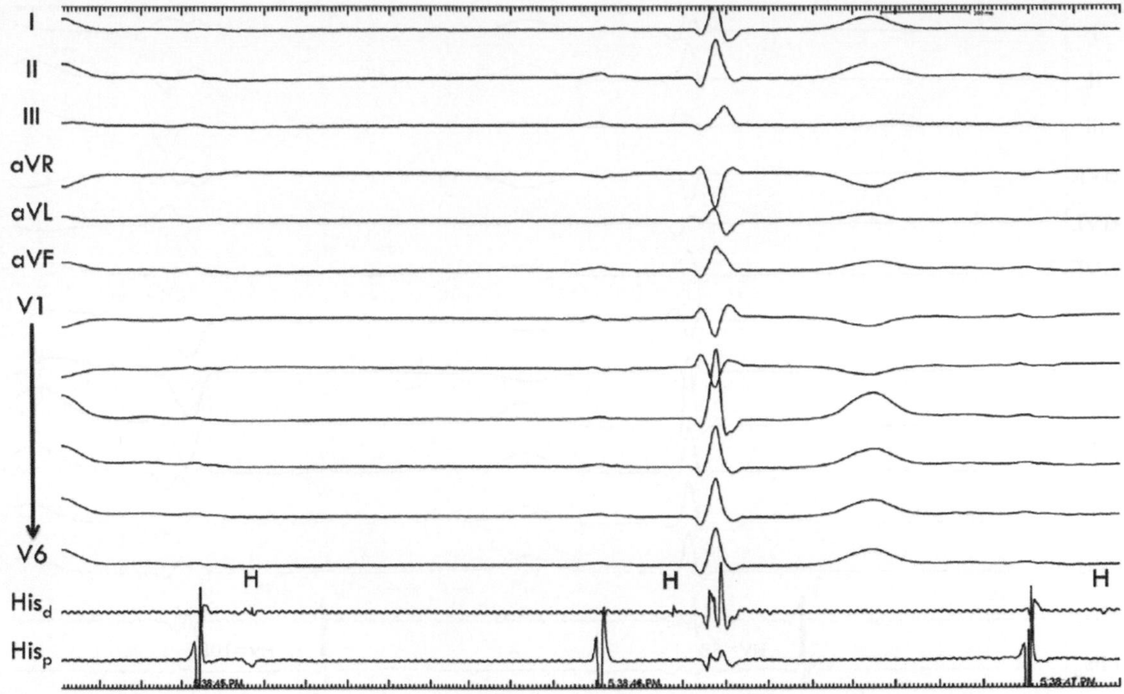

Fig. 2. 100-Speed surface 12-lead ECG with accompanying His electrograms, demonstrating 2:1 infra-Hisian block. H, His.

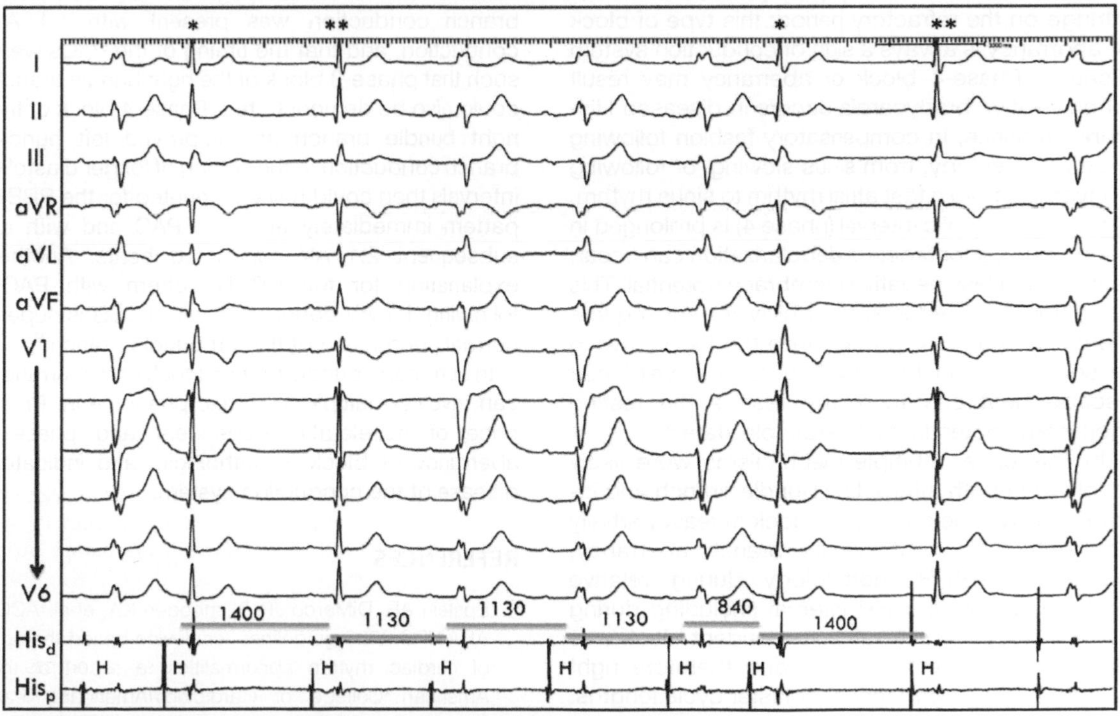

Fig. 3. 25-Speed surface 12-lead ECG with accompanying His (labeled H) electrograms, demonstrating alternating bundle branch block/aberrancy corresponding with differing H-H (measured in *blue lines*, with timing noted above each line in milliseconds) intervals. Note that the conducted beat following a pulmonary artery catheter is of differing RBBB morphology (*asterisk*) than the beats conducted with 2:1 AV block (*double asterisk*). See text for details.

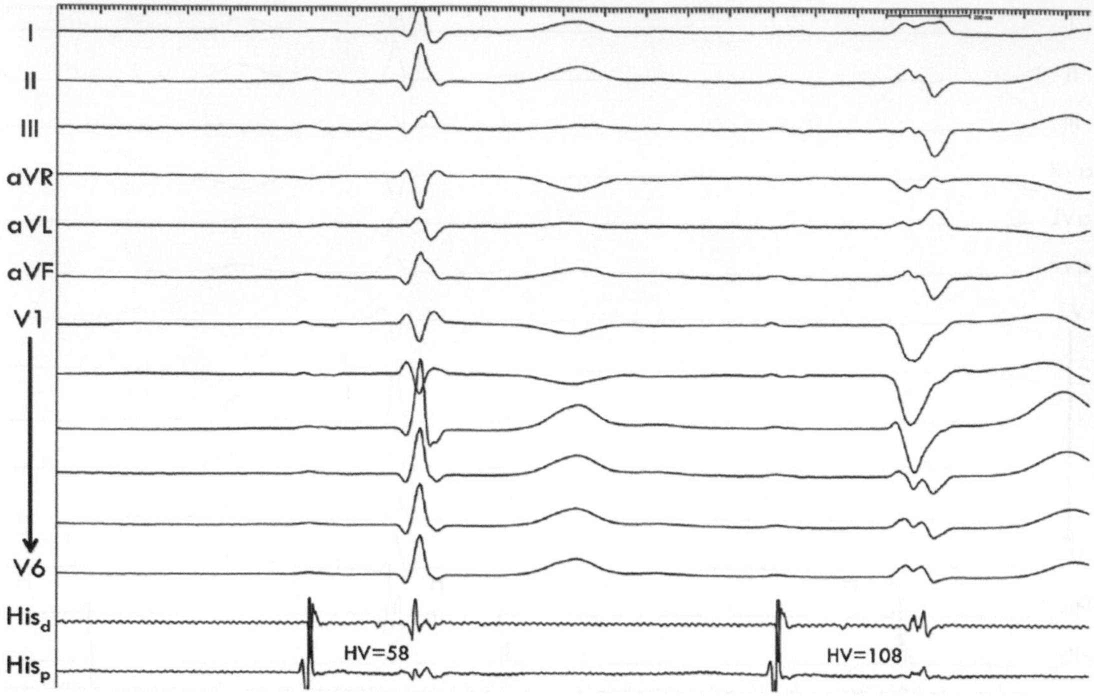

Fig. 4. 100-Speed surface 12-lead ECG with accompanying His electrograms during AV conduction with RBBB and LBBB.

premature or shorter-coupled impulses that do not infringe on the refractory period; this type of block or aberrancy is always a sign of conduction system disease. Phase-4 block or aberrancy may result when relative bradycardia occurs in diseased His-Purkinje tissue, in compensatory fashion following premature ectopy, from sinus slowing, or following conversion from a fast atrial rhythm to sinus rhythm. When the diastolic interval (phase 4) is prolonged in such tissue, spontaneous depolarization can occur, leading to a less negative membrane potential. This condition then reduces the ability for subsequent electrical impulses to depolarize the tissue, owing to sodium-channel inactivation. Only a well-timed escape beat can then fully restore the resting membrane potential to its excitable state.[8]

In this case, multiple mechanisms were likely involved in both alternating bundle branch and infranodal AV block. Phase-4 block at least partially accounted for right bundle branch aberrancy, given the RBBB morphology during relative prolongation of the HH interval (including during 2:1 AV block). Acceleration-dependent block was likely responsible for LBBB (and therefore right bundle branch conduction) at faster cycle lengths. With PACs occurring after 1:1 AV conduction, an RBBB morphology, more pronounced than that observed with 2:1 AV conduction, was reproducibly observed. This phenomenon could indicate that at least some, although slower, left bundle branch conduction was present with 1:1 AV conduction, and that the timing of the PACs were such that phase-3 block of the right bundle branch could also be demonstrated. Phase-4 block of the right bundle branch and improved left bundle branch conduction in the setting of longer diastolic intervals then could have accounted for the RBBB pattern immediately after the PAC and with all subsequent 2:1 AV conducted beats. Another explanation for the RBBB pattern with PACs following 1:1 AV conduction with LBBB is supernormal conduction of the left bundle branch.[9]

In summary, bundle branch block and aberrancy can involve multiple, dynamic phenomena. Presence of acceleration-dependent and phase-4 aberrancy or block is pathologic, and indicates disease of the conduction system.

REFERENCES

1. Epstein AE, DiMarco JP, Ellenbogen KA, et al. ACC/AHA/HRS 2008 guidelines for device-based therapy of cardiac rhythm abnormalities: a report of the American College of Cardiology/American Heart Association Task Force on Practice guidelines (Writing committee to revise the ACC/AHA/NASPE 2002 guideline update for implantation of cardiac pacemakers and antiarrhythmia devices) developed

in collaboration with the American Association for Thoracic Surgery and Society of Thoracic Surgeons. J Am Coll Cardiol 2008;51:e1–62.
2. Narula OS. Conduction disorders in the AV transmission system. In: Dreifus L, Likoff W, editors. Cardiac arrhythmias. New York: Grune and Stratton; 1973. p. 259.
3. Dhingra RC, Denes P, Wu D, et al. The significance of second degree atrioventricular block and bundle branch block: observations regarding site and type of block. Circulation 1974;49:638–46.
4. Dhingra RC, Palileo E, Strasberg B, et al. Significance of the HV interval in 517 patients with chronic bifascicular block. Circulation 1981;64:1265–71.
5. Cranefield PF, Klein HO, Hoffman BF. Conduction of the cardiac impulse: I. Delay, block, and one-way block in depressed Purkinje fibers. Circ Res 1971; 28:199–219.
6. Jalife J, Antzelevitch C, Lamanna V, et al. Rate-dependent changes in excitability of depressed cardiac Purkinje fibers as a mechanism of intermittent bundle branch block. Circulation 1983;67:912–22.
7. Josephson ME. Clinical cardiac electrophysiology: techniques and interpretations. 4th edition. Philadelphia: Lippincott Williams & Wilkins; 2008.
8. Singer DH, Lazzara R, Hoffman BF. Interrelationships between automaticity and conduction in Purkinje fibers. Circ Res 1967;21:537–58.
9. Chialvo DR, Michaels DC, Jalife J. Supernormal excitability as a mechanism of chaotic dynamics of activation in cardiac Purkinje fibers. Circ Res 1990;66:525–45.

Inappropriate Discharges After Implantable Cardioverter-Defibrillator Placement

Walter Li, MD[a,*], Ronn E. Tanel, MD[b]

KEYWORDS

• Implantable cardioverter-defibrillator • Inappropriate discharge • Twiddler syndrome

KEY POINTS

- Lead dislodgment is a common complication of a pacemakers and implantable cardioverter-defibrillators (ICDs), particularly in the pediatric patient population.
- Twiddler syndrome is a well-described but rare cause of lead dislodgment.
- Most cases of twiddler syndrome have occurred with pacemakers and result in a loss of capture, but occasionally twiddler syndrome can result in inappropriate ICD discharges.

CLINICAL HISTORY

A 16-year-old male presented to the emergency department after sustaining implantable cardioverter-defibrillator (ICD) shocks that awakened him from sleep. Several months earlier, he received an ICD placed for aborted cardiac arrest resulting from nonobstructive hypertrophic cardiomyopathy. During prior outpatient appointments, the patient was doing well with no progression in his cardiomyopathy, and interrogation of the device showed normal ICD function. He reported compliance with β-blocker therapy and had no significant changes to his health.

Interrogation of the patient's device revealed a St Jude Current VR RF single-chamber ICD. The device was programmed to provide therapies for ventricular tachyarrhythmia rates greater than 222 beats/min for 16 intervals. Lead impedance was within normal limits. Electrocardiograms of the ICD shocks were recorded by the device (**Fig. 1**), and a chest radiograph was obtained (**Fig. 2**).

CLINICAL QUESTION

What is the cause of this patient's inappropriate ICD discharges?

CLINICAL COURSE

Based on the chest radiograph, the patient was diagnosed with lead dislodgment likely attributable to twiddler syndrome. The patient denied manipulating the device. However, because of his obvious anxiety, the appearance of the twisted redundant lead within the pocket, and the lack of a better explanation, twiddler syndrome was the most likely reason for this lead dislodgment. Many patients with twiddler syndrome manipulate their device subconsciously, and the authors believe that such was the case for this patient.

The patient's device was revised and the lead was replaced. Multiple stay sutures were placed to fixate the lead to the surrounding tissues, and the patient recovered well with no complications during long-term follow-up.

Disclosure: Dr Li receives fellowship funding support from Medtronic and St Jude Medical.
[a] Division of Pediatric Cardiology, Department of Pediatrics, University of California, San Francisco, CA, USA;
[b] Division of Pediatric Cardiology, Department of Pediatrics, UCSF Medical Center, University of California, 521 Parnassus Avenue, Room C-350, Box 0632, San Francisco, CA 94143, USA
* Corresponding author.
E-mail address: walter.li@ucsf.edu

Card Electrophysiol Clin 4 (2012) 651–653
http://dx.doi.org/10.1016/j.ccep.2012.08.031
1877-9182/12/$ – see front matter

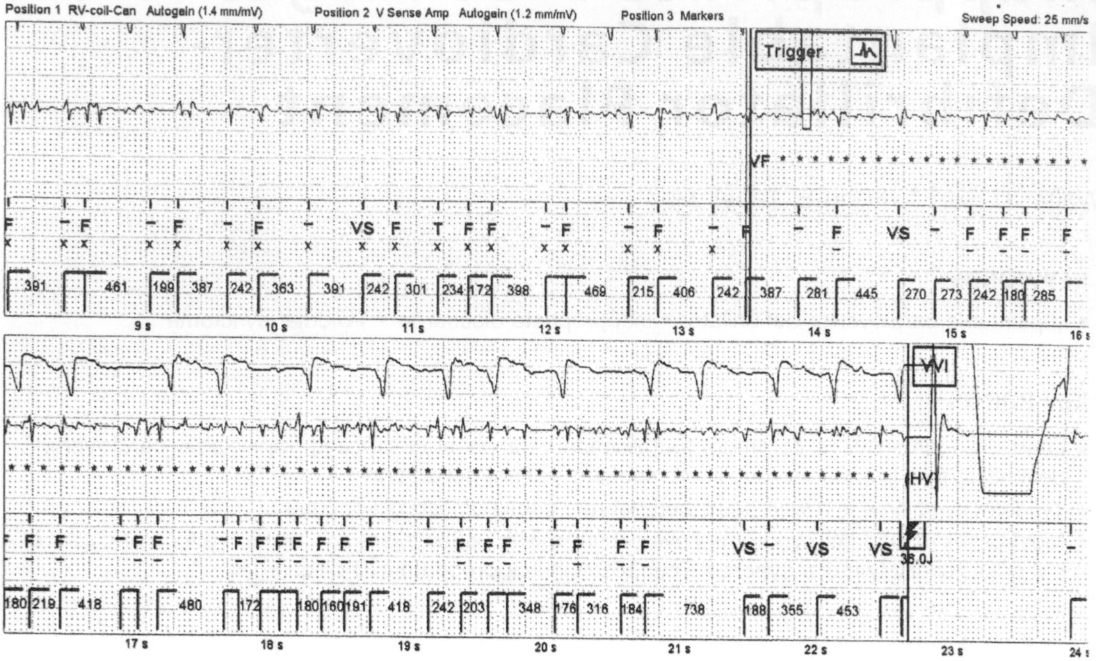

Fig. 1. Comparison of the ventricular lead tip to the RV-coil-Can electrograms shows oversensing that led to inappropriate ICD discharges.

DISCUSSION

Lead dislodgment is a common complication of pacemakers and ICDs,[1] particularly in the pediatric patient population.[2] Risk factors include heart failure, atrial tachyarrhythmias, and implantations performed by physicians trained under alternative pathways.[3] Another common cause of ventricular oversensing is lead fracture, which typically has markedly elevated lead impedance.

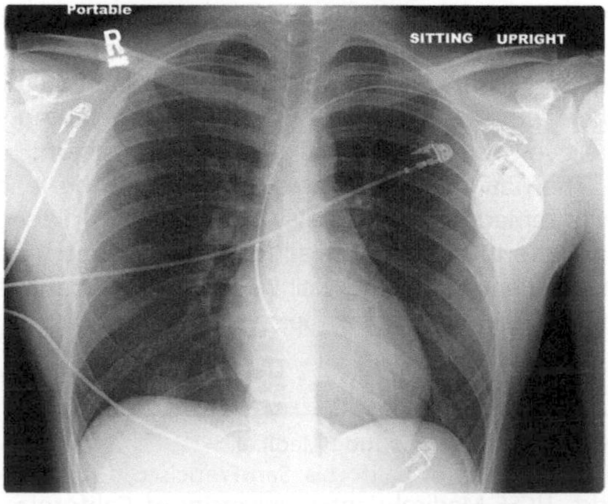

Fig. 2. Chest radiograph shows "twiddling" of the lead, which caused the lead to be retracted into the right atrium. Movement of the lead within the atrium caused oversensing, which led to inappropriate ICD discharges.

The chest radiograph showed the dislodged ventricular lead with the tip in the right atrium instead of the right ventricular apex. Close examination of the radiograph revealed a ventricular lead with excessive coiling and rotation near the ICD generator site. This case is an example of twiddler syndrome, a well-described[4–7] but rare cause of lead dislodgment.[8,9] Most cases of twiddler syndrome are observed in elderly patients, oversized generator pockets, soft-tissue laxity, loop of the lead outside the device pocket, or patients with psychiatric disorders. However, twiddler syndrome has also been described in pediatric patients.[10] Most cases of twiddler syndrome have occurred with pacemakers and result in a loss of capture, but occasionally it can result in inappropriate ICD discharges.[11]

REFERENCES

1. van Rees JB, de Bie MK, Thijssen J, et al. Implantation-related complications of implantable cardioverter-defibrillators and cardiac resynchronization therapy devices: a systematic review of randomized clinical trials. J Am Coll Cardiol 2011;58:995–1000.
2. Fortescue EB, Berul CI, Cecchin F, et al. Patient, procedural, and hardware factors associated with pacemaker lead failures in pediatrics and congenital heart disease. Heart Rhythm 2004;1:150–9.

3. Cheng A, Wang Y, Curtis JP, et al. Acute lead dislodgements and in-hospital mortality in patients enrolled in the national cardiovascular data registry implantable cardioverter defibrillator registry. J Am Coll Cardiol 2010;56:1651–6.
4. Bayliss CE, Beanlands DS, Baird RJ. The pacemaker-twiddler's syndrome: a new complication of implantable transvenous pacemakers. Can Med Assoc J 1968;99:371–3.
5. Chemello D, Subramanian A, Cameron D. Twiddler syndrome with 180 degrees rotation of an implantable cardioverter defibrillator generator resulting in malfunction of one of the shocking coils. Europace 2009;11:1259.
6. Tonino WA, Winter JB. Images in clinical medicine. The twiddler syndrome. N Engl J Med 2006;354:956.
7. Benezet-Mazuecos J, Benezet J, Ortega-Carnicer J. Pacemaker twiddler syndrome. Eur Heart J 2007;28: 2000.
8. Fahraeus T, Höijer CJ. Early pacemaker twiddler syndrome. Europace 2003;5:279–81.
9. Hill PE. Complications of permanent transvenous cardiac pacing: a 14-year review of all transvenous pacemakers inserted at one community hospital. Pacing Clin Electrophysiol 1987;10: 564–70.
10. Berul CI, Hill SL, Estes NA 3rd. A teenager with pacemaker twiddler syndrome. J Pediatr 1997;131: 496–7.
11. Spencker S, Poppelbaum A, Müller D. An unusual cause of oversensing leading to inappropriate ICD discharges. Int J Cardiol 2008;129:e24–6.

New Irregular Rhythm in a Patient with Baseline Left Bundle Branch Block

Marwan M. Refaat, MD[a], Byron K. Lee, MD, MAS[b,*]

KEYWORDS

• Bundle branch block • Implantable cardioverter-defibrillator • Ventricular tachycardia

KEY POINTS

- Transition from wide to narrow QRS complex has several mechanisms such as heart rate change, "peel-back" refractoriness, rate-dependent progressive shortening of bundle branch refractoriness, gap phenomena, supernormal conduction, loss of preexcitation, premature ventricular complex, or ventricular tachycardia (VT) ipsilateral to the bundle branch block and equal conduction delay in both of the bundle branches.
- The QRS complexes can be normal or near normal in width when the VT originates from the ventricular conduction system or near the ventricular conduction system.

CLINICAL PRESENTATION

A 63-year-old man with a history of Reiter syndrome, nonischemic idiopathic cardiomyopathy, and baseline left bundle branch block (LBBB) had a syncopal episode and episodes of nonsustained ventricular tachycardia (VT). He underwent biventricular implantable cardioverter-defibrillator (ICD) placement. Four months later, the patient presented with fatigue and episodes of palpitations. He was admitted for further management. Twelve-lead electrocardiograms (ECGs) recorded during his initial presentation are shown in **Fig. 1**.

CLINICAL QUESTION

What is the rhythm in this patient with baseline LBBB pattern?

ELECTROPHYSIOLOGY STUDY AND CLINICAL COURSE

The patient had an irregular tachycardia at 138 beats/min with QRS complexes much narrower than his baseline LBBB QRS. The QRS duration was generally 105 milliseconds, but there were some occasional wide complex beats. P waves could not be clearly identified on the baseline ECG. The rhythm on the initial 12-lead ECG was diagnosed as atrial fibrillation with occasional aberrant beats or premature ventricular complexes (PVCs). This diagnosis was later proved to be wrong.

The true diagnosis was VT, which was determined from the ICD interrogation that clearly showed atrioventricular dissociation (**Fig. 2**). The atrial beats march out at about 65 beats/min, whereas the ventricular beats are occurring at

Disclosures: None of the authors have any conflicts to disclose relevant to this article.

[a] Section of Cardiac Electrophysiology, Division of Cardiology, Department of Medicine, University of California, San Francisco, 500 Parnassus Avenue, San Francisco, CA 94143, USA; [b] Section of Cardiac Electrophysiology, Division of Cardiology, Department of Medicine, University of California, San Francisco, 500 Parnassus Avenue, Box 1354, MU 429, San Francisco, CA 94143, USA
* Corresponding author.
E-mail address: leeb@medicine.ucsf.edu

Card Electrophysiol Clin 4 (2012) 655–657
http://dx.doi.org/10.1016/j.ccep.2012.08.027

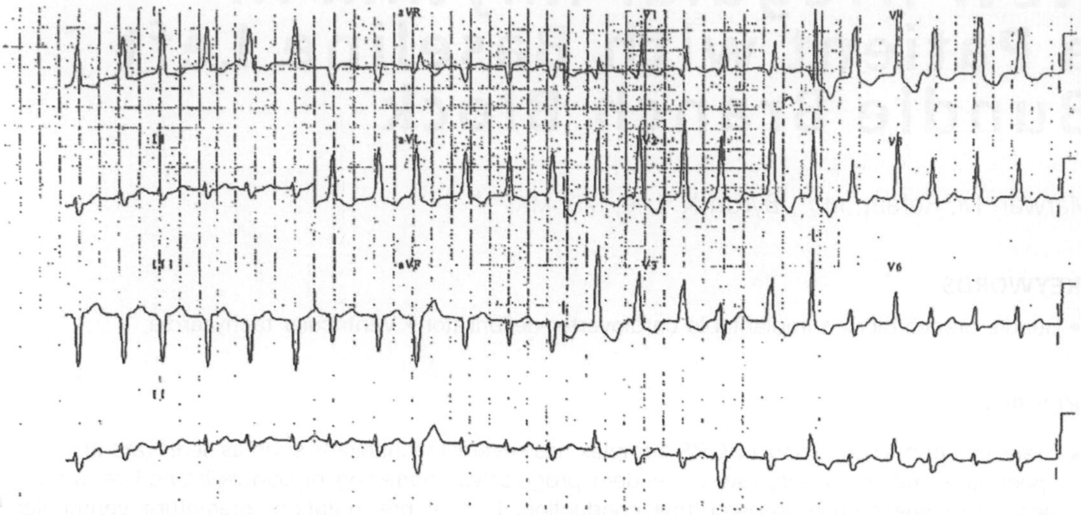

Fig. 1. Twelve-lead electrocardiograms of the patient's presenting rhythm show an irregular tachycardia at a rate of 138 beats/min with QRS complexes narrower than his baseline left bundle branch block. There are occasional wider complex beats.

about 140 beats/min but somewhat irregularly. There are more ventricular beats than atrial beats and there is no relationship between the atrial and ventricular rhythms, confirming that the ventricular rhythm must be VT.

The patient underwent an electrophysiology study, which revealed an easily inducible stable VT with earliest activation mapping to the septal superior anterior left ventricle, which terminated the VT.

DISCUSSION

This patient's baseline 12-lead ECG showed LBBB. By contrast, his presenting ECG showed a tachycardia with QRS complexes much narrower than his baseline LBBB. Transition from wide to narrow QRS complex has several mechanisms such as heart-rate change, "peel-back" refractoriness, rate-dependent progressive shortening of bundle branch refractoriness, gap phenomena, supernormal conduction, loss of preexcitation, PVC, or VT ipsilateral to the bundle branch block and equal conduction delay in both of the bundle branches.[1–3]

The patient had a baseline LBBB, no evidence of premature atrial complex, no delay in the right bundle, or change in conduction intervals. He had a left ventricular VT originating ipsilateral to

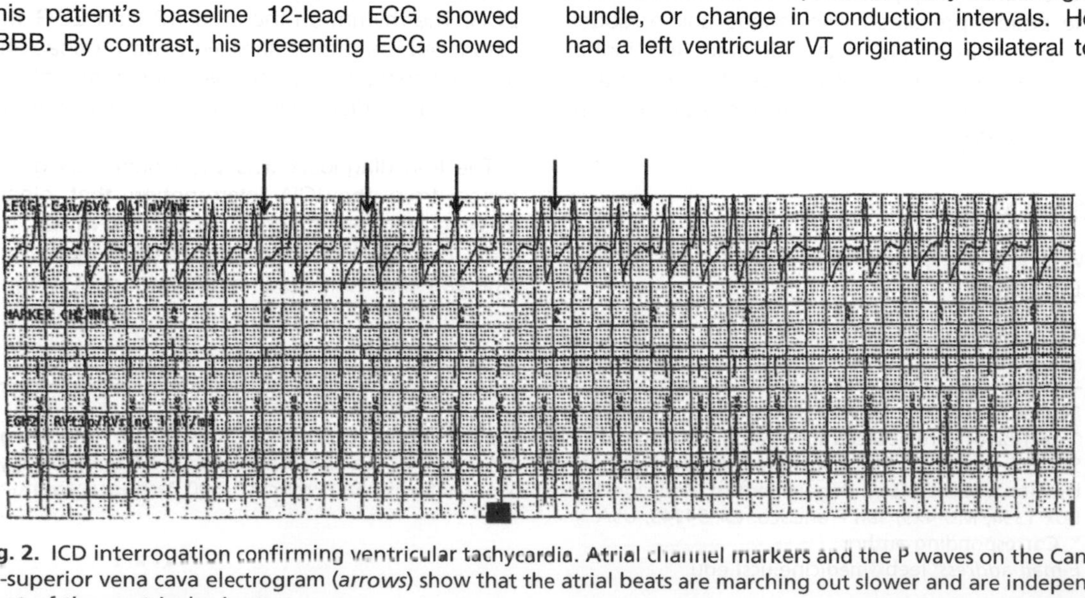

Fig. 2. ICD interrogation confirming ventricular tachycardia. Atrial channel markers and the P waves on the Can-to-superior vena cava electrogram (*arrows*) show that the atrial beats are marching out slower and are independent of the ventricular beats.

bundle branch block, which can cause normal or near normal QRS duration mimicking a supraventricular arrhythmia. In this instance, the rhythm was misdiagnosed as atrial fibrillation. The QRS complexes can be normal or near normal in width when the VT originates from the ventricular conduction system or near the ventricular conduction system. In summary, this case illustrates the physiology described previously in a patient with an LBBB who is detected to have a near normal QRS complex rhythm.

REFERENCES

1. Prystowsky EN, Klein GJ. Cardiac arrhythmias: an integrated approach for the clinician. New York: McGraw-Hill; 1994. p. 64–9.
2. Akhtar M, Damato AN, Batsford WP, et al. Unmasking and conversion of gap phenomenon in the human heart. Circulation 1974;49:624–30.
3. Massumi RA, Amsterdam EA, Mason DT. Phenomenon of supernormality in the human heart. Circulation 1972;46:264–75.

Index

Note: Page numbers of article titles are in **boldface** type.

Card Electrophysiol Clin 4 (2012) 659–662
http://dx.doi.org/10.1016/S1877-9182(12)00180-3

Printed and bound by CPI Group (UK) Ltd, Croydon, CR0 4YY
03/10/2024
01040348-0001